ATLAS OF TRAUMA SURGERY

Editors

Dale A. Dangleben, MD, FACS
Chief of Surgery and Trauma Medical Director
Penn State Health Holy Spirit Hospital
Camp Hill, Pennsylvania

Firas G. Madbak, MD, FACS, FCCM
Professor of Surgery
Division Chief, Acute Care Surgery
University of Florida College of Medicine
Jacksonville, Florida

Mc Graw Hill

Atlas of Trauma Surgery

1 2 3 4 5 6 7 8 9 DSS 31 30 29 28 27 26

ISBN 978-1-264-25842-0
MHID 1-264-25842-9

NOTICE

Medicine is an ever-changing science. As new research and clinical experience broaden our knowledge, changes in treatment and drug therapy are required. The authors and the publisher of this work have checked with sources believed to be reliable in their efforts to provide information that is complete and generally in accord with the standards accepted at the time of publication. However, in view of the possibility of human error or changes in medical sciences, neither the authors nor the publisher nor any other party who has been involved in the preparation or publication of this work warrants that the information contained herein is in every respect accurate or complete, and they disclaim all responsibility for any errors or omissions or for the results obtained from use of the information contained in this work. Readers are encouraged to confirm the information contained herein with other sources. For example and in particular, readers are advised to check the product information sheet included in the package of each drug they plan to administer to be certain that the information contained in this work is accurate and that changes have not been made in the recommended dose or in the contraindications for administration. This recommendation is of particular importance in connection with new or infrequently used drugs.

This book was set in Expressway by KnowledgeWorks Global Ltd.
The editors were Sydney Keen Vitale and Kim J. Davis.
The production supervisor was Catherine Saggese.
The digital production manager was Steve Brown.
Project management was provided by Radhika Jolly, KnowledgeWorks Global Ltd.
The cover designer was W2 Design.

This book is printed on acid-free paper.

Library of Congress Control Number: 2025950596

To my parents Arthur and Rita Dangleben who taught me the value of perseverance and integrity and laid the foundation for all I have achieved.

And to my children, may you always dream boldly and walk with strength.

Dale A. Dangleben

To the healthcare workers who risk everything to save lives under fire, whose courage persists through threats, pressure, and pain. Your humanity lights the darkest hours.

Firas G. Madbak

CONTENTS

CONTRIBUTORS

Steven R. Allen, MD, FACS
Professor and Chief
Division of Acute Care Surgery
Department of Surgery
University of Missouri-Columbia
Columbia, Missouri

Geoffrey A. Anderson, MD, MPH
Associate Professor of Clinical Surgery
Department of Surgery
University of Southern California
Los Angeles, California

Scott B. Armen, MD, FACS, FCCP, FCCM, COL, MC USAR
Charlene J. Smith Professor
Department of Surgery
Penn State University College of Medicine
Hershey, Pennsylvania

Mark Cipolle, MD, PhD, FACS, FCCM
Chief, Division of Trauma and Acute Care Surgery
Vice Chair for Research and Education Department of Surgery
Lehigh Valley Health Network
Allentown, Pennsylvania
Professor of Surgery
Morsani School of Medicine
University of South Florida
Tampa, Florida
Adjunct Professor of Surgery
Sidney Kimmel School of Medicine
Thomas Jefferson University
Philadelphia, Pennsylvania

Michael Coburn, MD
Professor and Russell and Mary Hugh Scott Chair in Urology
Baylor College of Medicine
Houston, Texas

Michael J. Collins, MD
Assistant Professor
Department of Surgery
Carilion Clinic–Virginia Tech Carilion School of Medicine
Roanoke, Virginia

Anthony Dakwar, MD, FACS, FASCRS
Assistant Professor of Surgical Oncology
Division of Colorectal Surgery
Department of Surgical Oncology
Roswell Park Comprehensive Cancer Center
Buffalo, New York

Dale A. Dangleben, MD, FACS
Chief of Surgery and Trauma Medical Director
Penn State Health Holy Spirit Hospital
Camp Hill, Pennsylvania

James W. Dennis, MD, FACS
Professor of Surgery
Chief, Division of Vascular Surgery and Endovascular Therapy
Vice Chair of Education and Academic Affairs
University of Florida College of Medicine–Jacksonville
Jacksonville, Florida

Jeffrey Glaser, MD, MBA, MB, FACS
Clinical Assistant Professor
Department of Surgery
Thomas Jefferson University
Philadelphia, Pennsylvania

Todd D. Husty, MD, FACS, CDR, MC, USN
Assistant Professor of Surgery
Uniformed Services University of the Health Sciences
Jacksonville, Florida

CONTRIBUTORS

Diana Jho, MD, MS, FAANS, FCNS
Associate Professor of Neurosurgery
Department of Neurosurgery
Penn State Health Holy Spirit Medical Center
Penn State Health Milton S. Hershey Medical Center
Camp Hill, Pennsylvania

Ginger L. Justice, MD
Trauma, Emergency General Surgery, and Surgical Critical Care
Wellstar Kennestone Hospital
Marietta, Georgia

Kathleen Koesarie, MD
General Surgery Resident PGY4
Conemaugh Memorial Medical Center
University of Pittsburgh School of Medicine 2021
Pittsburgh, Pennsylvania

Stanley J. Kurek, DO, FACS
Professor of Surgery, VCOM
Chief Medical Officer
Extant Healthcare, LLC
Richmond, Virginia

Anthony Lam, DO
General Surgeon, Clinical Instructor
Department of Surgery
Piedmont Medical Center
Rock Hill, South Carolina

Graham G. Laurence, MD, PhD
Staff Trauma Surgeon
Department of Surgery
Penn State–Holy Spirit Medical Center
Camp Hill, Pennsylvania

Daniel Lim, DO, FACS
Surgical Critical Care, Trauma and Acute Care Surgeon
Department of Surgery
Penn State Holy Spirit Hospital
Camp Hill, Pennsylvania

Ashley Ludwig, DO, FACS
Assistant Professor of Surgery
Medical Director, Trauma Surgical Unit
Associate Trauma Medical Director
Department of Surgery
Penn State University College of Medicine
Hershey, Pennsylvania

Sonia S. Majid, MD, MPH
Neurosurgical Resident
Department of Neurosurgery
Penn State Health Milton S. Hershey Medical Center
Hershey, Pennsylvania

Matthew D. Painter, MD, FACS
Assistant Professor
Department of Surgery
Wake Forest University School of Medicine
Winston-Salem, North Carolina

Adam Peton, DO
General Surgery Resident
Department of Surgery
Conemaugh Health System
Johnstown, Pennsylvania

Ali Salim, MD
Division of Trauma and Acute Care Surgery
Mass General Brigham
Professor of Surgery
Harvard Medical School
Boston, Massachusetts

Taylor Santor, MHS, PA-C
Physician Assistant Certified
Department of Neurosurgery
Penn State Health Holy Spirit Medical Center
Penn State Health Milton S. Hershey Medical Center
Camp Hill, Pennsylvania

Sebastian D. Schubl, MD, FACS, FSIS
Clinical Professor
Department of Surgery
University of California Irvine School of Medicine
Irvine, California

CONTRIBUTORS

David J. Skarupa, MD, FACS, FCCM, FACHE
Professor of Surgery
Division of Acute Care Surgery, Department of Surgery
University of Florida College of Medicine–Jacksonville
Associate Chief Medical Officer, UF Health–Jacksonville
Jacksonville, Florida

Daniel Steadman, DO
Vascular Surgery Fellow
Eastern Virginia Medical School
Norfolk, Virginia

Stephen Stopenski, MD
Clinical Associate Professor
Department of Surgery
Division of Trauma, Surgical Crucial Care, and Acute Care Surgery
University of Nevada, Reno
Reno, Nevada

Shyam Sukumar, MBBS
Associate Professor
Genitourinary Reconstruction
Scott Department of Urology
Baylor College of Medicine
Houston, Texas

Laura Velcu, MD
Trauma, Acute Care Surgeon
Department of Surgery
Pennsylvania State University
Camp Hill, Pennsylvania

Leon Ray White, DO, MS
Private Practice
Cleveland, Ohio

Renaldo Williams, MD
Surgical Critical Care Fellow
Brigham and Women's Hospital
Harvard Medical School
Boston, Massachusetts

Nathan Wong, MD
Department of Surgery
Christiana Care
Newark, Delaware

Grant Woodruff, DO
Chief Surgical Resident
University of Florida College of Medicine
Jacksonville, Florida

Chelsea Yap, DO
Chief Surgical Resident
University of Florida College of Medicine
Jacksonville, Florida

PREFACE

Trauma surgery is a demanding, high-stakes discipline that requires precision and an intimate understanding of anatomy and physiology. The unpredictable nature of traumatic injuries, whether from blunt force, penetrating trauma, or complex multisystem insults, demands that the trauma surgeon be not only technically skilled but also decisive, innovative, and prepared for the unexpected.

The *Atlas of Trauma Surgery* was born from a need we have encountered repeatedly throughout our years as trauma surgeons and mentors: a need for a comprehensive, yet practical, visual guide that bridges the gap between textbook learning and the dynamic reality of trauma care. This atlas is not merely a compilation of procedures. It is a visual narrative of surgical decision-making in trauma, grounded in real-world experience and designed for clarity, accessibility, and immediate application in the operating room.

This work is designed to be a quick-reference tool as much as a teaching guide. My intention is for the *Atlas of Trauma Surgery* to sit within arm's reach in trauma bays, operating rooms, and surgical libraries alike.

This work is also a tribute to the countless patients whose lives have intersected with trauma and to the tireless teams of surgeons, emergency physicians, nurses, anesthesiologists, medics, and support staff. Trauma surgery is not a solo art. It is a choreography of expertise, intuition, and action. If this atlas can contribute in even a small way to better outcomes, quicker decisions, or greater confidence among those who wield the scalpel in the service of others, then its purpose will be fulfilled.

We extend our deepest gratitude to our mentors, colleagues, and trainees who have challenged, taught, and inspired us throughout our careers. It is my hope that this *Atlas of Trauma Surgery* will serve as a lasting resource in your surgical journey, whether you are saving your first trauma patient or your thousandth.

Dale A. Dangleben, MD, FACS
Chief of Surgery and Trauma Medical Director
Penn State Health Holy Spirit Hospital
Camp Hill, Pennsylvania

NEUROSURGICAL INTERVENTIONS IN TRAUMA

1

Sonia S. Majid, MD, MPH
Taylor Santor, MHS, PA-C
Diana Jho, MD, MS, FAANS, FCNS

TIPS

1. **In all cranial traumas, always remember ABCs first to ensure the patient has a secured airway, adequate ventilation, and no hemodynamic instability.**
2. **It is important to remember the tier for management of increased intracranial pressure. In the absence of a mass lesion requiring emergent surgery or cerebrospinal fluid (CSF) diversion and after ABCs are addressed, multiple medical management options are available to manage elevated intracranial pressures including sedation, proper analgesia, hypertonic saline, hyperventilation (only temporary), barbiturates, and paralytics.**
3. **In traumas, it is often difficult to obtain a detailed patient history. This is why it is imperative to obtain labs prior to any intervention. Remember to always check coagulation studies and platelets prior to any surgical intervention.**

TRAUMATIC BRAIN INJURY

Introduction

Traumatic brain injury (TBI) is defined as damage to the brain resulting from external mechanical forces. The global incidence of TBIs is 939 cases per 100,00 people per year. Based on this, 69 million people worldwide suffer from TBIs annually. In the United States, an average of 1.4 million TBIs occur each year including 1.1 million emergency room visits, 235,000 hospitalizations, 99,000 permanent disabilities, and 50,000 deaths. Overall, males are about twice as likely as females to experience a TBI.

There are various classification modalities for TBIs. Closed brain injuries occur when there is no break in the skin and skull and are caused by a rapid forward and backward movement. Penetrating brain injuries occur when there is a break in the skin and skull such as with a bullet or other foreign object. TBIs include concussions, diffuse axonal injuries, contusion/intraparenchymal hemorrhages, traumatic subarachnoid hemorrhages, subdural hematomas, and epidural hematomas. There may be associated skull fractures or overlying scalp hematomas that may give a clue on the point of impact. There may also be associated edema within the brain tissue.

The Glasgow Coma Scale (GCS) was first presented in 1974 by Teasdale and Jennett as an aid in standardizing clinical assessment of the level of consciousness. The three components of the GCS assessment include eyes, verbal, and motor scores, with motor being the most important component determining outcomes. TBI is classified as mild, moderate, or severe based on structural imaging, length of loss of consciousness, duration of altered mental state, posttraumatic amnesia, and best GCS score within 24 hours.

The pathology and type of TBI will determine the best treatment modalities to maximize outcome. The Monro-Kellie doctrine describes the principle of homeostatic intracerebral volume, which stipulates that the total volume of the brain parenchyma, CSF, and blood remains constant due to the fixed volume of the skull. Medical and surgical treatment modalities attempt to manipulate these components to maximize recovery. Medical management for elevated intracranial pressures includes hyperosmolar therapies, raising the head of the bed to at least 30 degrees, sedation/paralysis, hyperventilation, hypothermia, and ensuring that the cervical collar is not on too tight. Surgical management of various TBIs includes placement of an intracranial pressure monitor or external ventricular drain, burr hole for chronic subdural hematoma evacuation, craniotomy for subdural or epidural evacuation, and decompressive craniectomy.

Intracranial Pressure (ICP) Monitors

Intraparenchymal Pressure Monitors

- **Operative tips**
  - Review all labs especially coagulation studies.
  - Review all radiographic images.
  - Remember to zero the system prior to placing the intraparenchymal probe into the brain parenchyma.
- **Introduction**
  - Indications
    - Severe head injury with a GCS ≤8 after cardiopulmonary resuscitation with an abnormal brain computed tomography (CT)

      OR
    - Severe head injury with a GCS ≤8 with a normal brain CT with two or more of the following:
      - Age >40
      - Systolic blood pressure <90 mm Hg
      - Decerebrate or decorticate posturing on motor exam
  - Monitoring intracranial pressure allows for goal-directed therapy to maintain ICP within normal range and maximize cerebral perfusion pressure (CPP).
- **Anatomy**
  - Commonly placed at Kocher's point, which is also the typical landmark for placement of eternal ventricular drains, but entry site may change depending on where it is determined that the pressure probe should be placed based on imaging studies.
  - Kocher's point
    - Measured 10-11 cm posterior to the nasion along the midline and 2.5-3 cm lateral to midline in the trajectory of 1 cm in front of the tragus.
    - Alternative landmarks are 1 cm anterior to the coronal suture and lined up with the ipsilateral mid-pupillary line.

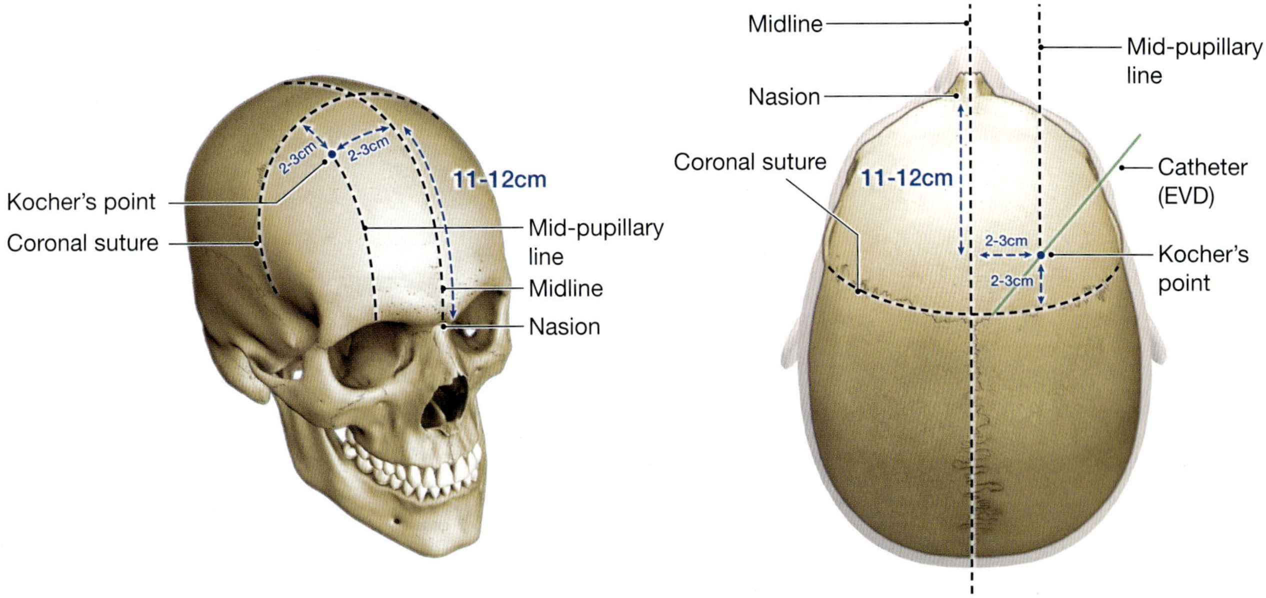

Figure 1-1

- **Operative steps**
  - A 1- to 1.5-cm linear anterior-to-posterior incision is made overlying Kocher's point.
  - A twist drill from the cranial access kit is utilized to create a small hole through the skull.
  - Bone dust is cleared and the dura pierced with either an 11-blade scalpel or trocar.
  - The system will need to be hooked up in order to zero the system prior to placing the probe into the brain parenchyma.

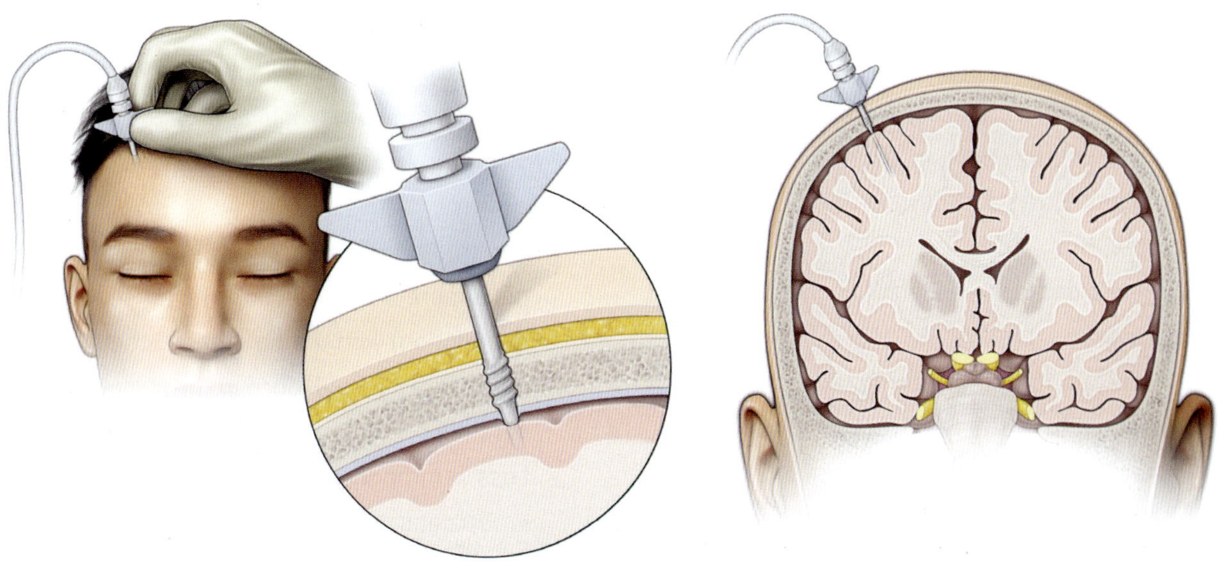

Figure 1-2

- If a skull bolt is used, twist the bolt into the skull and then place the probe through the bolt and into the brain tissue. Tighten the bolt around the probe to hold it securely in place.
- If the skull bolt is not used, tunnel the trocar to an area about 3-5 cm posterior to the incision and pass the probe anteriorly to the incision. A gentle bend is made in the probe wire at the desired depth, which is then inserted through the dura into the brain parenchyma. The tip of the probe should be placed about 2-3 cm into the brain parenchyma.
- The incision is sutured closed and the probe secured in place either with the bolt or with three points of sutures on the scalp. Dressing is then placed.
- The cable is again connected to the transducer box to obtain opening pressure.
- To ensure that the ICP recordings are working, venous outflow can be briefly occluded with gentle pressure on bilateral internal jugular veins, which should transiently increase ICP.

- **Complications**
  - Intracranial hemorrhage
  - Infection
  - Dislodgement
  - Misplacement
  - ICP drift where the probe becomes less accurate the longer it has been in place

Ventriculostomy/External Ventricular Drain (EVD)

- **Operative tips**
  - Review all lab work, especially coagulation studies.
  - Review radiographic imaging.
    - Placing the catheter directly into the hemorrhage may increase risk of catheter blockage but if planning to treat hemorrhage through the catheter, placing the catheter within the hemorrhage may be desired.
    - Plan to adjust the trajectory of the catheter based on ventricular anatomy and extent of midline shift.
    - Measure catheter trajectory length, scalp thickness, skull thickness, and distance to lateral ventricle on imaging studies to maximize accuracy of placement of the catheter.
  - Mark out lines for midline, entry point, line from midline to 1 cm in front of the tragus, and trajectory to the ipsilateral medial canthus to assist with placement.
  - If using entry sites other than Kocher's point, it may be helpful to use neuronavigation for placement.
- **Introduction**
  - Indications for placement are the same as for placement of an intraparenchymal pressure monitor (see above).
  - EVD can serve multiple purposes, including:
    - ICP monitoring
      - Allows for goal-directed therapies
    - CSF diversion
      - Allows for relief of CSF to decrease elevated ICPs
    - Intrathecal access
      - Allows access for intrathecal tissue plasminogen activator or antibiotics depending on the pathology
- **Anatomy**
  - The traditional and most common location for placement is over Kocher's point (see above for description) with the tip of the catheter located at the foramen of Monro in the ipsilateral lateral ventricle.
  - Less commonly used landmarks include:
    - Frazier's point
      - Located 6 cm above the inion and 3-4 cm off midline

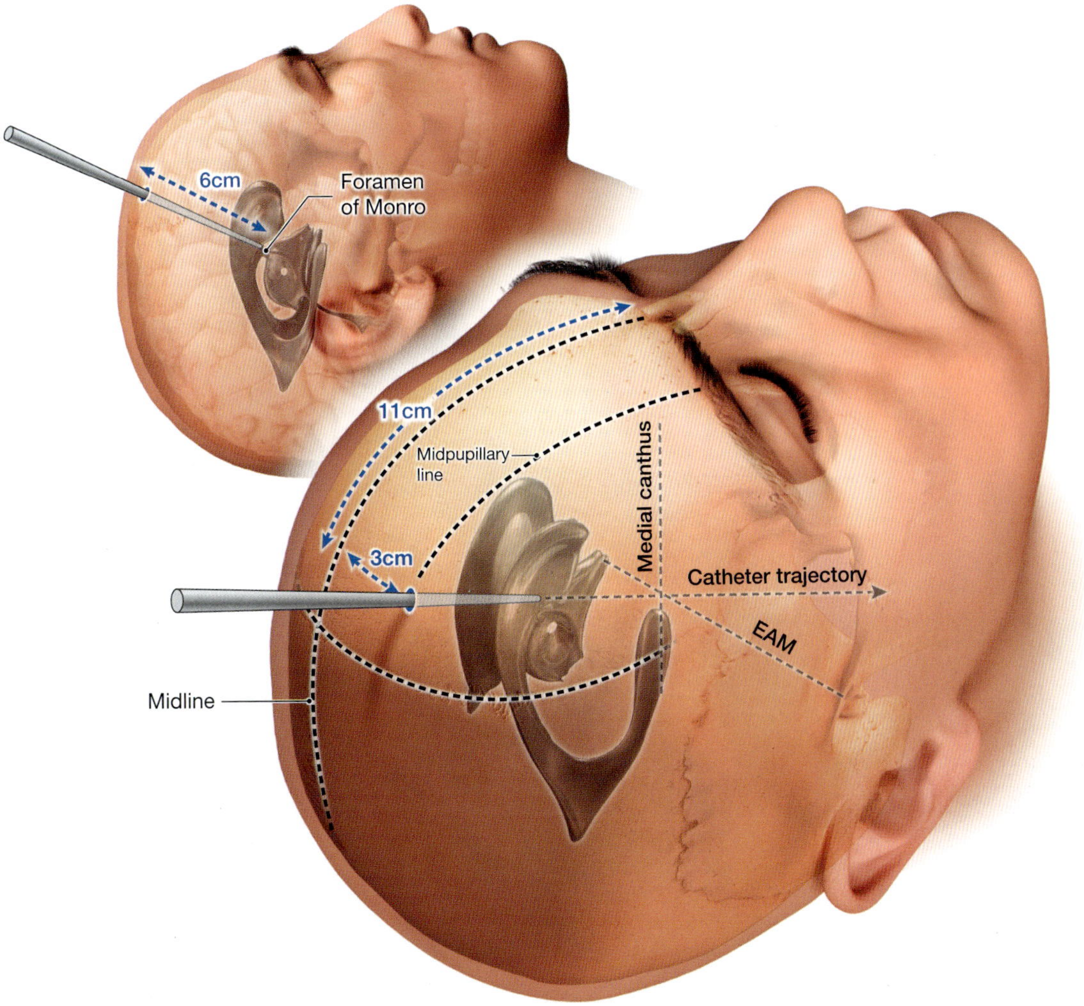

Figure 1-3

 - Trajectory of the catheter should be aimed toward the ipsilateral medial canthus.
 - Pass with the inner trocar to about 5 cm, and then soft pass the catheter to about 9-10 cm in length.
- Keen's point
 - Located 3 cm above and 3 cm posterior to the pinna of the ear
 - Trajectory of the catheter should be aimed toward the ipsilateral medial canthus.
 - Pass with the inner trocar to about 5 cm in depth, and then once CSF is observed, soft pass the catheter to about 9-10 cm in length.

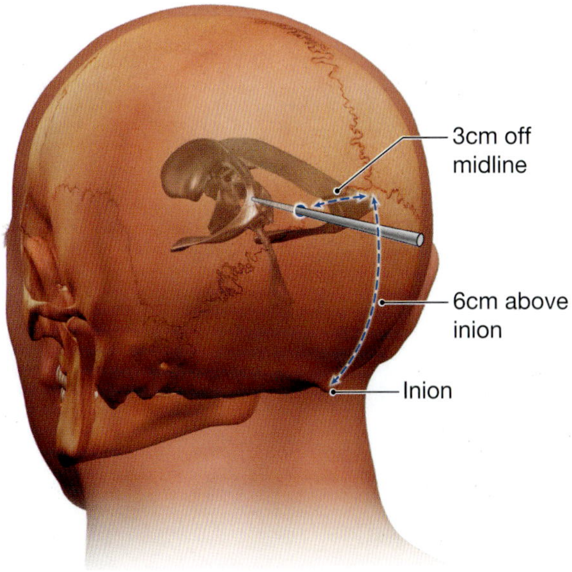

Figure 1-4

- **Operative steps**
  - Mark midline, Kocher's point, trajectory from midline to 1 cm in front of the tragus, and line from Kocher's point to the ipsilateral medial canthus.

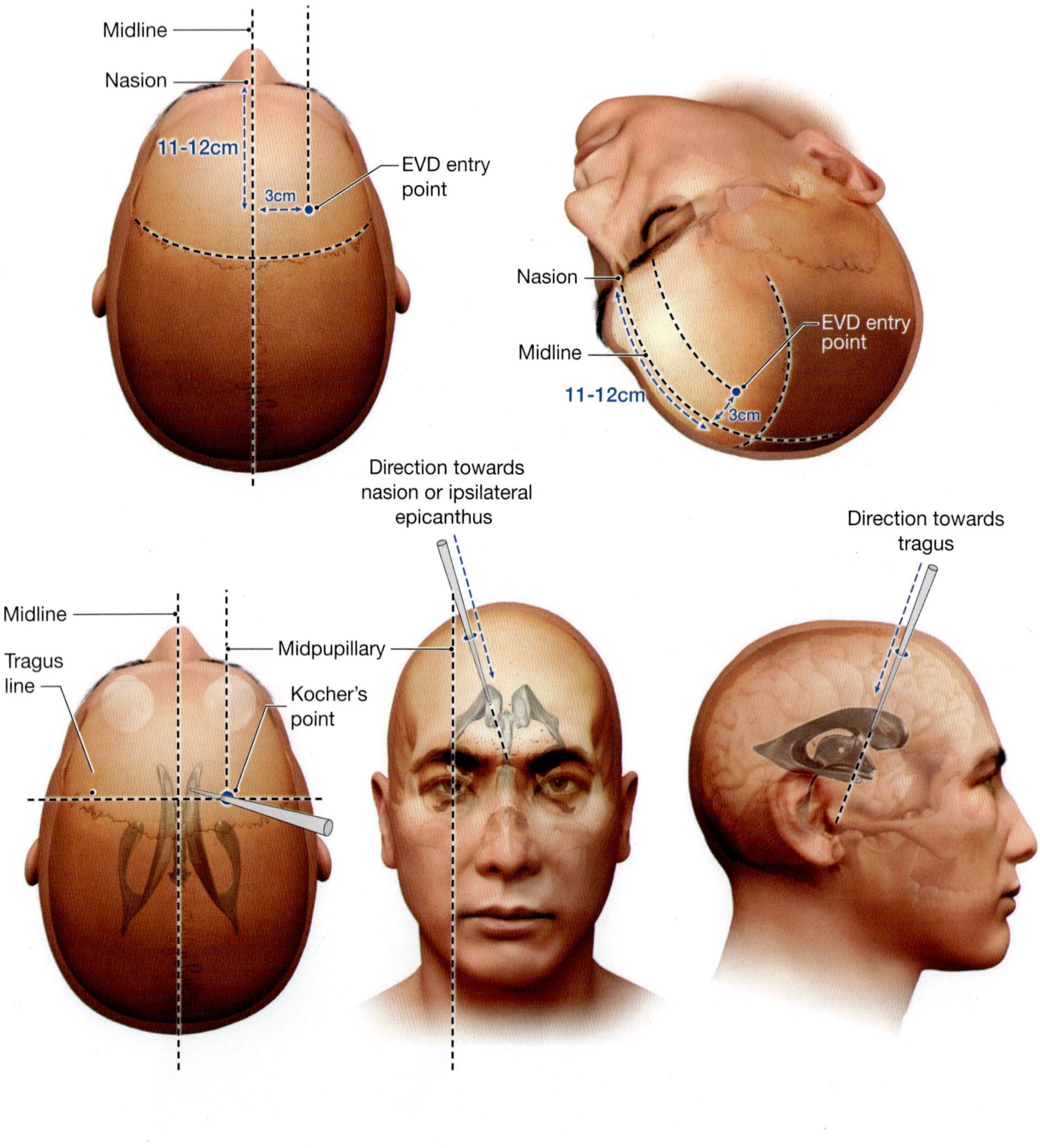

Figure 1-5

  - Make a 1.5- to 2-cm linear, anterior-to-posterior incision over Kocher's point.
  - A twist drill from the cranial access kit is utilized to create a small hole through the skull.
    - Drill the hole perpendicular to the skull and in the trajectory toward the ipsilateral medial canthus and 1 cm in front of the tragus. The hole through the skull may prevent optimal placement of the catheter if it is not drilled in the same trajectory as you would want the catheter to go.
    - Utilize an assistant at bedside to help stabilize the patient's head during the drilling process, especially if the cervical spine has not been cleared.
  - Pierce dura with the trocar or 11-blade scalpel.
  - Pass the ventricular catheter to about 6-7 cm at the outer table of the skull at the trajectory of the ipsilateral medial canthus and 1 cm in front of the tragus.
    - Modify the trajectory to the tip of the nose or contralateral medial canthus if there is a significant midline shift.

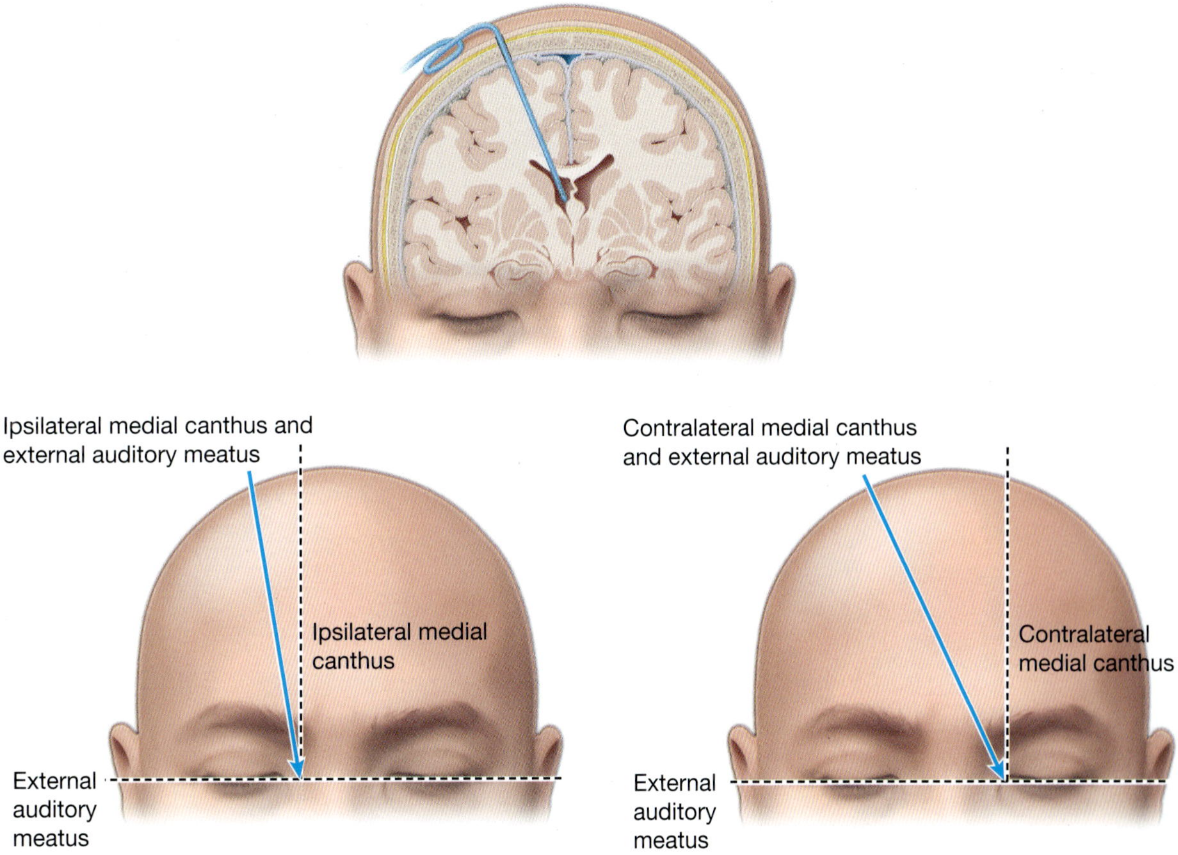

Figure 1-6

- After observing CSF flow from the catheter, place the trocar at the end of the catheter and tunnel the catheter posteriorly to an area about 5 cm away from the incision site.
    - With CSF flowing through the catheter, a quick estimate of ICP can be obtained by lifting the catheter straight and observing the level of CSF within the catheter. ICP will be the height of the CSF column above the tragus of the ear.
- Once tunneled, remove the trocar and either cap the ventricular catheter or connect it to the drainage bag.
- Suture the linear incision and place a purse-string suture around the exit site of the scalp using the ends of the suture to secure the catheter to the scalp.
- Secure the catheter to the scalp at three or more points with a skin stapler or with sutures, making sure that there is still flow from the catheter.
- Place a biopatch over the exit site and place Tegaderm over the entire area as dressing.
- Connect the catheter to the drainage bag if it has not been done already.
    - Bedside assistant should zero the system.
    - Obtain and record opening pressure.
    - Check the waveform and confirm drainage of CSF.
    - Set the drainage bag at the predetermined level above the tragus for continuous drainage or maintain the system clamped to monitor ICP.

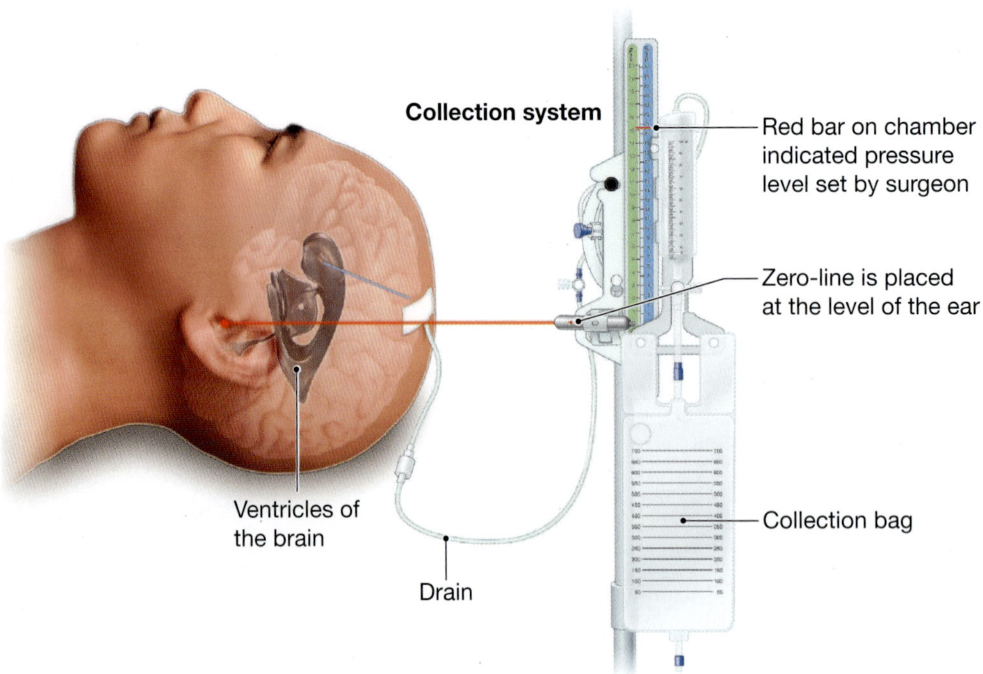

Figure 1-7

- **Complications**
  - Intracranial hemorrhage
  - Catheter blockage
  - Infection
    - Meningitis
    - Ventriculitis
    - Brain abscess
    - Subdural empyema
  - CSF leak
  - Misplacement
  - Dislodgement

Craniotomy for Evacuation of Epidural Hematoma (EDH)

- **Operative tips**
  - Review all lab work, especially coagulation studies.
  - Review imaging studies, especially relationship to landmarks around the skull.
  - Make sure to use plenty of tack-up sutures for the dura around the craniotomy as well as through the bone flap to prevent reaccumulation.
- **Introduction**
  - 20%-50% of cases may have history of a lucid interval where there is a brief period of full consciousness or the patient appearing back to their "normal self" following the initial confusion or decreased/loss of consciousness after the trauma, which can quickly decline as the EDH expands.
  - Indications for surgical evacuation
    - An EDH $\geq$30 cm^3 should be surgically evacuated regardless of the patient's GCS score.
    - An EDH <30 cm^3 *and* with less than a 15-mm thickness *and* with less than 5 mm of midline shift in a patient with a GCS score >8 *without* any focal deficits can be managed nonoperatively with close neurologic observation and serial imaging studies.
    - It is strongly recommended that patients with a GCS <9 with anisocoria undergo surgical evacuation as soon as possible.
  - 10%-30% will have delayed enlargement.

- **Anatomy**
  - EDH is a collection of blood between the inner table of the skull and the dura mater.
    - Does not cross suture lines in adults as the dura is adherent to the sutures of the skull
  - EDH is biconvex or lenticular in shape compared to an acute subdural hematoma.

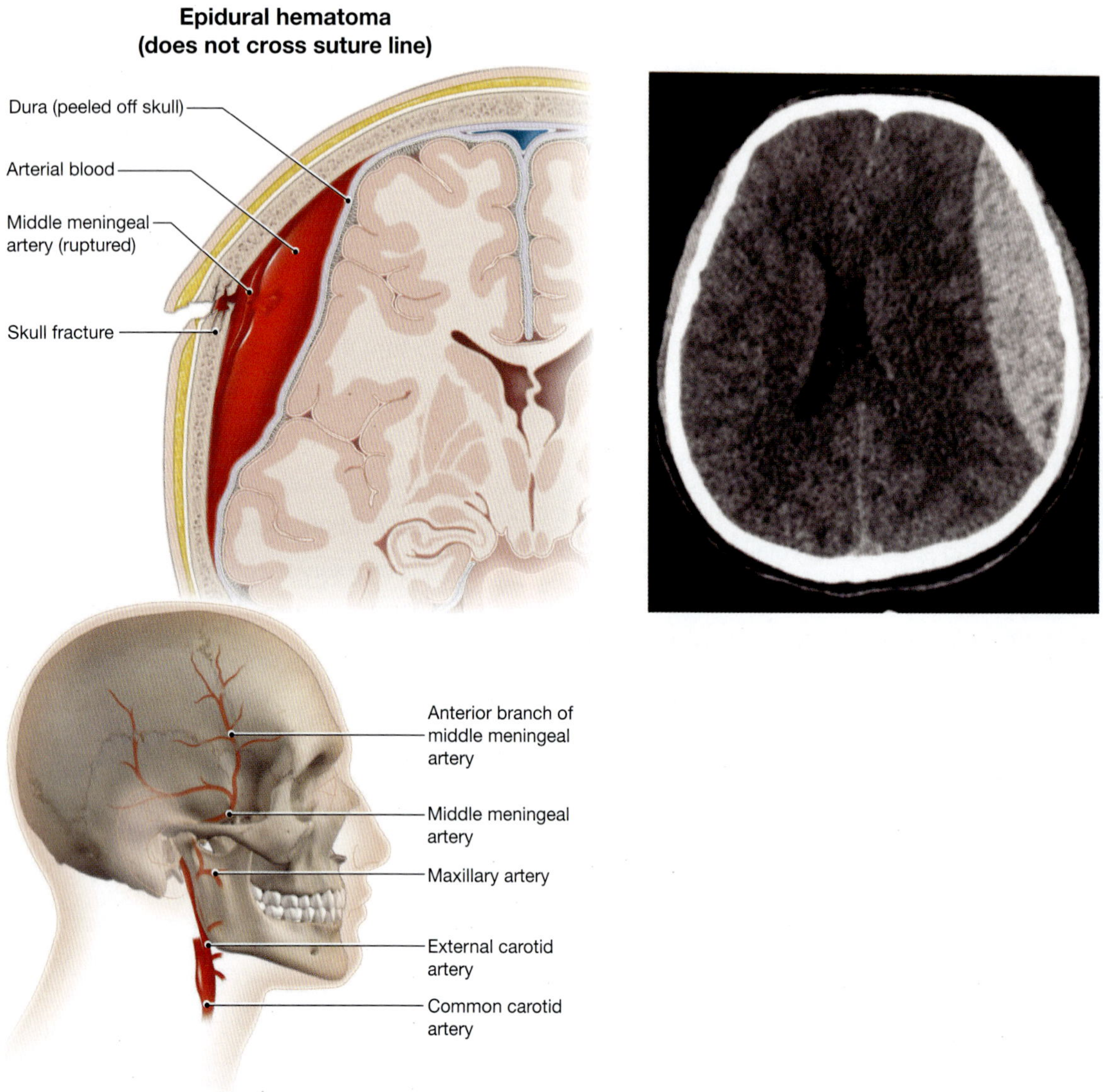

Figure 1-8

  - It is associated with injury to the middle meningeal artery and branches, with 70%-80% located in the temporoparietal location.
- **Operative steps**
  - Patient is positioned supine with a gel roll under the ipsilateral shoulder and head turned to the contralateral side. Maintain cervical spine precautions if necessary. If EDH is located more posteriorly, may position lateral or prone. May use gel head holder versus a horseshoe headframe versus a clamp with pins headframe.

- Based on imaging studies, determine either a linear versus a curvilinear incision overlying the location of the EDH. The craniotomy should be planned to maximize anterior-to-posterior decompression.

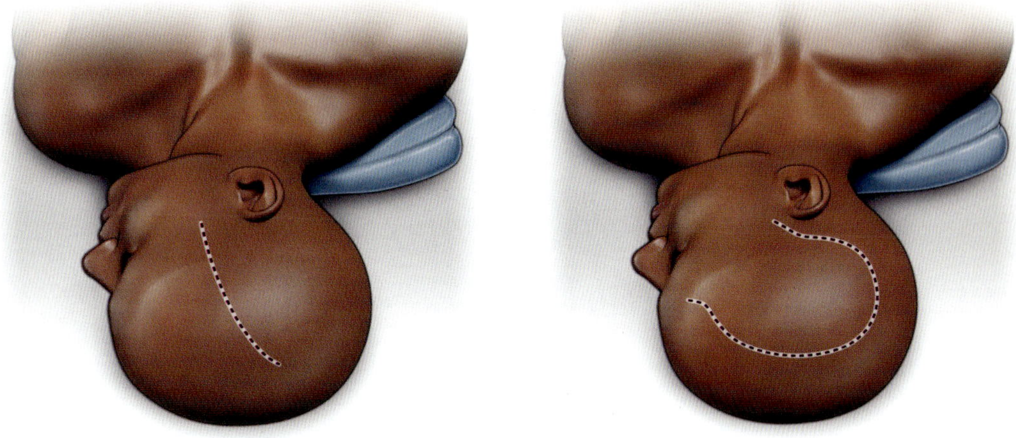

Figure 1-9

- Elevate the bone flap. There may be an associated skull fracture that may need to be incorporated into the bone flap and plated.

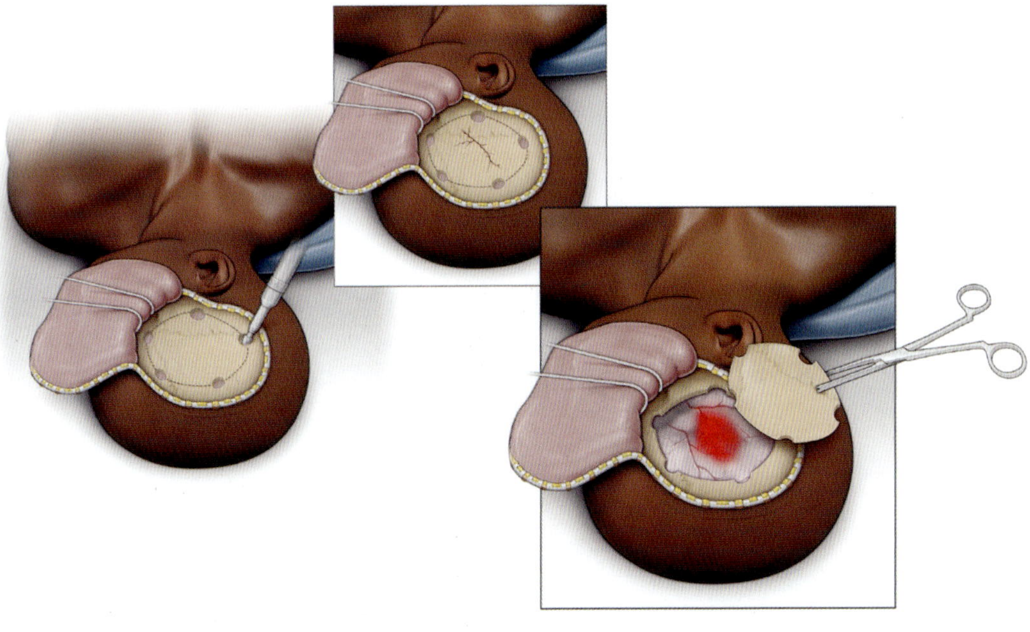

Figure 1-10

- Once the bone flap is elevated, the EDH should be visible under the bone. EDH can be removed using a copious amount of irrigation, suction, and various instruments.
- Identify the source of bleeding as quickly as possible. Control the bleeding with either direct cautery to the vessel or with bone wax if the bleeding is coming from the squamous portion of the temporal bone.

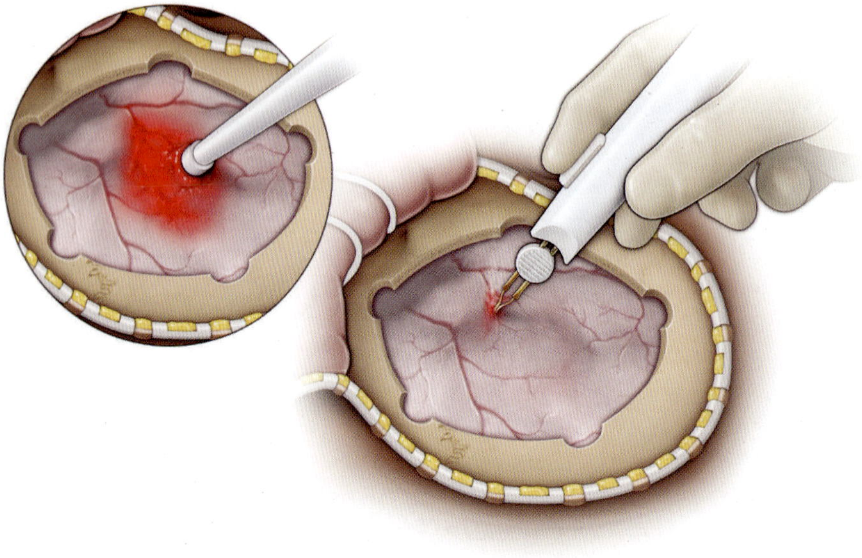

Figure 1-11

- After bleeding is controlled, dural tack-up sutures are placed around the edges of the craniotomy as well as through the bone flap to decrease risks of reaccumulation. There cannot be too many dural tack-up sutures.

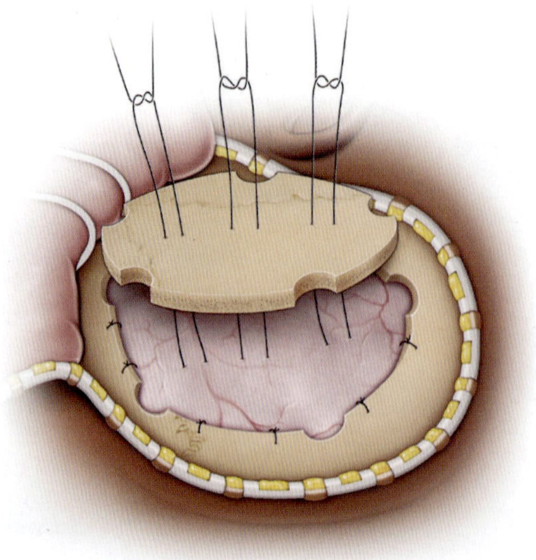

Figure 1-12

- Bone flap is secured in anatomic position utilizing cranial plating systems.
- Can consider placing a drain either within the epidural space or under the temporalis muscle.
- Approximate the temporalis fascia, galeal layer, and skin layer for closure.

- **Complications**
  - Reaccumulation of EDH if hemostasis is not achieved or not enough dural tack-up sutures were placed.
  - Infection

Craniotomy for Evacuation of Acute Subdural Hematoma

- **Operative tips**
  - Review all lab work, especially coagulation studies.
  - Review imaging studies, especially relationship to landmarks around the skull.
- **Introduction**
  - An acute subdural hematoma (aSDH) is a collection of blood under the dura mater and overlying the brain parenchyma. They appear hyperdense on CT head.
  - Indications for surgical evacuation
    - Hematoma >10 mm in thickness or midlines shift >5 mm regardless of the patient's GCS
    - Hematoma <10 mm in thickness and midline shift <5 mm with any of the following:
      - GCS decrease ≥2 points from injury on admission
      - Pupils asymmetric or fixed and dilated
      - ICP >20 mm Hg
- **Anatomy**
  - Crescentic in shape

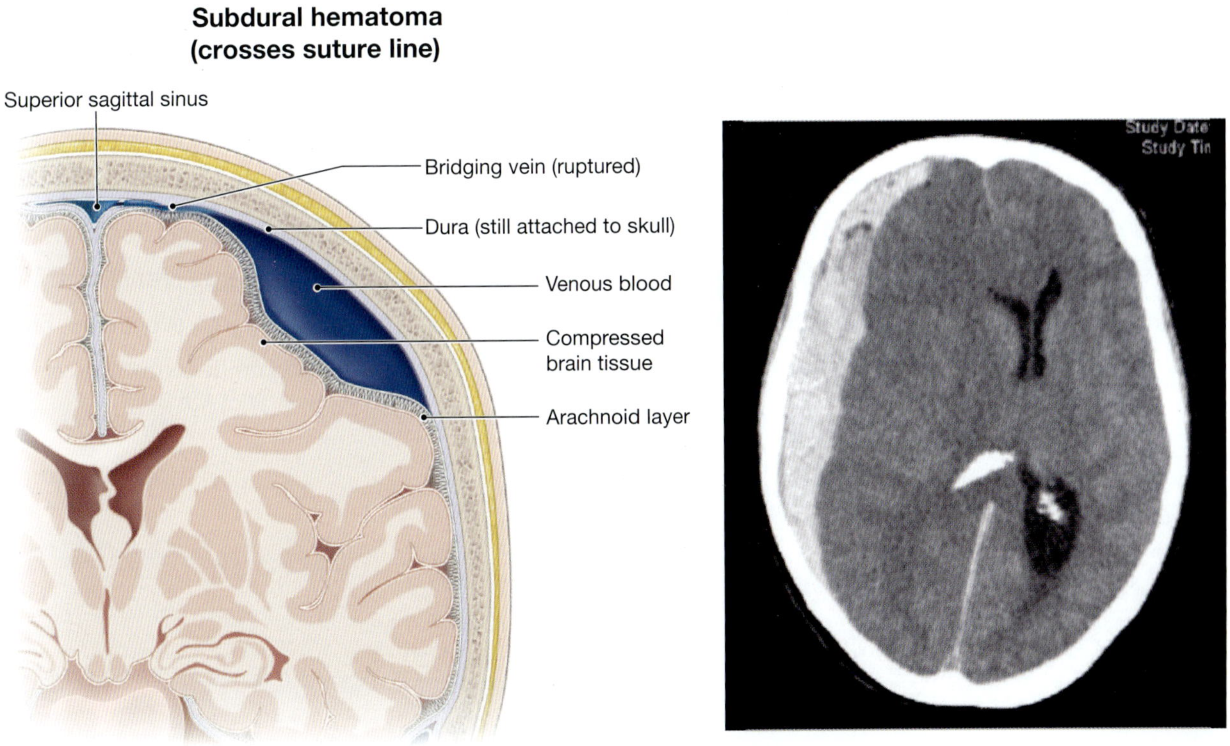

Figure 1-13

- Crosses suture lines as the hematoma located under the dura
- Typically associated with venous injury, though source of bleeding may not be obvious during surgery

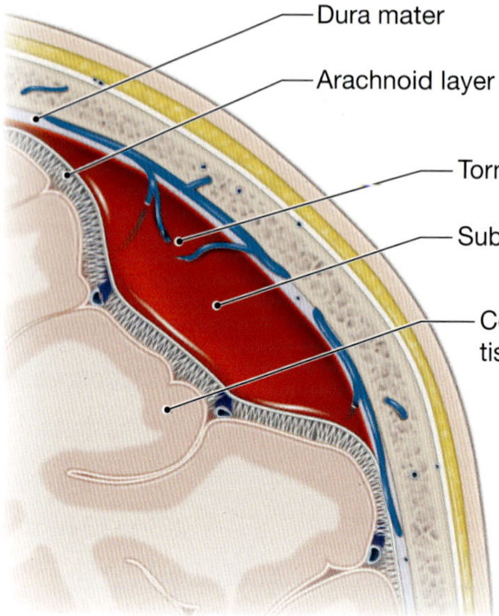

Figure 1-14

- **Operative steps**
  - Patient is positioned supine with a gel roll under the ipsilateral shoulder and head turned to the contralateral side. Maintain cervical spine precautions if necessary. If aSDH is located more posteriorly, may position lateral or prone. May use gel head holder versus a horseshoe headframe versus a clamp with pins headframe.
  - Based on imaging studies, determine either a linear versus a curvilinear incision overlying the location of the aSDH. The craniotomy should be planned to maximize anterior-to-posterior decompression. If there is associated underlying brain edema, consider a large craniectomy for decompression along with evacuation of the aSDH. (See section on decompressive craniectomy.)

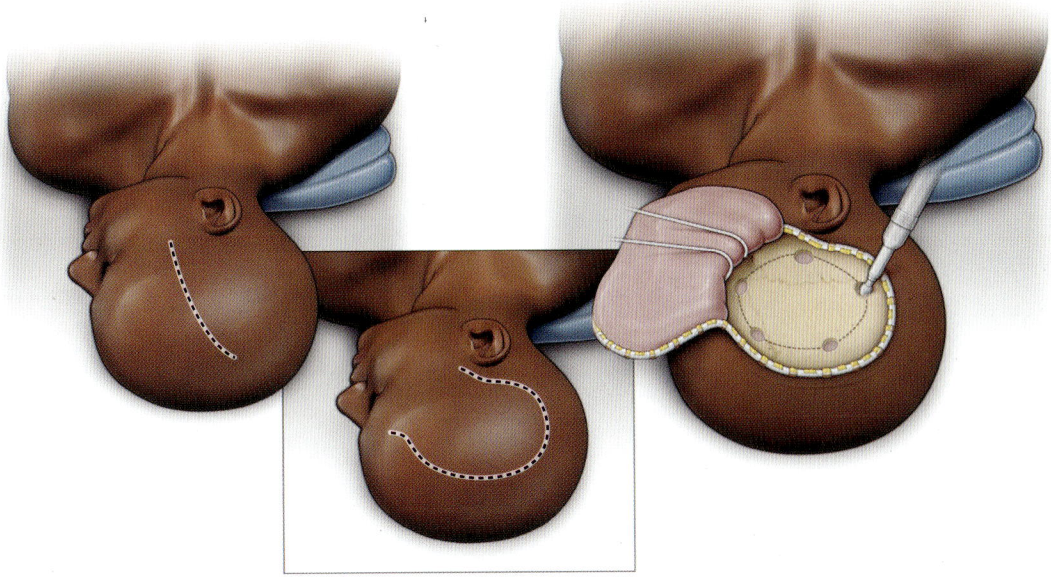

Figure 1-15

- Elevate the bone flap.
- Once the bone flap is elevated, dura will be observed. Cauterize the surface of the dura to minimize bleeding with dural opening.
- Dura may be opened in C-shape or stellate fashion. Place a dural stitch and open the dura with an 11- or 15-blade scalpel for the initial cut. Then use curved Metzenbaum scissors to continue the dural opening, making sure not to cut any cortical bridging veins. Leave a cuff of dura along the edges of the craniotomy to prevent retraction of the dura and to allow for closure of the dura. Tack-up dural sutures around the bony edges of the craniotomy may be helpful in decreased venous ooze but are not absolutely necessary.

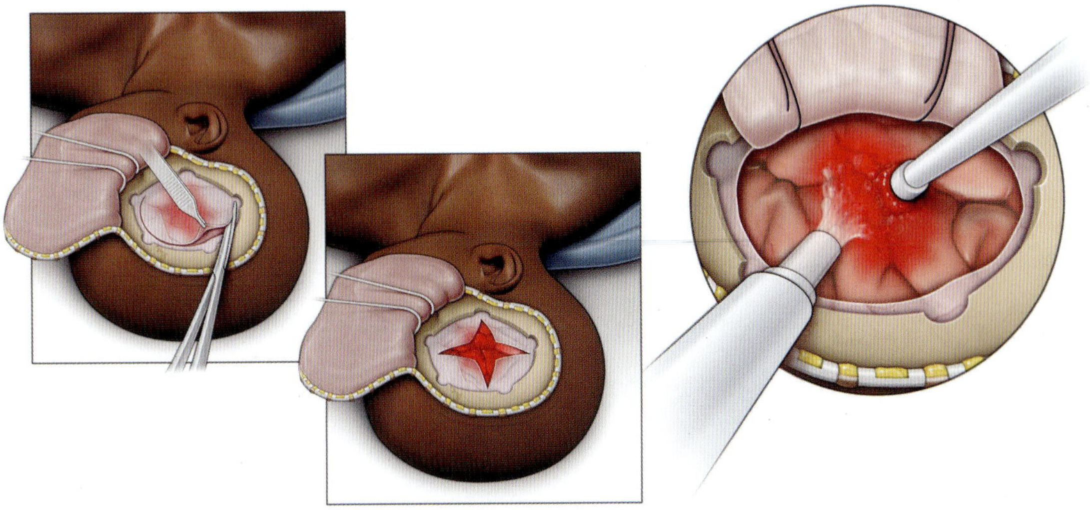

Figure 1-16

- Evacuate the aSDH with a combination of copious amount of irrigation, suction, and various instruments.
- Once the clot is evacuated, observe for any sites of active bleeding such as a cortical vein. If identified, cauterize with bipolar cautery or use hemostatic agents and gentle pressure with cotton patties.
- If a subdural drain is going to be placed, lay the drain under the dura prior to dural closure. The subdural drain can be placed to drain to gravity or to very gentle suction depending on the preference of the surgeon.
- Once hemostasis is achieved, the dura can be closed primarily. If a drain is present, make sure the opening is loose around the drain. Synthetic dura material and fibrin glue may be used to assist with dural closure.
- If replacing the bone, the bone flap is secured in an anatomic position utilizing cranial plating systems.

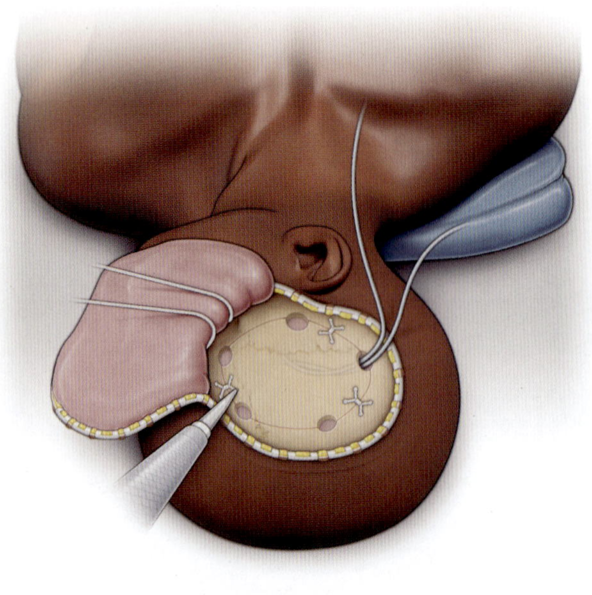

Figure 1-17

- If a subdural drain was not placed, a subgaleal drain may be placed under the temporalis muscle to decrease risks of reaccumulation.
- Approximate the temporalis fascia, galeal layer, and skin layer for closure.

- **Complications**
  - Reaccumulation of aSDH
  - Infection
  - Postoperative pneumocephalus
  - Seizures

Burr Holes for Evacuation of Chronic Subdural Hematomas (cSDH)

- **Operative tips**
  - Review all lab work, especially coagulation studies.
  - Review imaging studies, especially relationship to landmarks around the skull.
  - Recommend placement of a subdural drain with burr hole evacuation.
  - Burr hole evacuation does not allow for significant coagulation or removal of membranes.
  - If a craniotomy is performed for cSDH evacuation, do not aggressively remove the inner membrane as this will increase the risks of seizures that are difficult to control following surgery. Coagulate as much of the membranes as possible, especially along the dura.
- **Introduction**
  - cSDH is a common disease prevalent in the elderly population.
  - The incidence of cSDH ranges from 1.72 to 20.6 per 100,000 persons per year.
  - Risks factors include advanced age, male gender, and antiplatelet or anticoagulant use.

- The pathophysiology underlying the formation of cSDH is unclear but has been hypothesized to be secondary to an inflammatory response, transformation from acute hematoma, or an increased osmotic pressure gap between the hematoma and blood vessels.
- aSDHs turn subacute in nature between 10 and 14 days from the initial trauma and will appear isodense to brain on head CT. cSDHs are typically older than 14 days and appear hypodense on head CT.
- cSDH is more liquid than an acute hematoma and is classically described as motor oil in appearance.
- Clinical presentation is variable but mainly caused by increased intracranial compression through expansion of the hematoma. Symptoms include headaches, seizures, mental status changes, weakness, sensory deficits, dysarthria, gait disturbance, nausea, and vomiting.
- Considerations for surgical evacuation include symptoms and size of the cSDH including localized mass effect and extent of midline shift.
- Other options for surgical management include bedside subdural drain or subdural evacuating port (SEPs) placement and mini-craniotomy versus full-size craniotomy similar to those for aSDH.
- Risks factors associated with seizures with cSDH include alcohol abuse, mental status change, previous stroke, and density of hematoma on CT scan.

- **Anatomy**
  - cSDHs often are encapsulated in membranes with an inner membrane along the brain surface and an outer membrane adherent to the undersurface of the dura.

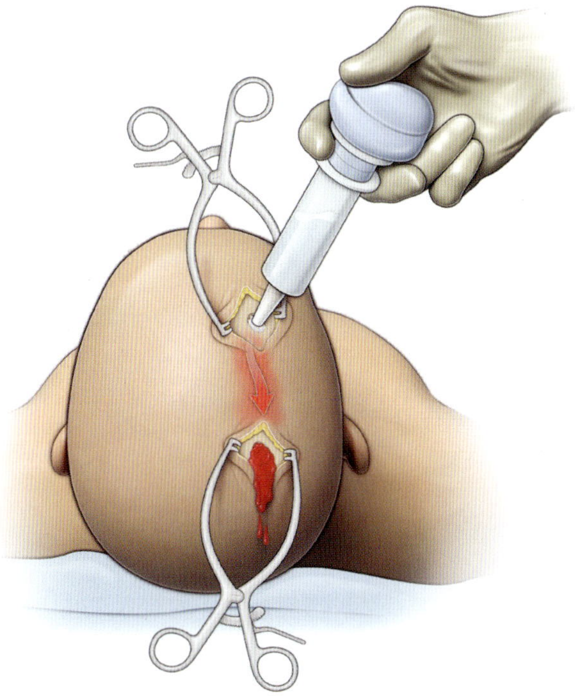

Figure 1-18

- **Operative steps**
  - Patient is positioned supine with a gel roll under the ipsilateral shoulder and head turned to the contralateral side. May use gel head holder versus a horseshoe headframe versus a clamp with pins headframe.
  - Two linear incisions approximately 2-3 cm in length are made along the frontal and parietal convexities depending on the location of the cSDH. Alternatively, a single burr hole may be used, but care must be taken to ensure adequate drainage of any irrigation used.

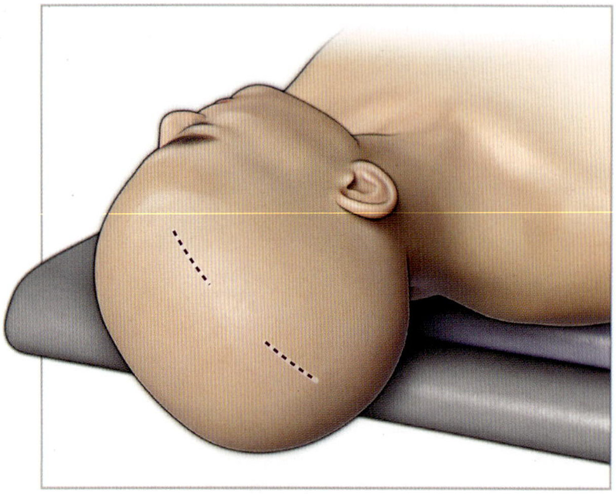

Figure 1-19

- A burr hole is placed at each incision, and the dura is coagulated and opened in a cruciate fashion. Dural leaflets are cauterized.
- If the outer membrane has not been punctured, cauterize and open the outer membrane to allow for drainage of cSDH. Copious amounts of irrigation should be used through both burr holes until the fluid starts to drain clear. Some surgeons may use a red rubber catheter to help irrigate cSDH fluid from recesses not easily accessible such as lateral and posterior to the burr holes.

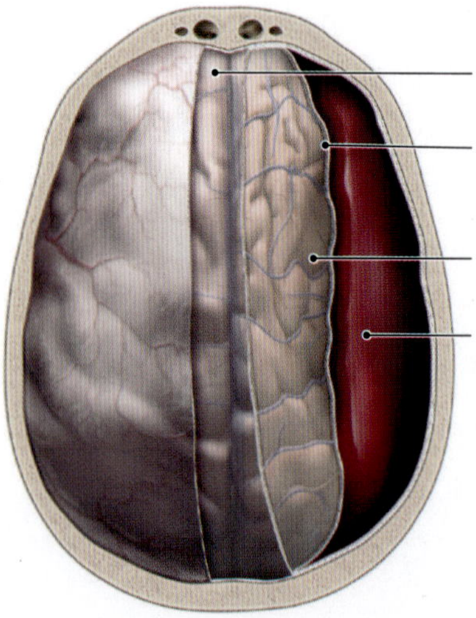

Figure 1-20

- Pass a subdural drain from one burr hole to the other. Tunnel under the skin to an exit site about 3-5 cm away from the incisions and secure onto the scalp. The subdural drain can be placed to drain to gravity or to very gentle suction depending on the preference of the surgeon.
- Burr hole covers may be placed and the skin incisions closed.

- **Complications**
  - Accumulation of aSDH
    - Placement of subdural drain reduces the recurrence rate
  - Infection
  - Postoperative pneumocephalus
  - Seizures

Decompressive Hemicraniectomy

- **Operative tips**
  - Review all lab work, especially coagulation studies.
  - Review imaging studies, especially relationship to landmarks around the skull.
  - A 14- to 15-cm width for the craniectomy is optimal size.
  - Make sure the craniectomy includes the parietal boss to ensure that the craniectomy is large enough.
  - Make sure to remove skull down to the floor of the middle fossa to decompress the temporal lobe to decrease risk of uncal herniation.
  - Bite down the sphenoid wing with a Leksell rongeur. There may be bleeding from the sphenoid wing, which can be controlled with bone wax.
  - Plan ahead of time where the drains will be exiting the scalp.

- **Introduction**
  - Indications for surgery
    - Elevated ICP refractory to medical management
    - Early signs of cerebral edema, significant midline shift, or herniation

- **Anatomy**
  - Utilize at least three burr holes to turn the craniectomy bone flap.
  - Burr hole placement
    - Use a MacCarty keyhole burr hole or sphenopterional point ("modified keyhole").

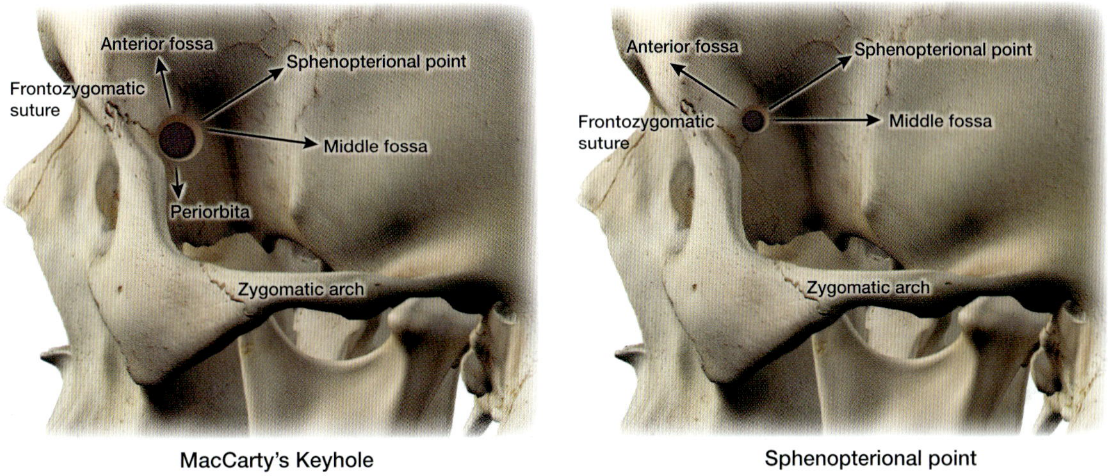

Figure 1-21

- Place a burr hole near the floor of the middle fossa just above the zygomatic arch.
- Another burr hole near the preauricular depression keyhole can be made.

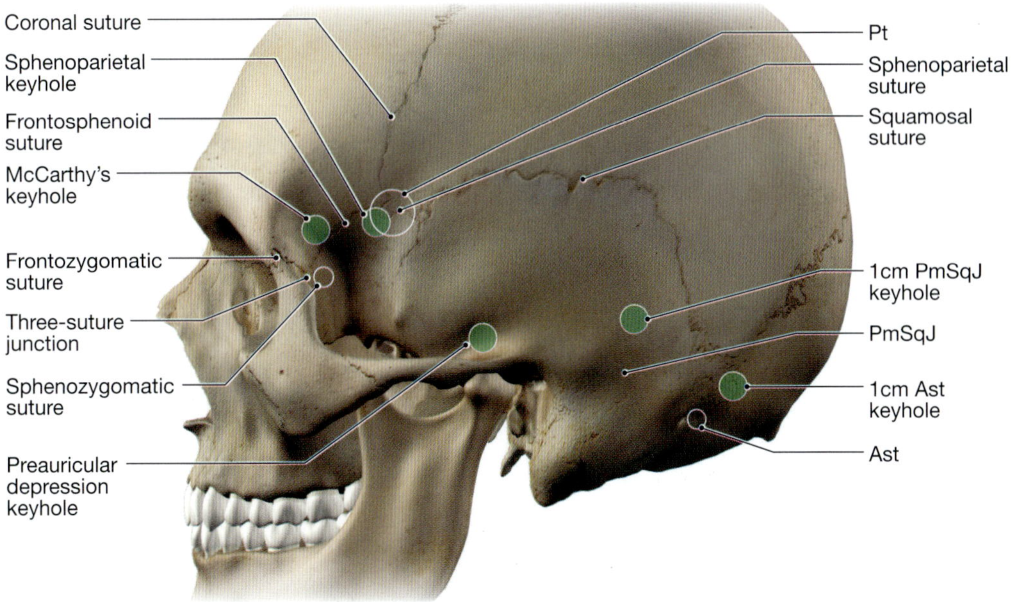

Figure 1-22

- A burr hole over the frontal lobe can help mark the superior and anterior point of the craniotomy.
- Another burr hole along the superior parietal region may be placed but not absolutely necessary.
- A final burr hole at the parietal-occipital region of the craniectomy site will help demarcate the posterior aspect of the craniectomy.

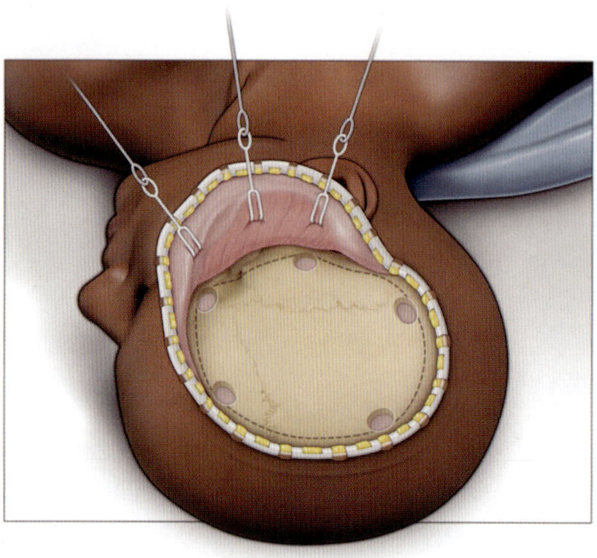

Figure 1-23

- **Operative steps**
  - Patient is positioned supine with a gel roll under the ipsilateral shoulder and head turned to the contralateral side. May use gel head holder versus a horseshoe headframe versus a clamp with pins headframe.
  - A large curvilinear incision is made about 1 cm from the midline curving around the parietal boss and either in front of the tragus or behind the ear.

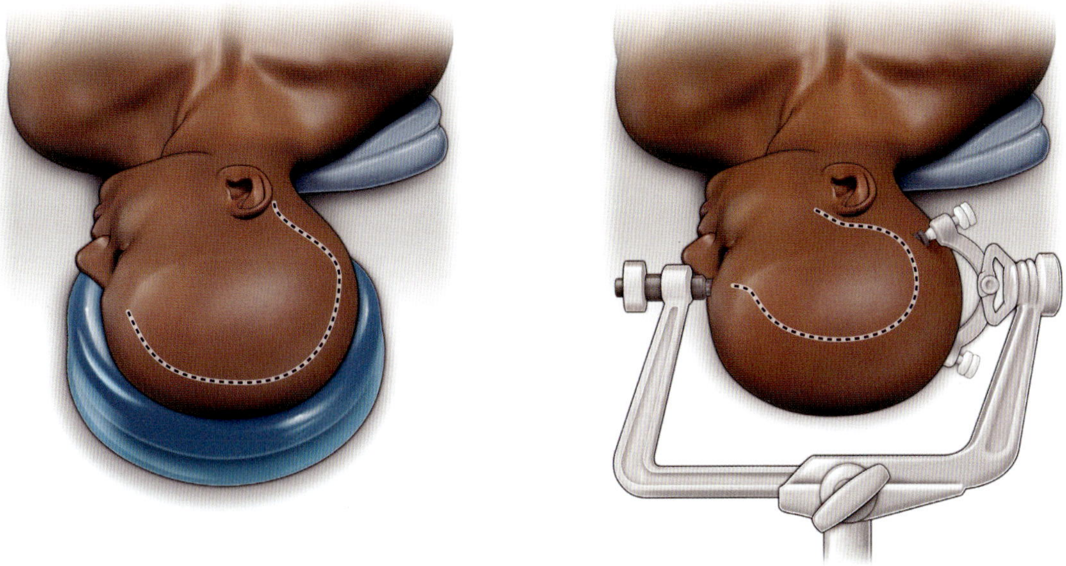

Figure 1-24

- Elevate the periosteum and the temporalis muscle from the skull and retract the myocutaneous flap anteriorly. The myocutaneous flap should extend anteriorly to the MacCarty keyhole and inferiorly to the root of the zygoma.

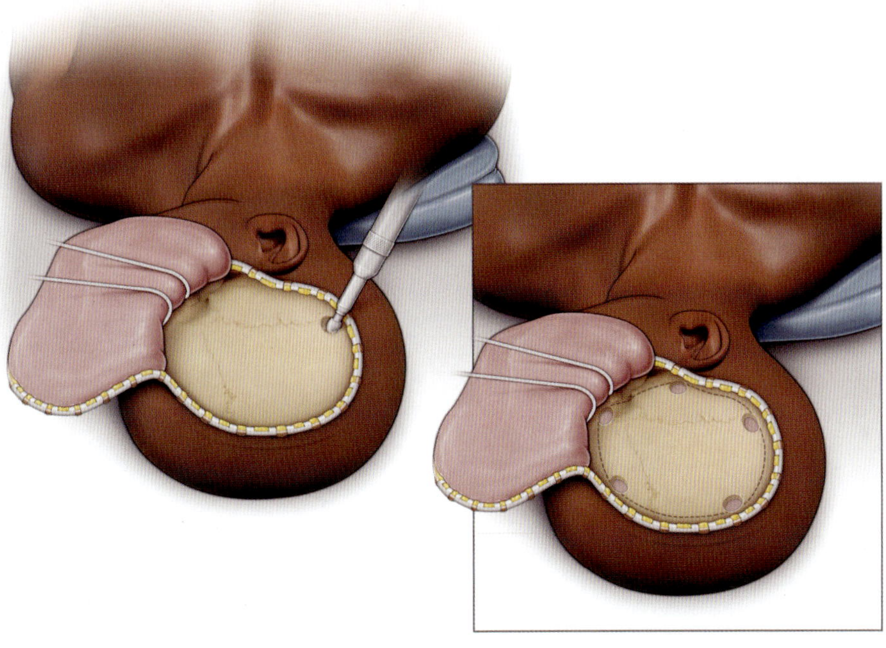

Figure 1-25

- Place your burr holes and connect with a craniotome.

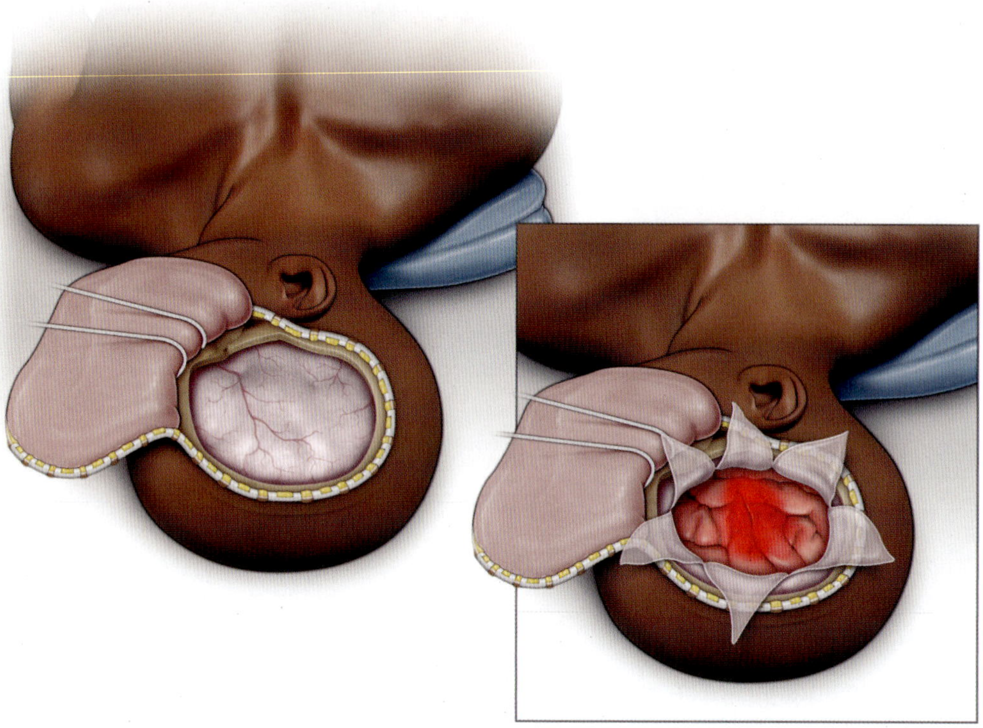

Figure 1-26

- Elevate the bone flap and place in sterile container for storage for future cranioplasty.
- Use a Leksell rongeur to bite down the temporal bone to be flush with the floor of the middle fossa, and also bite down the sphenoid wing for adequate decompression of the temporal lobe.

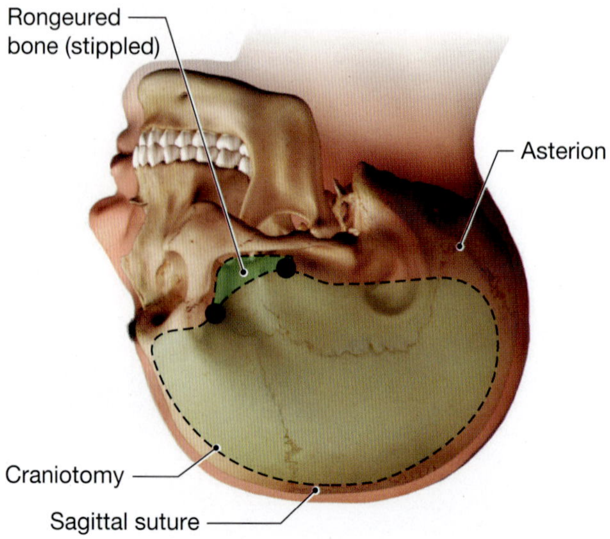

  - Cauterize the dura with the bipolar to reduce bleeding with opening of the dura.
  - Open the dura in a stellate fashion with numerous flaps, ensuring that there is no tension on the brain tissue along the edges of the flaps.
  - If an aSDH or intraparenchymal hemorrhage is present, it can be evacuated with copious irrigation, bipolar electrocautery, hemostatic agents, and various other instruments.
  - Synthetic dural replacement material can be gently laid on top of the brain parenchyma and the dural flaps gently laid on top of it.
  - Synthetic film may be placed between the temporalis muscle and dural layer to prevent adhesion and allow for easier dissection for future cranioplasty.
  - Place a subgaleal drain under the temporalis muscle and tunnel to exit the skin about 3-5 cm away from the incision. Secure the drain in place. Some surgeons may use two subgaleal drains to prevent epidural hematoma collection.
  - Approximate the temporalis fascia and close the skin with simple running sutures versus skin staples.
- **Complications**
  - Epidural/subgaleal hematoma
  - Infection
  - Seizures
  - Herniation of brain outside of the skull bone defect
  - Development of hydrocephalus requiring placement of a ventriculoperitoneal shunt
  - Subdural effusions
  - Resorption of bone flap
  - Syndrome of the trephined

2

CAROTID ARTERY

Daniel Steadman, DO
James W. Dennis, MD, FACS
Chelsea Yap, DO

TIPS

1. **For a near bloodless plane on a neck exploration, keep your incision along the anterior border of the sternocleidomastoid muscle, then along the medial border of the internal jugular vein.**
2. **Proximal control should first be obtained in an uninjured plane away from the site of the trauma or hematoma, which may require extension of the incision down to the sternal notch or into a median sternotomy.**
3. **The facial vein is the gateway structure of the neck; it is the key landmark that should be identified and ligated to gain access to the carotid bifurcation.**

Introduction

All injuries to the carotid artery should be addressed because they can lead to devastating morbidity and mortality in otherwise healthy patients. Old military data show simple ligation will result in at least a 30% incidence of major stroke and is the last resort when no repair is feasible. Traumatic injuries to the carotid are divided into blunt and penetrating injuries. Physical exam is of utmost importance in penetrating trauma and is 95% sensitive in detecting arterial injuries that require repair in zone II (see discussion of neck zones below). Hard signs of vascular injury to the carotid (active hemorrhage, pulse deficit, expanding/pulsatile hematoma, bruit/thrill, or distal ischemia or central neurologic deficits) should be explored in the operating room. Penetrating injuries to zones I and III typically need computed tomographic angiography (CTA) of the neck to confirm the diagnosis. The management of neck trauma is further dictated by the patient's hemodynamics. If the patient is hemodynamically normal and there are no hard signs of vascular injury on exam, then a CTA of the neck is obtained to assess for occult injuries to the vasculature and other critical aerodigestive structures of the neck. There is no clear consensus on whether CTA is reliable for excluding aerodigestive injuries as studies have demonstrated mixed results.

There is currently growing support for the "no zone" evaluation of neck injuries as contrasted with the traditional zone method described above. As previously mentioned, with the advent of CTA, hemodynamically stable patients can be evaluated with a radiographic study in combination with the standard trauma physical examination, regardless of the zone of injury, thus changing the zone approach toward guiding management.

Thus, the "no zone" algorithm for penetrating neck trauma focuses on identifying hard signs of injury and assessing patient stability rather than looking to the zone of injury for management. In addition, research has demonstrated that traditional "zoning" of a neck injury is not entirely accurate because almost 20% of zone II injuries were shown to enter zone I or III internally; however, the more concerning issues are zone I or III injuries that enter zone II, which automatically would be considered surgical. Regardless, the zone approach is still useful for helping clinicians quickly and effectively describe the anatomic location of the injury.

In blunt trauma, a CTA is indicated in a symptomatic patient or when a blunt cerebrovascular injury (BCVI) is suspected based on certain mechanisms of injury. These include hyperextension/rotation, hyperflexion, hanging, the presence of neurologic deficits, diffuse axonal injury, skull base fractures, LeFort II/III fractures, cervical spine fractures (especially C1-3), or a cervical seatbelt sign. Studies have demonstrated that a postcontrast acquisition of the neck included in a whole-body CT protocol is an acceptable initial means of screening multitrauma patients for the presence of BCVI. Most trauma centers have a CTA protocol that integrates BCVI screening into whole-body computed tomography (CT) with a single bolus of contrast, ensuring that the circle of Willis is included. Some variability exists among trauma centers for specific BCVI imaging, however, as many will obtain CTA studies selectively based on algorithmic criteria.

Blunt carotid artery injuries are most typically dissections of the internal carotid 1-2 cm above the bifurcation. Most dissections are best managed with anticoagulation or antiplatelet therapy alone if therapeutic anticoagulation is initially relatively contraindicated as in cases where there is concurrent brain or solid organ injury. If such medications are contraindicated, then endovascular therapy may be useful. Secondary pseudoaneurysms or arteriovenous fistulas may undergo either open repair or endovascular repair if not amenable to open surgery.

Anatomy

A detailed understanding of neck anatomy is crucial because there are many critical anatomic structures condensed into this relatively small area. The classic three zones of the neck first described at Cook County Hospital in the 1960s are still useful in the evaluation and treatment of penetrating injuries. Zone I is from the base of the neck to the cricoid cartilage; zone II is from the cricoid cartilage to the angle of the mandible; zone III is from the angle of the mandible to the base of the skull. The majority of penetrating injuries are found in zone II and are amenable to open surgical repair. Penetrating injuries to zone III are rare but usually involve the internal carotid. Open repair tends to be challenging because obtaining distal control can be difficult. Any surgeon operating in the neck needs to be thoroughly familiar with structural anatomy including locations of the cranial nerves that are at risk of iatrogenic injury.

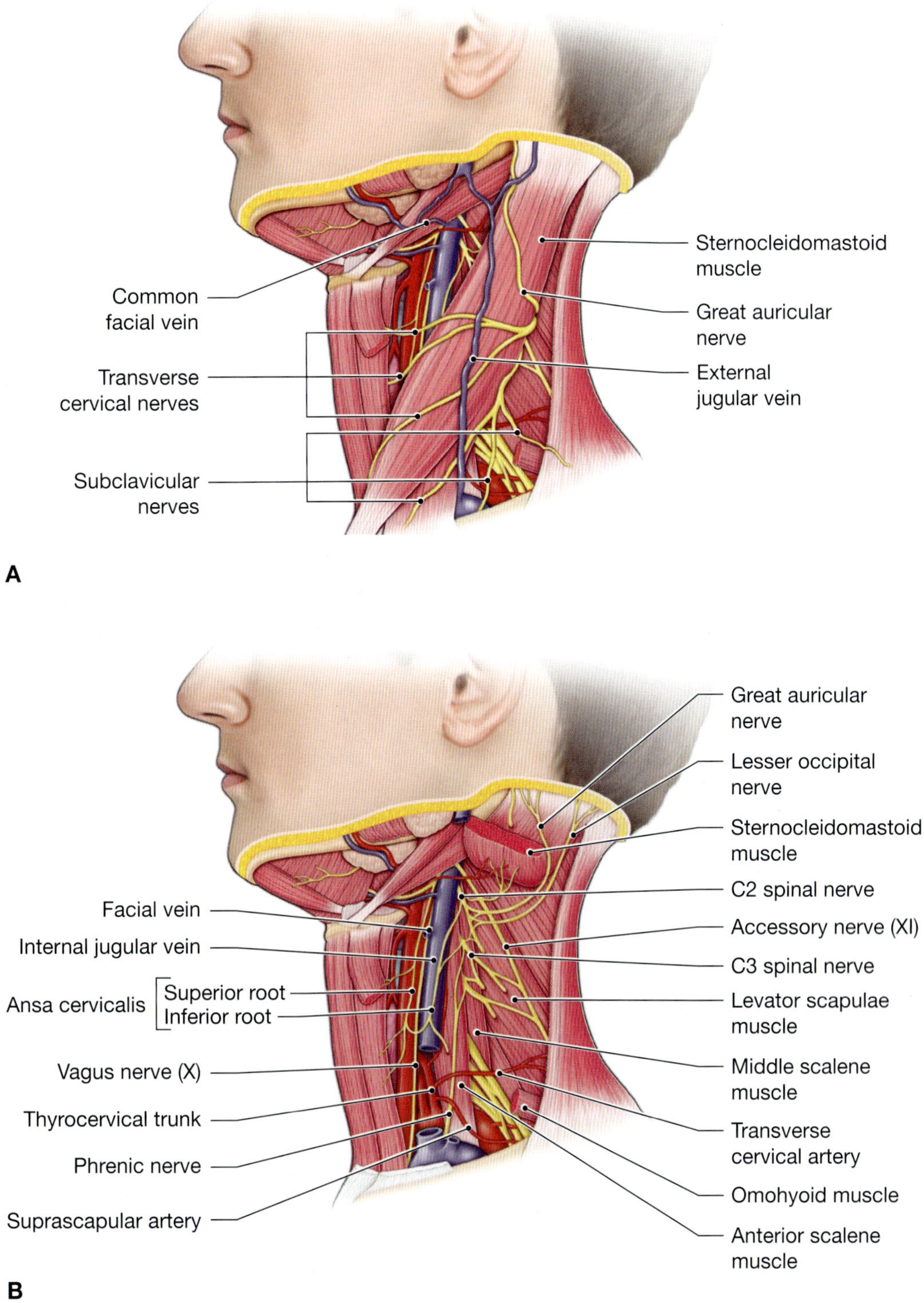
Common facial vein
Transverse cervical nerves
Subclavicular nerves
Sternocleidomastoid muscle
Great auricular nerve
External jugular vein
A
Facial vein
Internal jugular vein
Ansa cervicalis
Superior root
Inferior root
Vagus nerve (X)
Thyrocervical trunk
Phrenic nerve
Suprascapular artery
Great auricular nerve
Lesser occipital nerve
Sternocleidomastoid muscle
C2 spinal nerve
Accessory nerve (XI)
C3 spinal nerve
Levator scapulae muscle
Middle scalene muscle
Transverse cervical artery
Omohyoid muscle
Anterior scalene muscle
B

Figure 2-1

Operative Steps

- Proper positioning is important. Place a shoulder roll along with full extension of the head with rotation toward the contralateral side.
- The oblique incision begins on the side of the injury along the anterior border of the sternocleidomastoid (SCM). This is extended down through the platysma to the level of the internal jugular vein.
- This is the most commonly used incision to access the carotid artery. The incision is extended along the anterior edge of the SCM muscle.

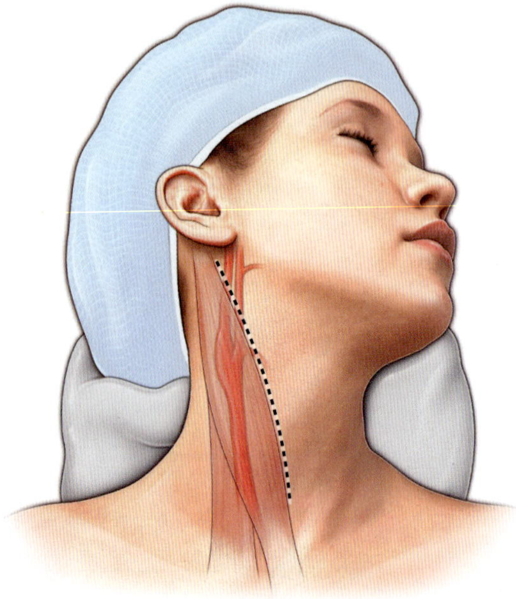

Figure 2-2

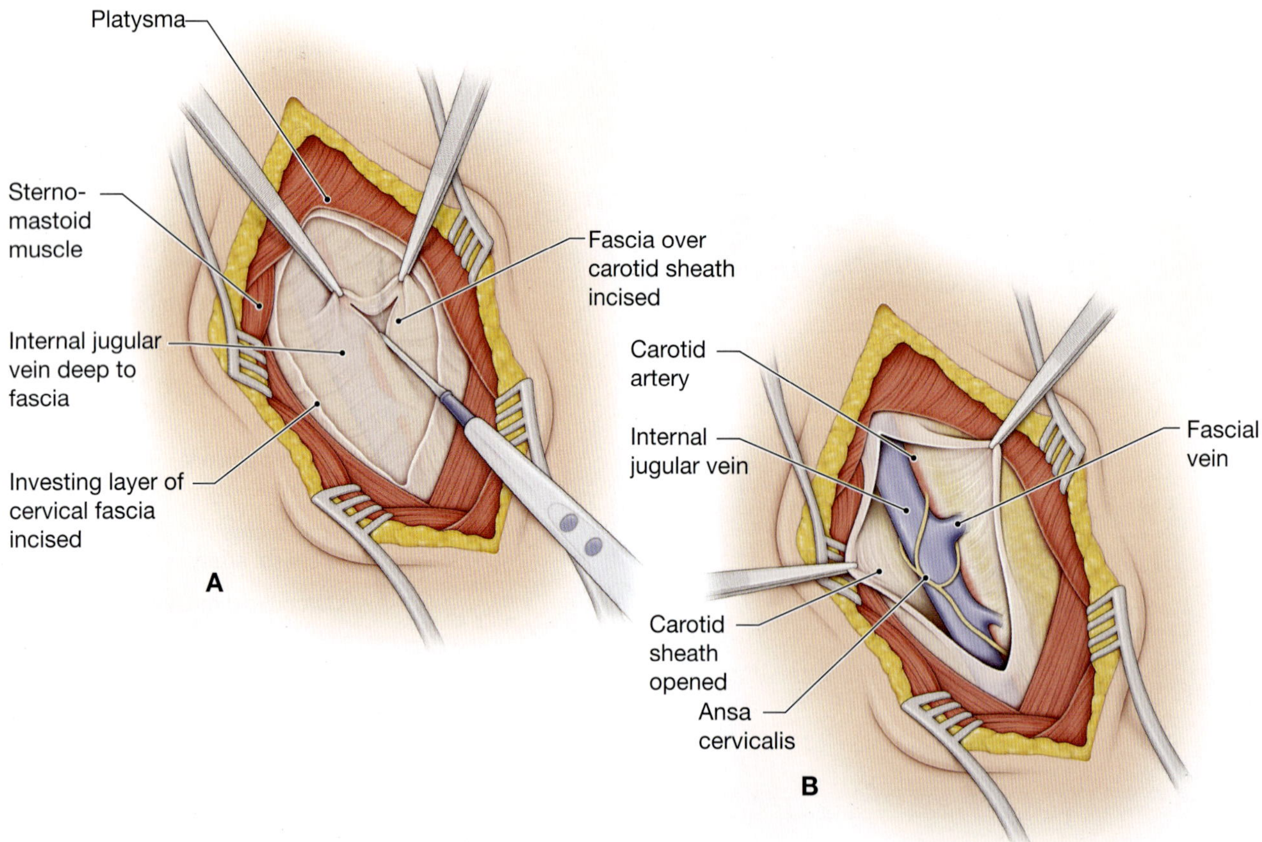

Figure 2-3

Penetrating Injuries

- For penetrating transcervical trajectories, a "U" incision is made for bilateral exploration. The superior subplatysmal flaps are developed transversely and reflected cephalad, exposing the important structures on both sides of the neck.
- The internal jugular vein is the most commonly injured structure in the neck. Bleeding from this structure should be controlled first with direct pressure. A side-biting clamp can then be placed to allow primary venorrhaphy. This is usually performed with a 5-0 Prolene suture in a running fashion. Ligation can also be performed in a damage control setting if the vein cannot be repaired expeditiously. If the internal jugular vein is not injured, then it should be unroofed to the level of the common facial vein and reflected laterally.
- Proximal and distal control of the carotid is the essential first step if there is a high suspicion for major arterial injury.
- The facial vein is an important structure to identify during a neck dissection. It is ligated to obtain access to the internal and external carotid, making it the "gateway structure" to the carotid bifurcation, which usually lies just posterior to it.

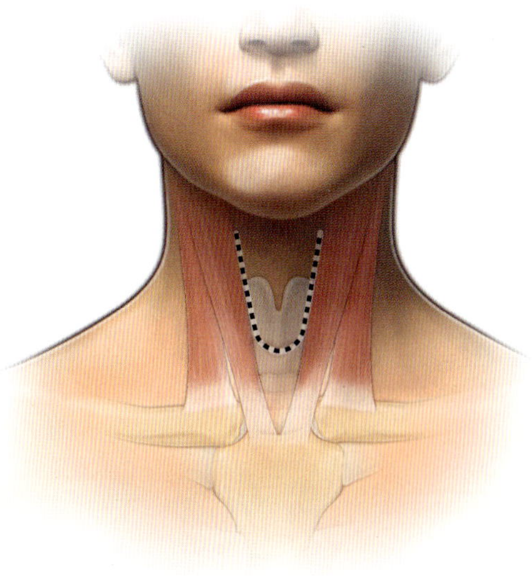

Figure 2-4

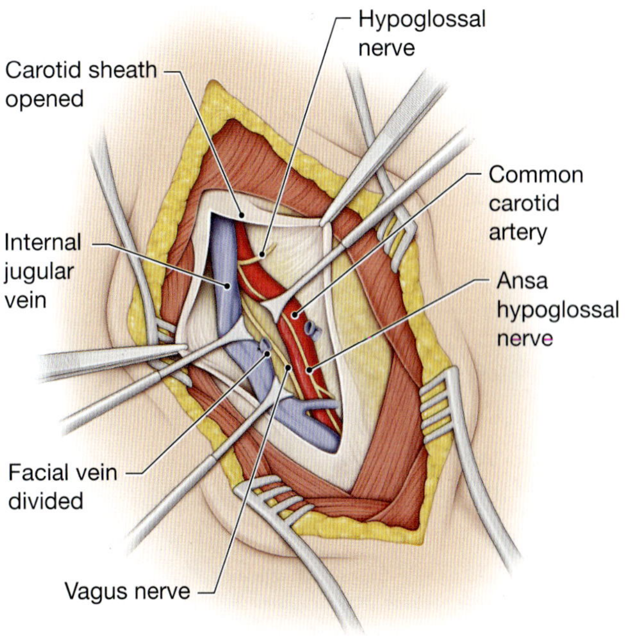

Figure 2-5

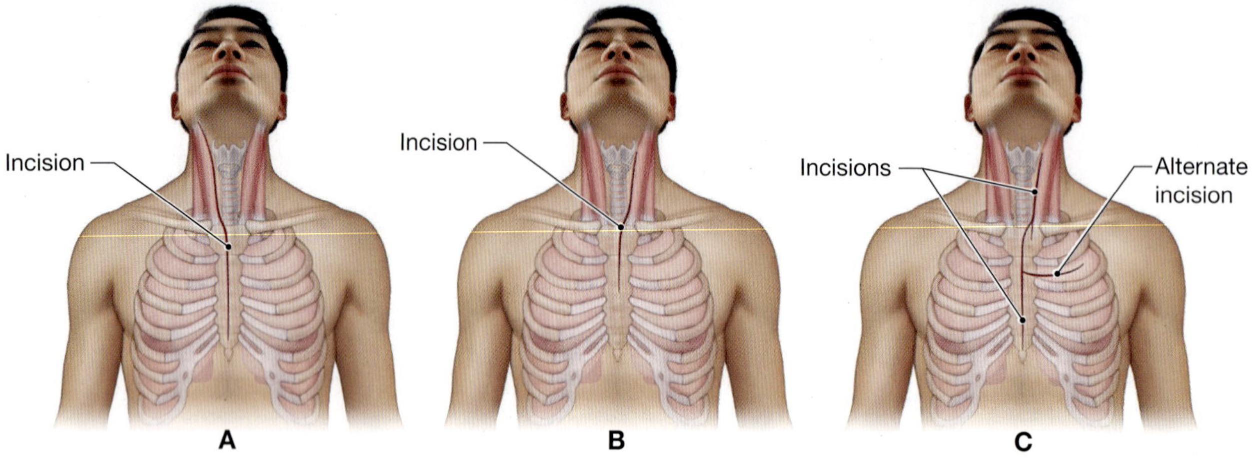

Figure 2-6

- Proximal control of the common carotid, usually first with a vessel loop, is best accomplished in a virgin plane away from the area of hematoma if possible, being sure to avoid the vagus nerve usually positioned posteriorly in the carotid sheath. Extension of the incision to the sternal notch or a median sternotomy may be required for zone I injuries of the proximal internal carotid system.

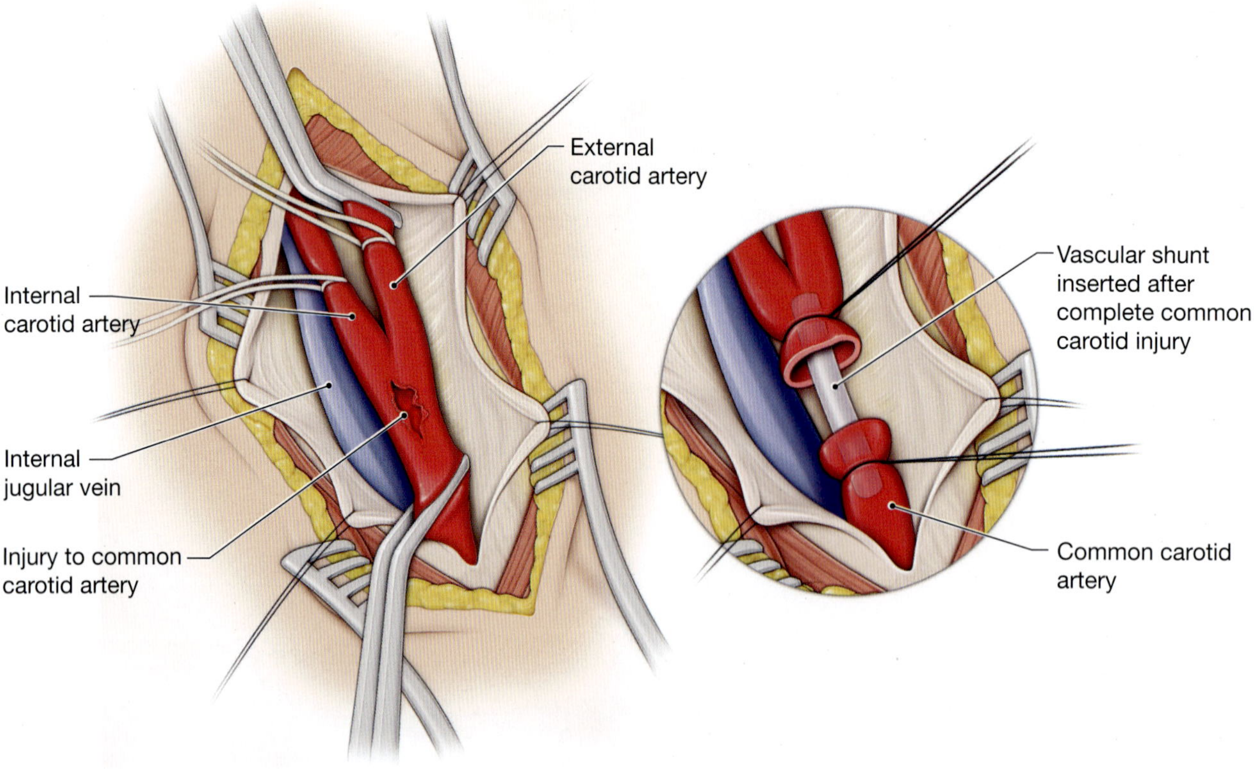

Figure 2-7

- Next, distal control must be secured. This typically occurs within the hematoma and may require extension of the incision to the mastoid process. Be sure to curve the incision at least 1 cm away from the angle of the mandible to avoid injury to the marginal mandibular branch of the facial nerve. Ligation of the facial vein will then allow for identification and control of the internal and external carotid arteries.
- The view will likely be obscured by a cervical hematoma and damaged tissue, so control of back bleeding is likely first achieved with direct pressure. Quick dissection will then allow clamp placement for more definitive control. If a clamp cannot be safely placed, then a Fogarty balloon can be inserted into the internal carotid artery (ICA) lumen followed by inflation of the balloon distal to the injury to allow for control of the hemorrhage. The superior thyroid artery is the first branch of the external carotid artery and will be encountered; this vessel can be ligated if needed to improve exposure.
- While dissecting out the carotid artery, it is important to remain in a periadventitial plane. This will help prevent injuries to important structures like the vagus nerve in the posterior carotid sheath or the hypoglossal nerve at the superior portion of the incision.
- It is important to maintain adequate blood pressure after clamping the carotid, with a mean arterial blood pressure of at least 100 mm Hg.
- The external carotid can be ligated with impunity if it is injured.
- Ligation of the common carotid can also be performed in rare situations. This is usually tolerated due to cerebral perfusion through the intact internal carotid from back pressure from the external carotid.
- As with any vascular injury, prior to any repair, the full extent of the injury must be determined. The surgeon must perform a longitudinal arteriotomy to define the extent of damage to the intima seen with the naked eye. Repairs beyond any damaged tissue should be the goal, regardless of technique.
- A direct thrombectomy may be needed, usually with a #4 Fogarty catheter proximally and a #3 Fogarty distally (using extreme care and gentle technique). Advance the distal catheter a few centimeters to avoid creating damage to the inaccessible portion of the carotid. This part of the case should be done with extreme caution because if it is done too aggressively, a pseudoaneurysm of a carotid-jugular fistula may occur.
- Heparinized saline is appropriate to flush the local artery proximally and distally with care to avoid any air in the circuit.

- There are multiple repair options for the ICA.
  - Primary repair or an end-to-end anastomosis (this generally works best in the case of stab wound with a clean laceration).
  - Patch angioplasty with bovine pericardium, Dacron, or vein. Vein is usually not used unless contamination is present.
  - Interposition graft with synthetic material (common carotid) or vein (ICA).
  - Transposition of the internal carotid to the distal external carotid.

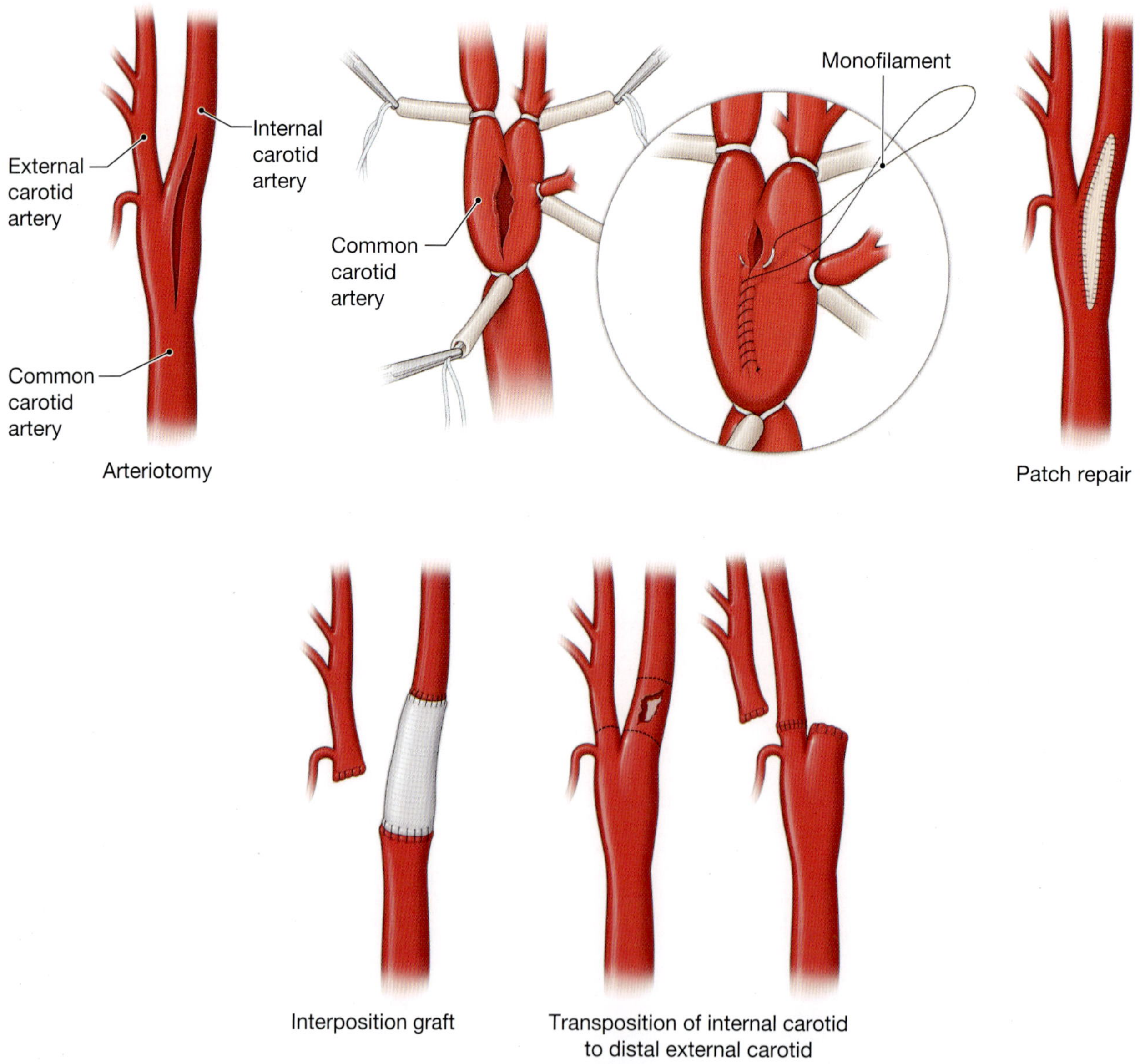

Figure 2-8

- Temporary indwelling shunts are useful to maintain brain perfusion during the repair if possible. This can be done in conjunction with the above reconstruction techniques in a similar fashion to that done with an endarterectomy (patch angioplasty) or by the graft being threaded over the shunt with the distal anastomosis and the majority of the proximal anastomosis performed around it.

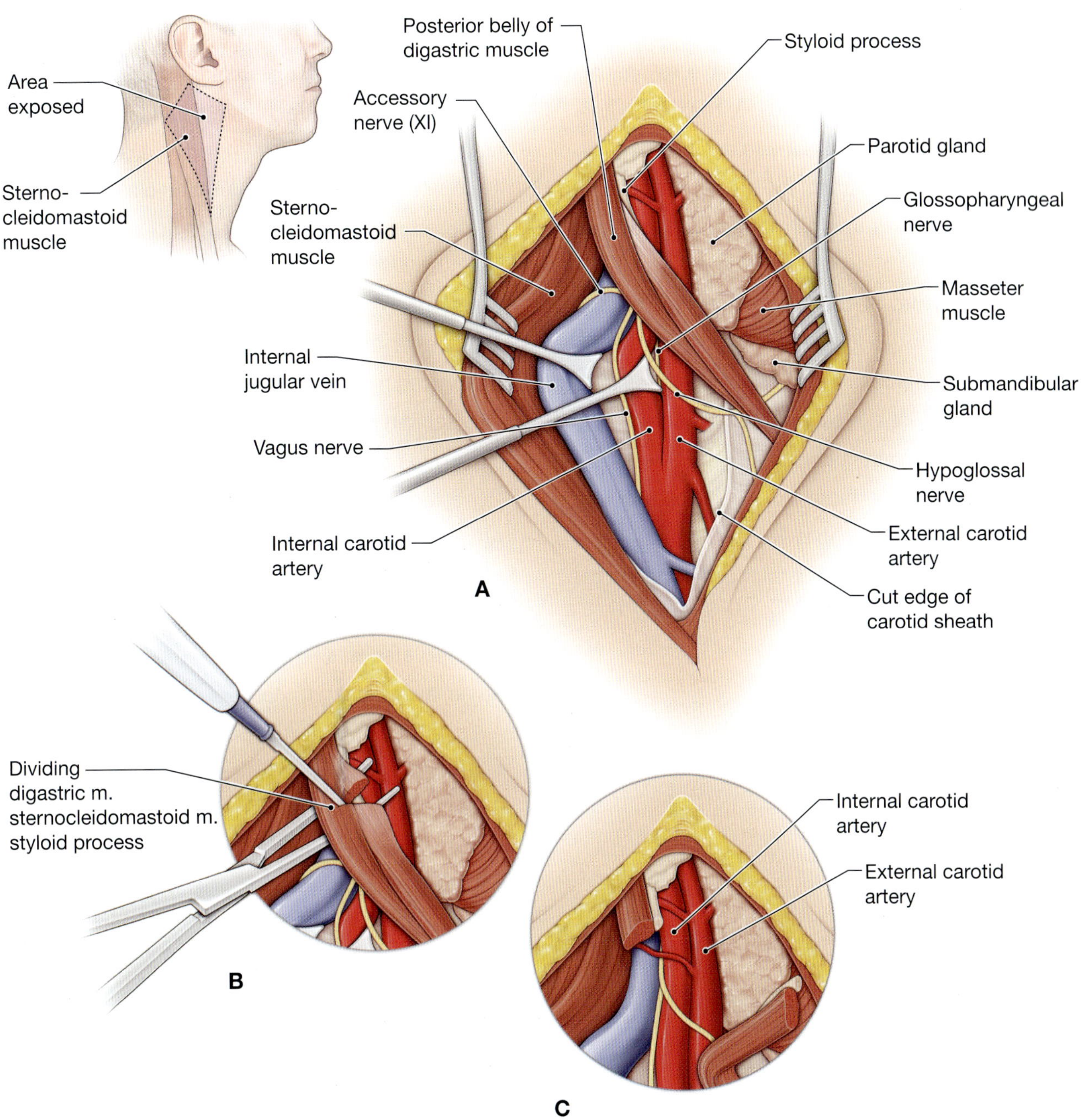

Figure 2-9

- For high internal carotid injuries that are difficult to access, there are multiple maneuvers that may aid in gaining access to the injury. First, extend the incision to the mastoid process. The posterior body of the digastric muscle can be transected next if needed. If that is not sufficient, subluxation of the jaw can allow further distal exposure. If the injury still cannot be accessed, the only option is to occlude the bleeding vessel in any way possible. A Fogarty catheter balloon can be placed into the lumen and then slowly inflated to tamponade any bleeding.
- In a damage control setting, the ICA can be ligated. However, this carries a significant risk and may lead to ischemia to the brain and significant morbidity and mortality. This may be the only option in the instance of a zone III injury, as this part of the ICA is difficult to access. Some authors argue that all injuries to the ICA that do not exhibit good backflow should be ligated because the patient has likely already experienced an ischemic stroke. If back pressure can be obtained and the mean is >70 mm Hg, stroke is very rare. Reperfusion after prolonged ischemia has a small risk (2%-5%) of converting an ischemic stroke to a hemorrhagic one.

Complications

Injury to Nerves

- Vagus (X) nerve
    - Located in the posterior carotid sheath
    - Hoarseness
    - Most commonly injured during carotid endarterectomy (accidentally clamping vagus nerve along with carotid artery)
    - Can also represent damage to recurrent laryngeal nerve (branch of vagus)
- Hypoglossal (XII) nerve
    - Located anterior to external carotid then medial to ICA
    - Tongue deviation toward injury
    - Difficulty with speech and mastication
- Marginal mandibular (VII) nerve
    - Located 1-2 cm below the mandible
    - Ipsilateral lip droop or mouth droop
    - Usually from retraction during exposure of high lesions
- Glossopharyngeal (IX) nerve
    - Located high, posterior and medial to the ICA
    - Disabling dysphagia
    - During high carotid dissection (lies deep to posterior belly of the digastric)
- Ansa cervicalis
    - Location variable
    - No serious deficits
    - Innervates strap muscles
- Spinal accessory (XI) nerve
    - Located high entering SCM/trapezius
    - Shoulder muscle weakness
- Greater auricular
    - High, anterior to SCM
    - Ear numbness

Blunt Trauma

- Carotid dissection
  - Treat with anticoagulation (heparin or dual antiplatelets) if grade >1 intimal defect.
  - If symptomatic or unable to anticoagulate, consider a covered stent.
  - Repeat imaging at 7-10 days or prior to discharge and then at 3 months after injury.
  - If worsened, then consider a covered stent.
- Carotid occlusion
  - If already has neurologic injury, then no intervention (unlikely to get better).
  - Consider anticoagulation if patient is a candidate based on other injuries.

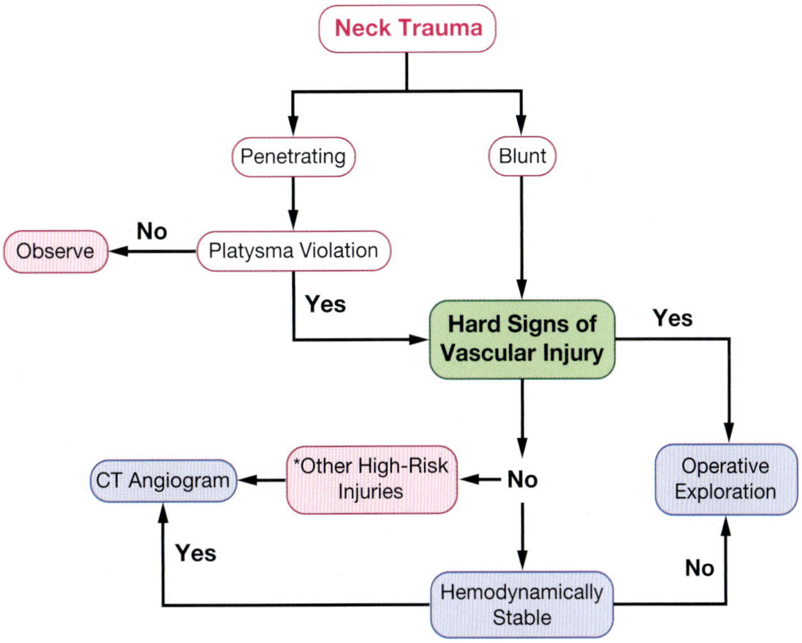

***High-risk injuries:**
- **Hyperextension/rotation, hyperflexion, or hanging**
- **Neurologic deficits**
- **Diffuse axonal injuries**
- **Skull base fractures**
- **C spine fractures (especially C1-C3)**
- **Cervical seatbelt sign**

Figure 2-10

3 SUBCLAVIAN ARTERY

Chelsea Yap, DO
James W. Dennis, MD, FACS
Daniel Steadman, DO

TIPS

1. **A thorough knowledge of the complex anatomy of the base of the neck and thoracic outlet is crucial when exploring and repairing vascular structures in this area. Central to this is the location of the major arteries, veins, and nerves in relation to the clavicle and scalene muscles.**
2. **Any arterial injury proximal to the axillary artery should first be considered for an endovascular approach if clinically possible.**
3. **Despite successful vascular repair, long-term morbidity is usually related to associated nerve injury.**
4. **Intravenous access should be obtained on the contralateral side of the suspected injury.**

Introduction

Subclavian artery trauma accounts for less than 5% of all traumas yet carries a high risk of death and permanent neurologic deficits. Young males are the most common victims, with the vast majority due to penetrating injuries. Blunt trauma to subclavian vessels is far less common due to their deep location and protection by the clavicle. When it does occur, it is usually associated with a clavicle fracture or fall from a great height. Safe and rapid exposure has always been the primary roadblock in open repair, which has led surgeons to seek endovascular options when possible. As with all vascular injuries, early diagnosis and treatment are essential in the care of a patient with subclavian artery trauma.

Hard signs of subclavian artery injury found on physical exam are similar to those of the extremity, including an absent pulse or ischemia in the ipsilateral upper extremity, an audible bruit, an expanding supraclavicular hematoma, and significant active hemorrhage. Soft signs or indirect findings include a brachial plexus palsy, a fracture of the first rib, and severe crush injury to the upper chest. The presence of an upper extremity pulse, however, does not rule out a subclavian artery injury, which can be present with a contained pseudoaneurysm, arteriovenous (AV) fistula, or limited intimal disruption. Hemodynamic instability of a patient or presence of active bleeding will dictate whether the patient needs to be taken emergently to the operating room. When feasible, bilateral upper extremity blood pressures should be recorded, and a standard chest X-ray is often helpful and should routinely be obtained upon presentation. Hemodynamically stable patients with concern for subclavian vessel injury should undergo immediate computed tomographic angiography (CTA) of the neck, chest, and upper extremity. Most subclavian artery injuries are considered grade 3 in the American Association for the Surgery of Trauma grading system, and subclavian vein injuries are classified as grade 2 (Table 3-1).

TABLE 3-1. American Association for the Surgery of Trauma Thoracic Vascular Injury Scale

Grade	Description of Injury
I	Intercostal artery/vein
	Internal mammary artery/vein
	Bronchial artery/vein
	Esophageal artery/vein
	Hemizygous vein
	Unnamed artery/vein
II	Azygos vein
	Internal jugular vein
	Subclavian vein
	Innominate vein
III	Carotid artery
	Innominate artery
	Subclavian artery
IV	Thoracic aorta, descending
	Inferior vena cava (intrathoracic)
	Pulmonary artery, primary intraparenchymal branch
	Pulmonary vein, primary intraparenchymal branch
V	Thoracic aorta, ascending and arch
	Superior vena cava
	Pulmonary artery, main trunk
	Pulmonary vein, main trunk
VI	Uncontained total transection of
	thoracic aorta or pulmonary
	Hilum

Source: Adapted with permission from Moore EE, Malangoni MA, Cogbill TH, et al. Organ injury scaling. IV: Thoracic vascular, lung, cardiac, and diaphragm. *J Trauma.* 1994;36(3):299-300.

Depending on the type of vascular injury and the location found on CTA, either direct open repair may be considered or endovascular treatment may be performed in a stable patient. Due to the difficulty with exposure, endovascular repair has been found to be safe and effective in select patients. Usually, a stent graft extending intraluminally from normal proximal to normal distal vessel is the preferred technique. These stent grafts work exceedingly well with pseudoaneurysms, AV fistulas, and minor injuries with limited extravasation of contrast and avoid the morbidity of lengthy open procedures. Intimal flaps or minor irregularities require a judgment call regarding whether any treatment is needed. Long-term follow-up of similar injuries in extremity arteries has shown that these occult injuries usually heal or do not worsen. Occlusions of the artery from trauma can be crossed in a number of cases and flow restored with a stent graft. The indications and angiographic findings in one large study are shown in Table 3-2.

With blunt injuries, a pseudoaneurysm is the most common type of injury to the subclavian artery. Types of injuries seen in penetrating subclavian artery injuries are pseudoaneurysms, occlusion or transection, AV fistula, intimal flap, or a combination of pseudoaneurysm and AV fistula.

TABLE 3-2. Indication for Angiography and Their Findings in 37 Patients

	Number (%)
Indications for angiogram	
Pulse discrepancy	19 (38)
Bruit	10 (20)
Large hematoma	1 (2)
Moderate hematoma	4 (8)
Pulsatile hematoma	1
Widened mediastinum on chest radiograph	1
Delayed presentation of brachial plexus deficit	1
Angiographic finding	
False aneurysm (FA)	13 (26)
Occlusion/transection	13 (26)
Arteriovenous fistula (AVF)	5 (10)
Intimal flap	4 (8)
FA and AVF	2 (4)

Source: Reproduced with permission from Sobnach S, Nicol AJ, Nathire H, et al. An analysis of 50 surgically managed penetrating subclavian artery injuries. *Eur J Vasc Endovasc Surg.* 2010;39(2):155-159.

Anatomy

Successful treatment of these subclavian injuries requires a detailed understanding of the anatomy surrounding the vessels and nearby vital structures.

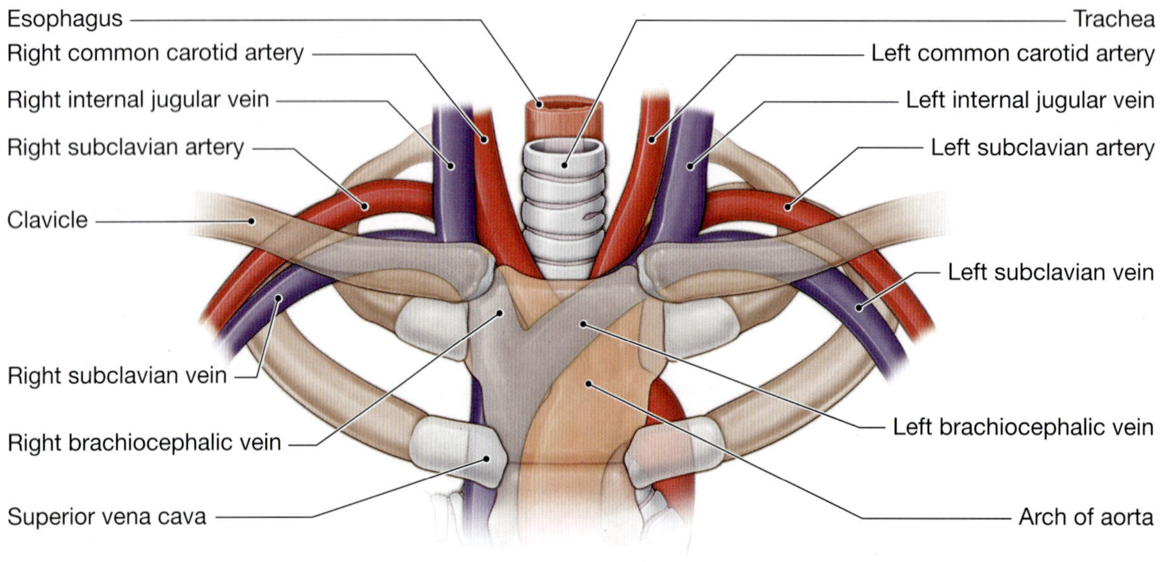

Figure 3-1

Some Important Anatomic Facts

1. The subclavian artery generally is located posterior and superior to the vein.
2. The vein runs anterior to the anterior scalene muscle and the artery posterior to it.
3. The phrenic nerve is found on the anterior surface of the anterior scalene muscle.
4. The thoracic duct enters the venous system on the left where the subclavian vein and internal jugular vein merge.
5. There is great anatomic variation on the magnitude of the cephalad loop of the proximal subclavian artery above the clavicle.
6. The proximal left subclavian near its origin is the only great vessel that cannot be explored safely through a median sternotomy because it is too posterior.

Segments of the Subclavian Artery

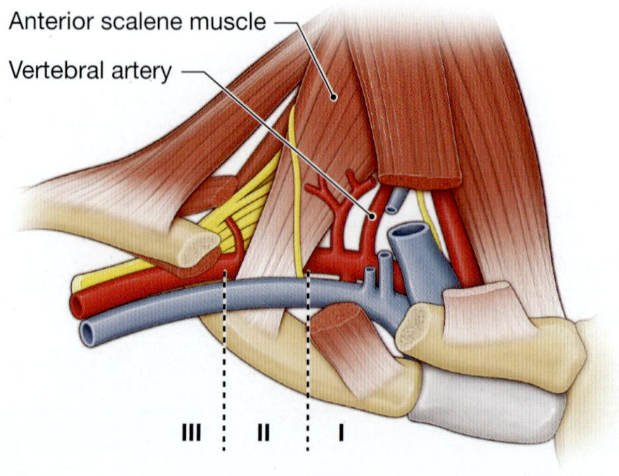

Figure 3-2

Operative Incisions

The CTA will identify a subclavian artery injury and its exact type and location. If an endovascular approach is not possible or feasible, the incision used for an open repair is also determined by its findings. A standard median sternotomy is excellent for exposure of the proximal right subclavian artery (segments 1 and 2) as well as the innominate artery from which it originates. The proximal left subclavian artery (segments 1 and 2) is best approached via a high anterolateral thoracotomy through the third or fourth intercostal space where its origin from the thoracic aorta can be visualized. Injuries to the third segment can be approached with a supraclavicular incision on the affected side and still usually have adequate room for proximal control. If in doubt, a combination of the two incisions can be made to assure safe exposure. A trapdoor incision (shown as extension of median sternotomy over left chest) has also been described as occasionally necessary but is technically difficult and associated with chronic morbidity. Thus, it has been all but abandoned. A lateral infraclavicular incision may also be needed for distal control in some cases.

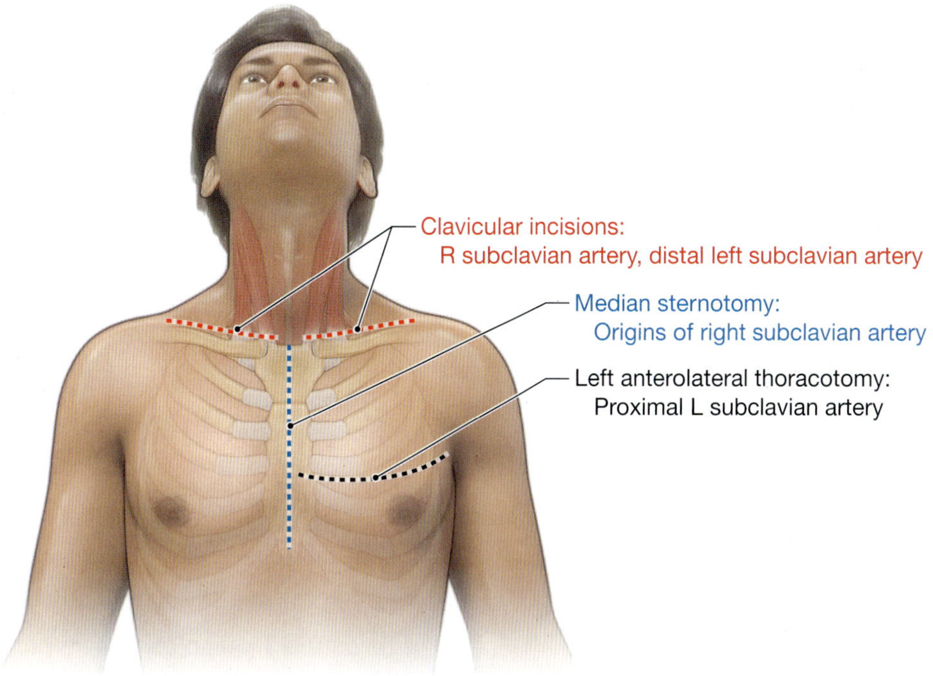

Figure 3-3

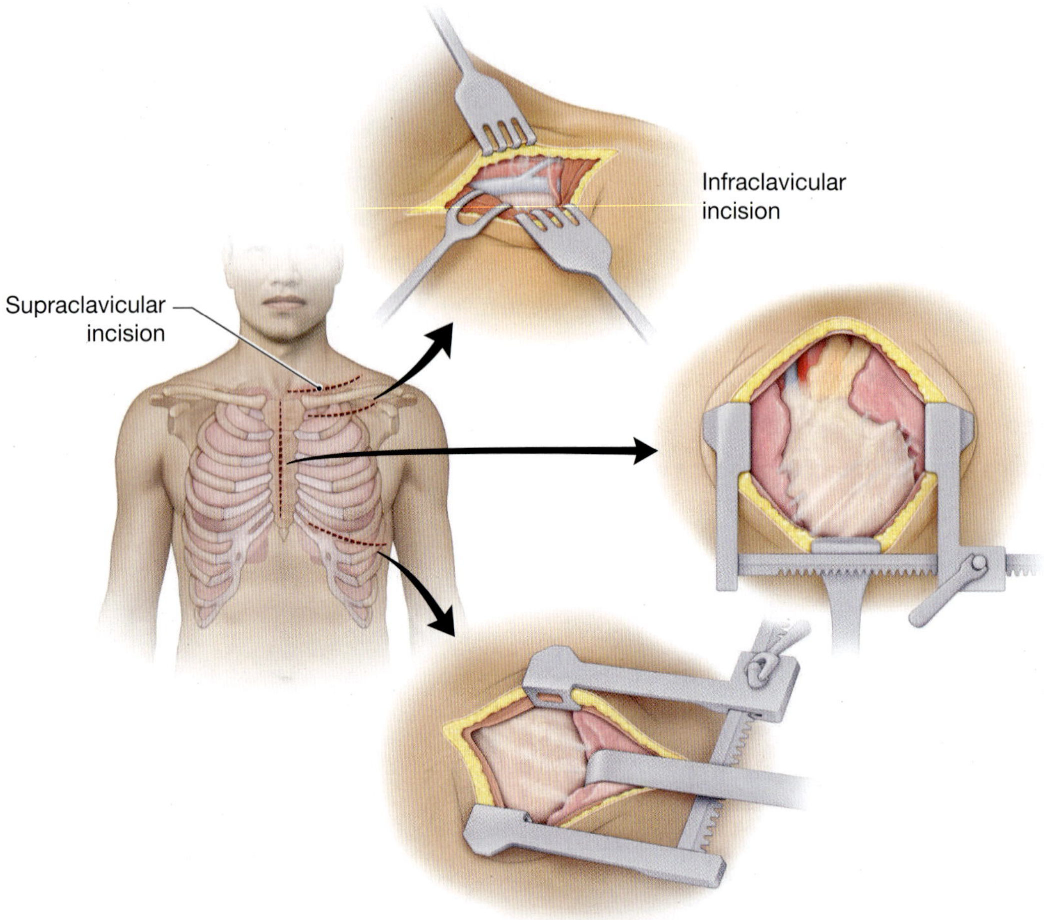

Figure 3-4

Incisions to Access Injuries

General Considerations

- Proper positioning is important and begins with placement of a shoulder roll vertically along the thoracic spine so the patient's shoulders drop back.
- Support the head and rotate it to the contralateral side from the injury, extending the neck.
- Be sure to widely prep the entire chest and drape the ipsilateral upper extremity so there is access to adduct and abduct as needed intraoperatively.
- Any arterial line and intravenous lines should be placed on the noninjured side.
- If operating emergently or unsure of where the injury is, the safest way to obtain proximal control is through a median sternotomy or use a high third intercostal space left anterolateral thoracotomy if the left subclavian in injured by exam at an undetermined level.
- Open surgical repair of subclavian injuries usually involves debridement of any injured arterial wall followed by either primary repair or an interposition graft.
- Prosthetic grafts are usually preferred due to better size match, but vein grafts should be used in cases of contamination from the aerodigestive system.

- The upper extremity has a more robust collateral network than the lower extremity and will usually remain viable if a ligation is done in extreme cases.
- Major venous injuries should also be repaired if possible, although ligation of the subclavian vein will lead to arm edema but no limb loss in most cases.

Right Proximal Subclavian Artery Exposure

- A midline sternotomy must be performed in order to access the proximal right subclavian artery and should extend from the sternal notch to the xiphoid using the sternal saw.
- The right sternohyoid and sternothyroid muscles are divided, and the scalene fat pad is exposed.
- Major branches including the thyrocervical trunk, vertebral artery, and internal mammary artery are identified as needed and dissected from surrounding tissue, and the anterior scalene muscle is exposed.
- The phrenic nerve should be identified and protected as it courses lateral to medial across the anterior scalene muscle. The anterior scalene is divided just above insertion on the first rib, and the proximal right subclavian artery is exposed.

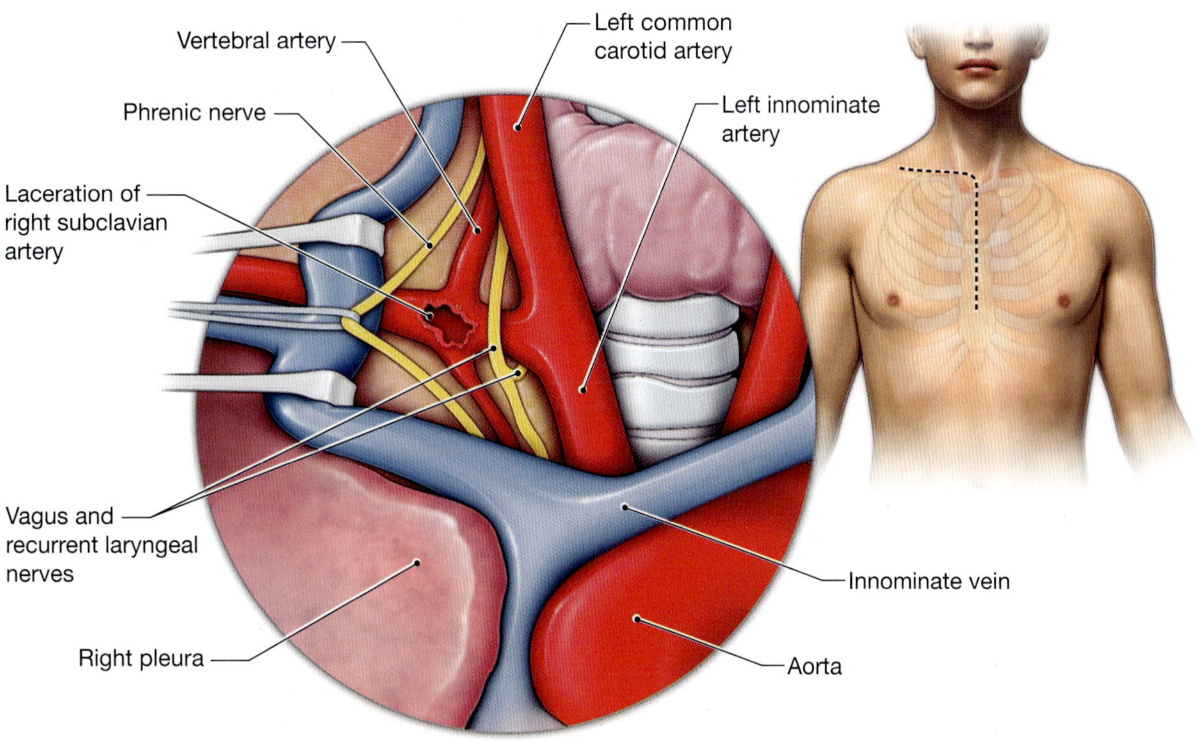

Figure 3-5

Left Proximal Subclavian Artery Exposure

- The left subclavian artery arises from the aortic arch posteriorly and therefore is best accessed through a left anterolateral thoracotomy in the third or fourth intercostal space.
- The left upper lobe of the lung is retracted, the origin of the subclavian from the distal aortic arch is found, and control of the subclavian artery is obtained.
- Usually, a separate supraclavicular incision is also made for distal control.
- The artery can be repaired through incision following mobilization and ligation of branches as needed.
- Foley catheter balloon tamponade can be used initially to control difficult bleeding, especially in the retroclavicular area.
- Exposure of the second portion of the subclavian artery is done via a supraclavicular incision. Start at the sternal notch and extend the incision laterally to the mid clavicle.
- Make the incision one fingerbreadth above and parallel to the clavicle (about 8-10 cm).

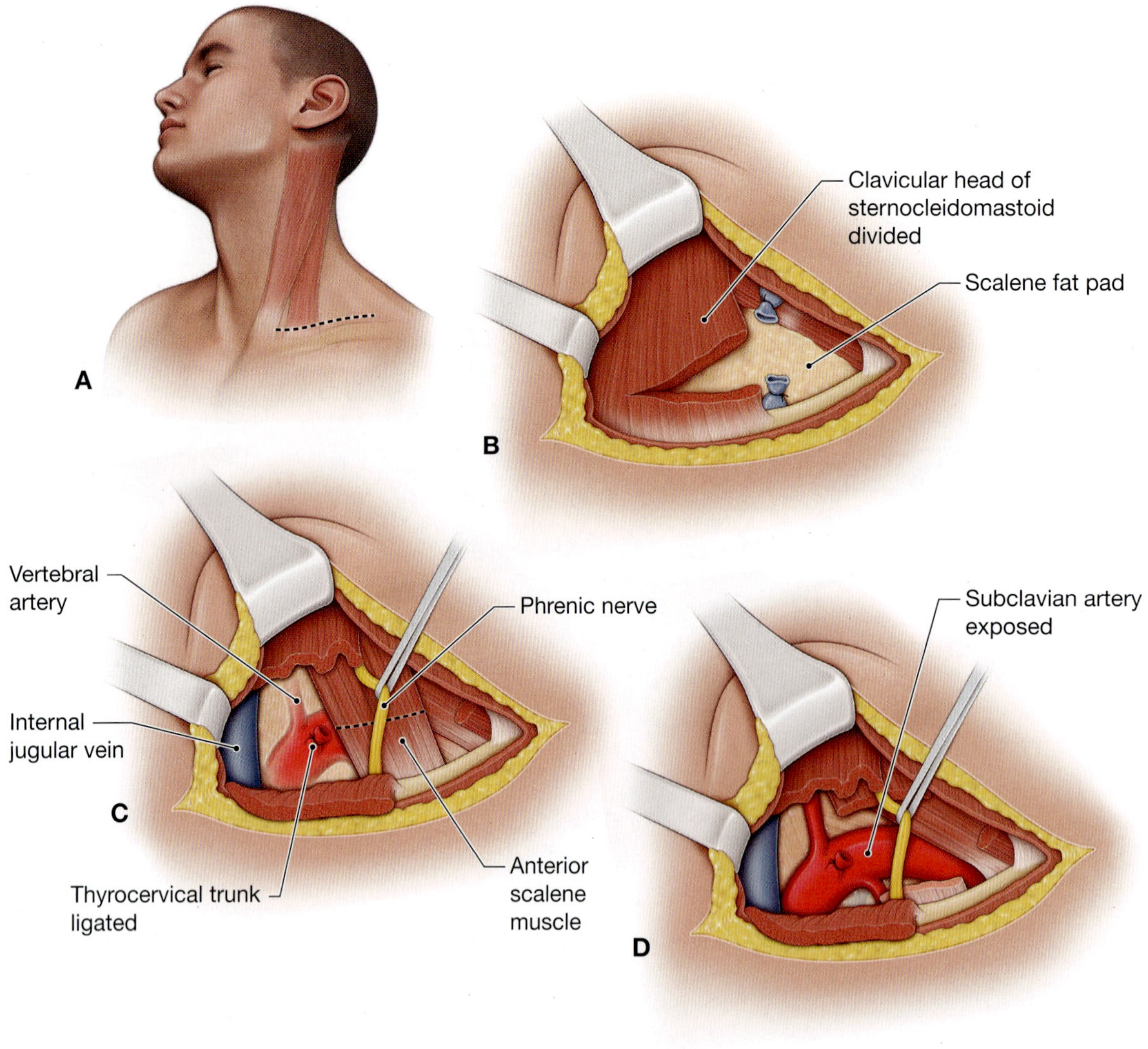

Figure 3-6

Left and Right Distal Subclavian Artery Exposure

- The platysma muscle is divided, and the clavicular head of the sternocleidomastoid and the omohyoid laterally are dissected. The muscles are divided as close to the clavicle as possible.
- If the internal jugular vein is obstructing view, it is medially retracted. The subclavian vein will be visualized, and behind the anterior scalene lies the subclavian artery.
- The scalene fat pad is mobilized from lateral to medial to locate the phrenic nerve.
- The phrenic nerve crosses the anterior scalene from superior and lateral to inferior and medial. After the nerve has been isolated, it is gently retracted out of the way with a vessel loop, and the anterior scalene is divided as inferiorly as possible at the point of insertion on the first rib. This should be done with scissors, not cautery, because it minimizes bleeding and is close to the brachial plexus.
- Dividing and ligating the thyrocervical trunk will make it easier to mobilize the subclavian artery.

Directly on the Clavicle

- An incision is made directly on the clavicle to expose the medial two-thirds of the bone.
- With cautery, a line is scored on the anterior surface of the clavicle and a periosteal elevator is used to peel the periosteum off the clavicle. Using bone cutters or a saw, the clavicle is divided as far lateral as possible.
- The medial fragment is grasped with a towel clip and pulled firmly out of its bed.
- Immediately deep to the clavicle is the subclavius muscle. Dividing this muscle will expose the prescalene fat pad and the phrenic nerve.

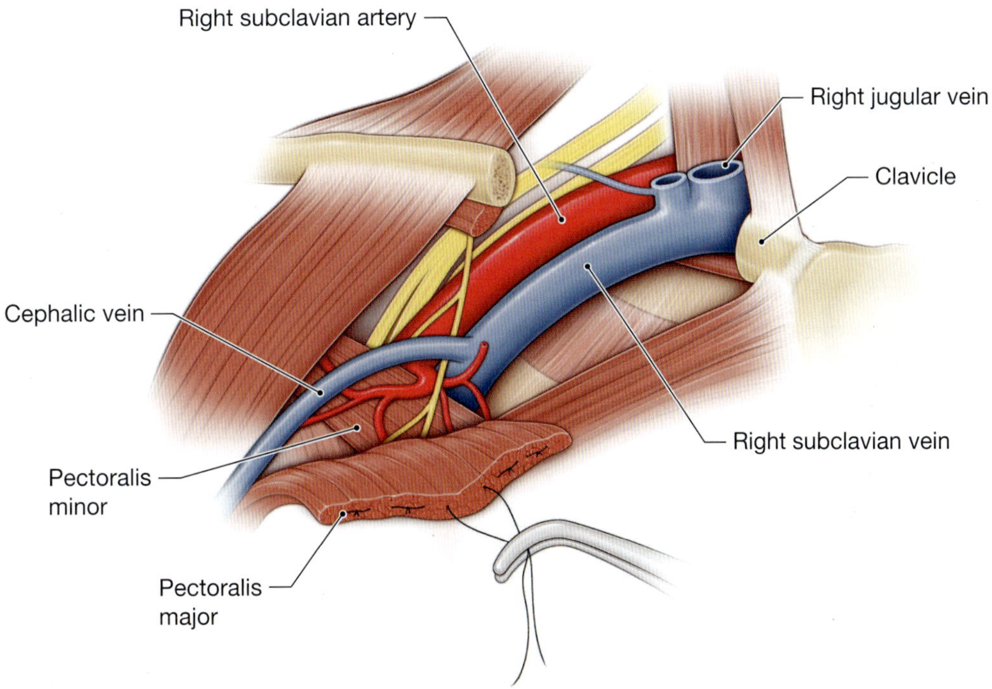

Figure 3-7

Damage Control or Definitive Repair

In an open case for subclavian artery injury, damage control surgery for the critically ill patient should include temporary shunting with a wide variety of prosthetic tubing and, rarely, ligation of the artery with or without packing. Ligation is well tolerated if the major collateral pathways around the shoulder are still intact. Once the patient has been resuscitated, definitive arterial repair should be performed 24-48 hours later. An interposition graft is most commonly used to repair subclavian artery damage with either a reversed saphenous vein graft or polytetrafluoroethylene (PTFE) graft. Mobilizing the subclavian artery is difficult, and there is seldom enough length for an end-to-end repair.

Endovascular Approach

Endovascular techniques are successful in over 90% of cases in a stable patient and should be the first consideration in institutions with advanced endovascular capabilities. Catheter-based techniques can be applied to the upper extremity junctional zone for traumatic injuries and are particularly useful to treat AV fistulas and pseudoaneurysms. These can be approached from either the femoral artery or the ipsilateral brachial artery. A retrograde brachial approach is often used due to the shorter distance from access site to the injury. Even patients with hemodynamic instability and hard signs of vascular injury, such as pulsatile bleeding, expanding hematoma, absent distal pulses, or a bruit or thrill, can be considered for endovascular repair or control in an operating room with hybrid technology. If a patient is stable, CTA or duplex ultrasound can be obtained to confirm injury location; however, if the patient is unstable, they should proceed directly to either the operating room or a hybrid suite for emergent angiography and endovascular intervention. Bare metal stents and self-expanding and balloon-expandable covered stents have all been reported to be effective in managing axillo-subclavian injuries, with the newest versions of covered stents now the device of choice. One of the greatest benefits of the endovascular approach is avoiding emergent operative dissection in an area unfamiliar to many surgeons and avoidance of iatrogenic brachial plexus injuries.

Complications

Due to the proximity of the brachial plexus to the subclavian artery, injury to the brachial plexus accounts for the majority of complications of open repair. Nerve deficits are the most common long-term morbidity in these injuries. Complete lacerations are managed with primary repair of the nerves; however, these patients experience major neurologic deficits following repair. Incomplete lacerations and contusions can be managed conservatively with physiotherapy and splinting. The recurrent laryngeal nerve can also be damaged during subclavian artery dissection, leading to hoarseness. Thoracic duct injuries are also a potential complication to an open repair. These can be at first managed with a diet of medium-chain triglycerides; however, if the patient continues to have a high-output leak, it can be managed definitively with a ligation of the thoracic duct. As with any other vascular anastomosis, after a graft repair of the subclavian artery, there is risk for pseudoaneurysm, thrombosis, stenosis, and graft sepsis. Graft sepsis should be managed with antibiotics; however, if the patient is unstable or not improving, the patient may require reoperation.

The endovascular approach carries its unique set of complications including access site hematoma, late pseudoaneurysm formation, stent-graft stenosis, and thrombosis. Long-term follow-up is mandatory to identify endoleaks, stent fractures, and migration.

Decreased blood flow through the vertebral artery after an endovascular stent placement can also occur, and covering the artery should be avoided if the patient lacks a normal contralateral vertebral artery. Often, endovascularly treated patients benefit from long-term antiplatelet therapy if associated injuries are not present that contradict this therapy.

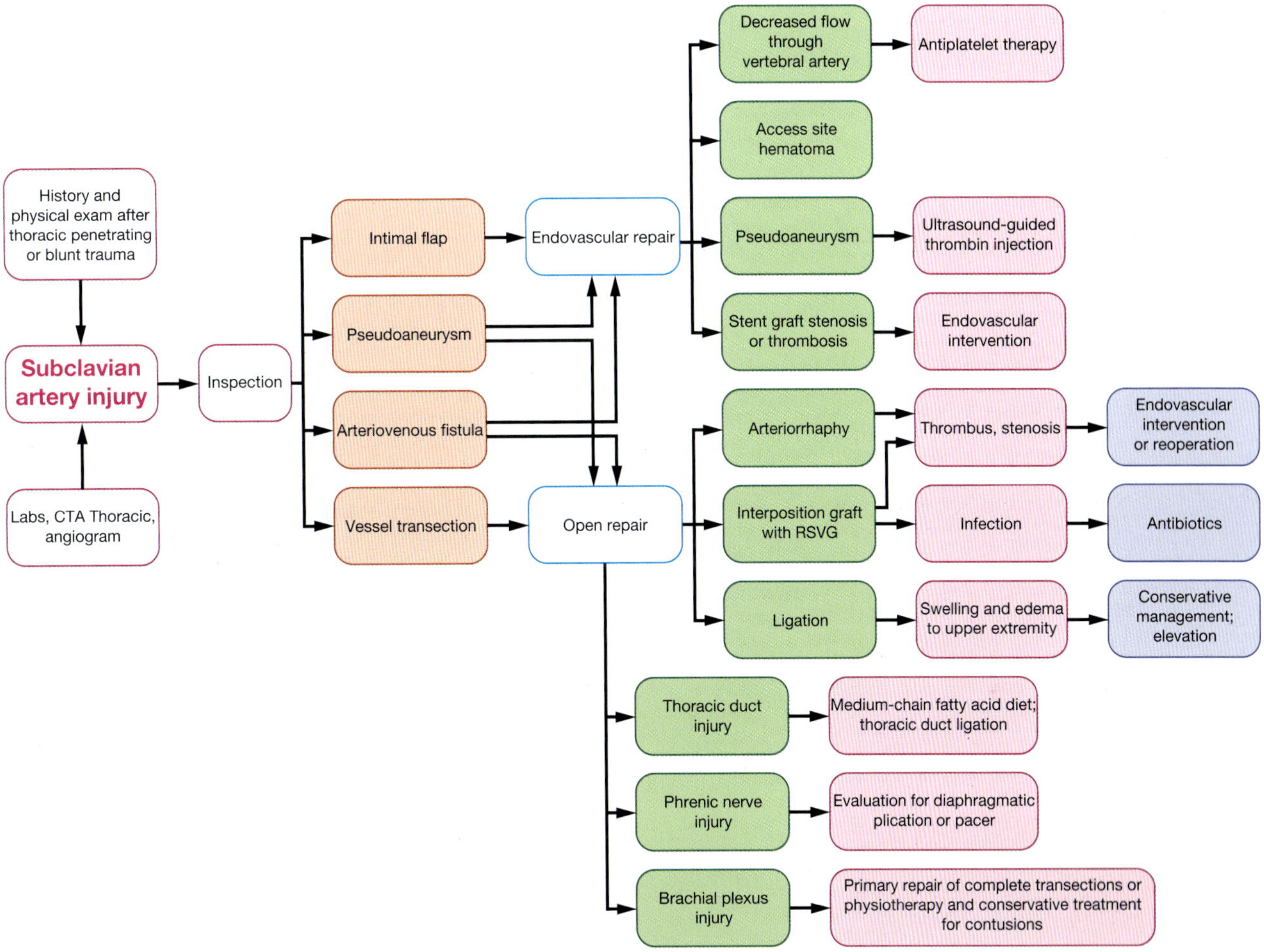

Figure 3-8

THORACIC VASCULAR TRAUMA: THORACIC AORTA

4

Chelsea Yap, DO
James W. Dennis, MD, FACS
Daniel Steadman, DO

TIPS

1. **Endovascular techniques should be the first consideration, as opposed to open surgery, in stable patients with both penetrating and blunt injuries.**
2. **Successful thoracic endovascular aortic repair requires rapid accurate preoperative planning along with adequate staff and specialized equipment available 24 hours a day.**
3. **Any clamping of the thoracic aorta for an extended time risks spinal cord ischemia and paralysis.**

Introduction

Traumatic injury to the thoracic aorta can result from either blunt or penetrating mechanisms. Blunt injury typically results from rapid deceleration and ranges from an intimal tear to a complete rupture, with the majority occurring at the aortic isthmus where the relatively mobile descending thoracic aorta joins the fixed arch and at the level of the ligamentum arteriosum. Traumatic rupture of the thoracic aorta is a life-threatening injury that result from blunt thoracic trauma and is the second most common cause of death after traumatic brain injury. The highest mortality usually occurs within the first few hours after injury; almost 90% of patients die at the scene, and approximately one-third of patients who arrive at a hospital succumb before intervention.

The timing of when to intervene on blunt aortic injuries has been a matter of debate as a result of competing priorities; these injuries often present with other associated injuries such as solid organ or head injuries. Management depends on the nature of the associated injuries and the grade of aortic injury seen on computed tomographic aortography (CTA). Generally, associated injuries must first be addressed and stabilized, and where indicated, the aortic repair should immediately follow. Exceptions include patients with grade 4 aortic injuries resulting in active extravasation of contrast or massive hemothorax with hemodynamic instability. Stable patients who arrive to the hospital alive with lower grade injuries that require repair can safely have delayed aortic repair after the resuscitation phase is complete. The initial medical management of a traumatic aortic lesion should include close hemodynamic monitoring along with anti-impulse and antihypertensive therapy, typically with β blockade (eg, esmolol continuous infusion). The exact timing of the aortic repair depends on the overall condition of the patient, the grade of aortic injury, and the severity of associated injuries. For the past two decades, endovascular repair has been the procedure of choice if possible for all the benefits listed below. Additionally, the ability to forgo systemic anticoagulation makes it particularly attractive in patients with concomitant intracranial or high-grade solid organ injuries.

Penetrating thoracic aortic injury is often not found on a computed tomography scan but instead during an exploratory operation on an unstable patient with active hemorrhage. Primary repair may be possible or a short interposition prosthetic graft may be needed in cases of segmental loss of the artery. Some penetrating wounds to the chest can also form a contained pseudoaneurysm that is identified by CTA. In a stable patient, an endovascular stent graft coverage of the injury would be the treatment of choice if an endovascular specialist is available. Physical findings are mostly lacking due to the deep location of the thoracic aorta in the chest.

TABLE 4-1. Comparison of Open Vs. Endovascular Approach

Results-metanalysis		
	ENDO	**OPEN**
Mortality	7.6%	15.2%
Paraplegia	0%	5.5%
Stroke	0.81%	5.1%
Tech success	96.5%	98.5%
Blood trans	2.3 units	7.3 units
OR time	2.7 h	4.4 h

Source: Data from Tang GL, Tehrani HY, Usman A, Katariya K, Otero C, Perez E, Eskandari MK. Reduced mortality, paraplegia, and stroke with stent graft repair of blunt aortic transections: a modern meta-analysis. *J Vasc Surg.* 2008 Mar;47(3):671-5. doi: 10.1016/j.jvs.2007.08.031. Epub 2007 Nov 5. PMID: 17980541.

Anatomy

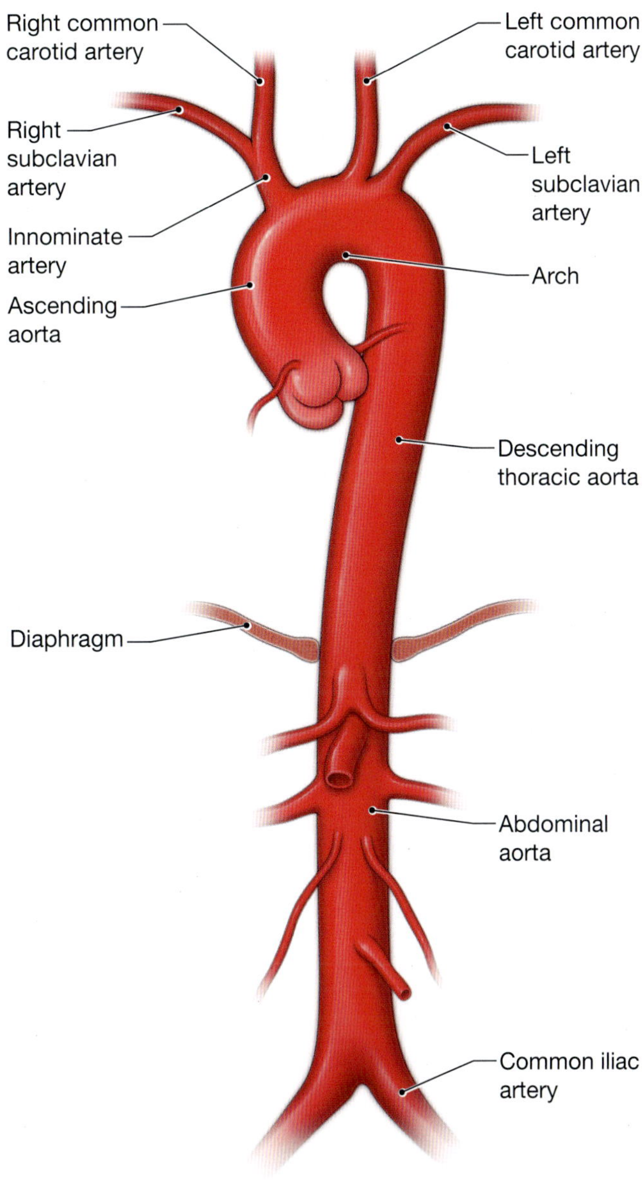

Figure 4-1

TABLE 4-2. American Association for the Surgery of Trauma Organ Injury Scale

Grade	AAST Injury Scale - Thoracic Aorta	Grade	AAST Injury Scale - Thoracic Aorta
I Initial tear	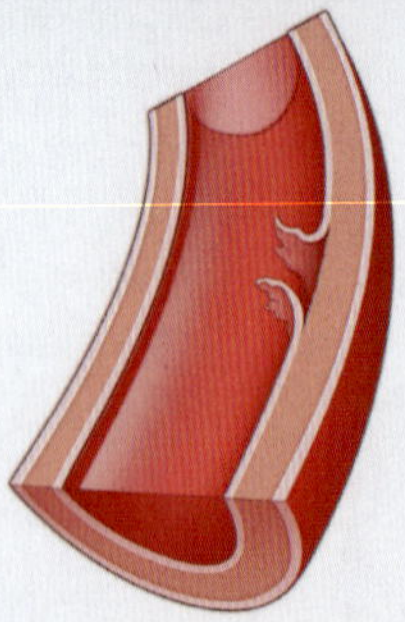	III Pseudoaneurysm	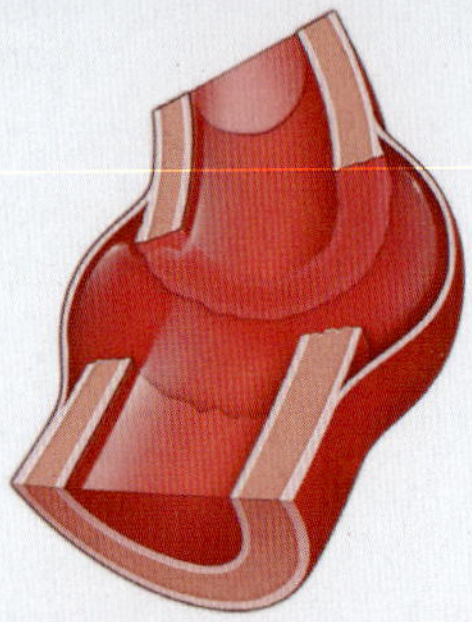
II Intramural hematoma	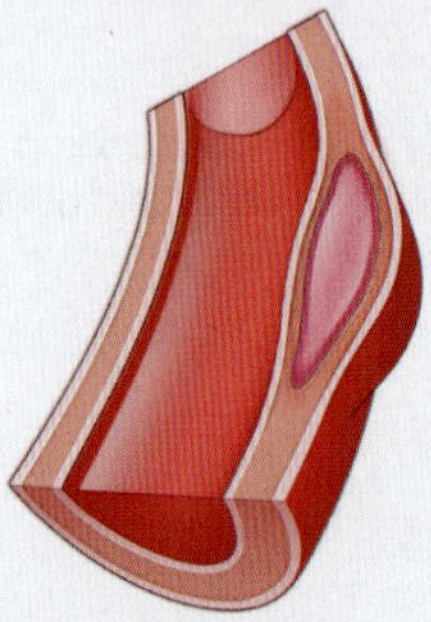	IV Rupture	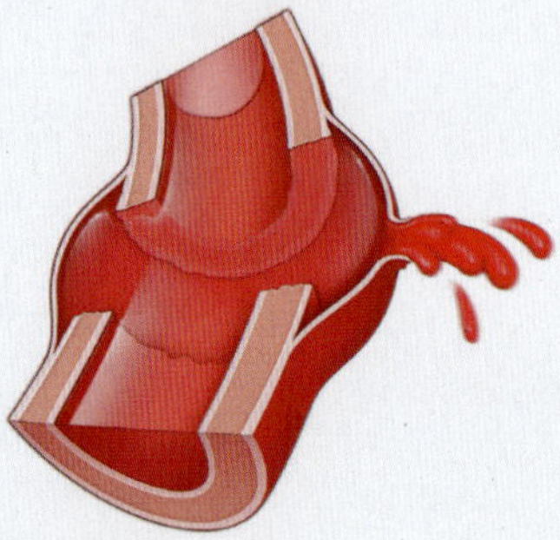

Operative Incisions

Anterolateral Thoracotomy

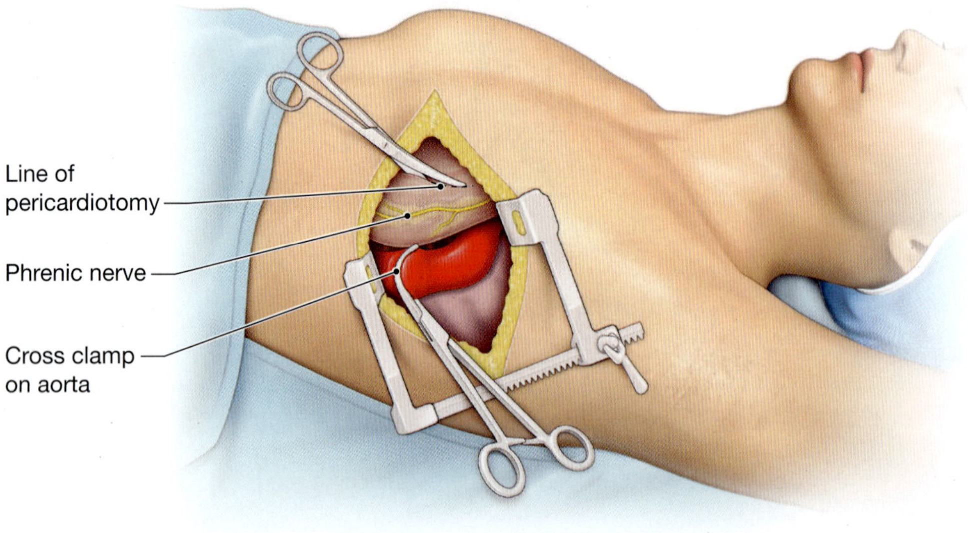

Figure 4-2

Left Posterolateral Thoracotomy

- Patient should be positioned in right lateral decubitus, the left arm should be raised to be anterior and cephalad, and a double-lumen endotracheal tube should be placed.
- The incision should start along the inframammary crease in the fourth intercostal space and extend posterolaterally to below the tip of the scapula until the posterior axillary line.
- The subcutaneous tissue and trapezius muscle are divided and the serratus anterior and latissimus dorsi muscles can then be retracted. In emergent situations, the latissimus can be divided for more rapid access.
- The external and internal intercostal muscles are divided, staying superior to the lower rib to avoid the neurovascular bundle.
- The ipsilateral lung is isolated by the anesthesiology team, and the pleura is entered.
- The rib spreader is placed and the lung is mobilized anteriorly, allowing posterior pleural dissection behind the aorta.

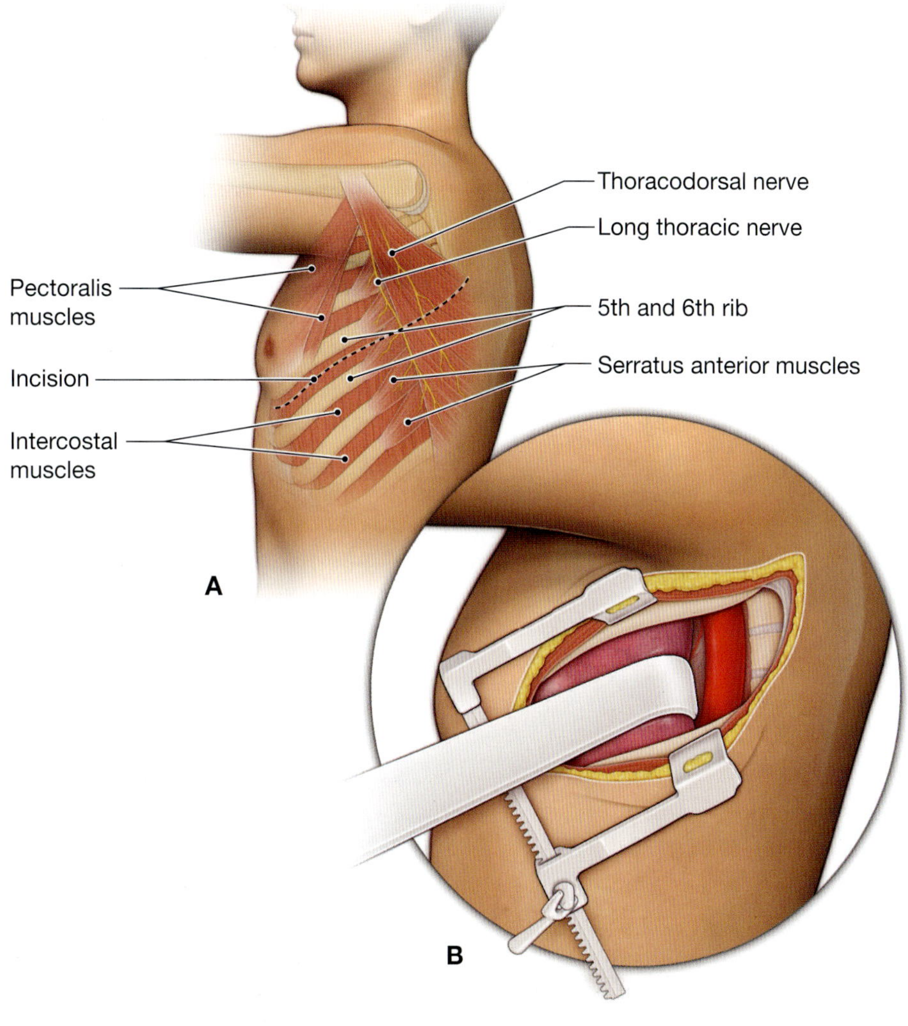

Figure 4-3

Operative Steps

Open approaches to repair a descending thoracic aortic injury include clamp repair ("clamp and sew"), atrial-femoral bypass, and cardiopulmonary bypass. A median sternotomy is used to expose the ascending aorta and arch, whereas the descending thoracic aorta is approached via a posterolateral thoracotomy. An emergency thoracotomy can be extended using a transverse sternotomy into a bilateral anterolateral thoracotomy (clamshell) for optimal exposure in patients with localized injuries. The management of blunt aortic injuries is usually accomplished with endovascular techniques with excellent success rates depending on proper planning and the vascular anatomy. Small access vessels can be a limiting factor for endovascular repair, and this is managed using a retroperitoneal exposure of the common iliac artery and placement of a temporary conduit.

- Clamp and sew technique: The aorta is clamped above and below the injury, and the graft is quickly sutured in place.
- Passive shunt: Blood from the proximal aorta is pumped into the aorta distal to the injury.
- Active bypass with blood from the left atrium is circulated through a roller pump and perfused into the femoral artery through a retrograde catheter.

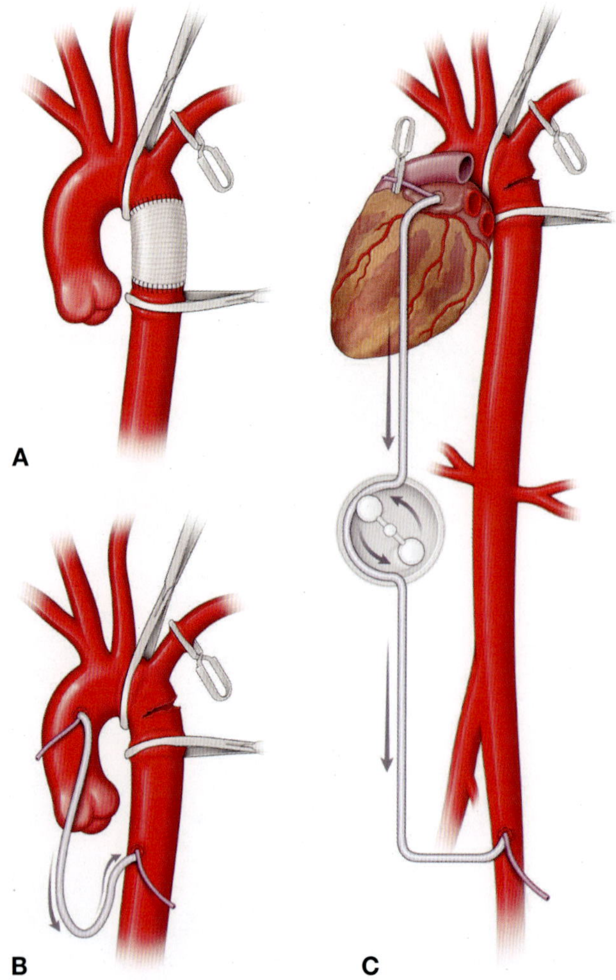

Figure 4-4

Endovascular Approach

- The patient is positioned supine with abdomen and bilateral groins prepped and draped.
    - If right radial or brachial arteries are going to be used for access, the right arm should be prepped.
- The common femoral artery is the most common access site.
- A femoral cutdown is typically performed on the device access site, and a percutaneous sheath is placed via the contralateral femoral artery.
- Stent graft is placed.

There are many variations of grafts available. **Aortic zones are based on the Ishimura classification system. The type of graft used is based on the zone of injury and what vascular branches are involved.**

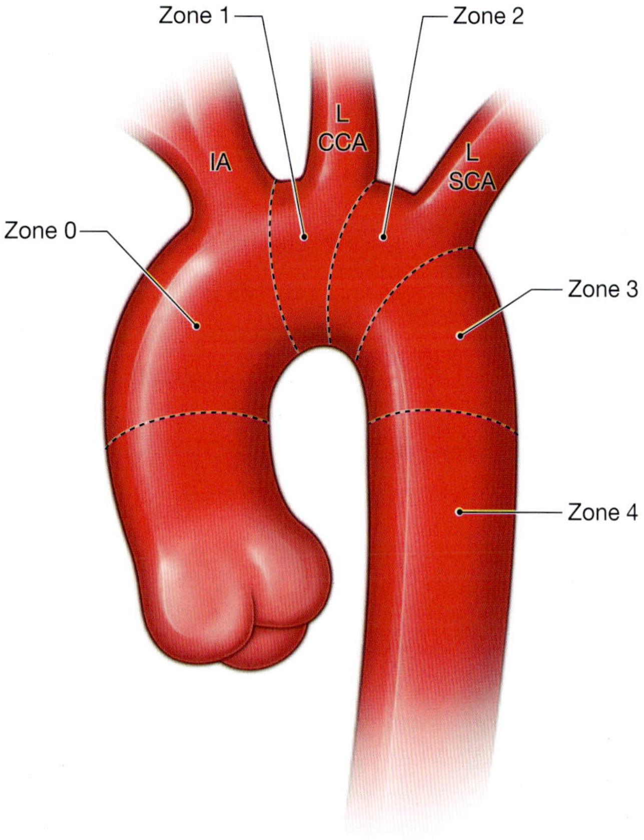

Figure 4-5

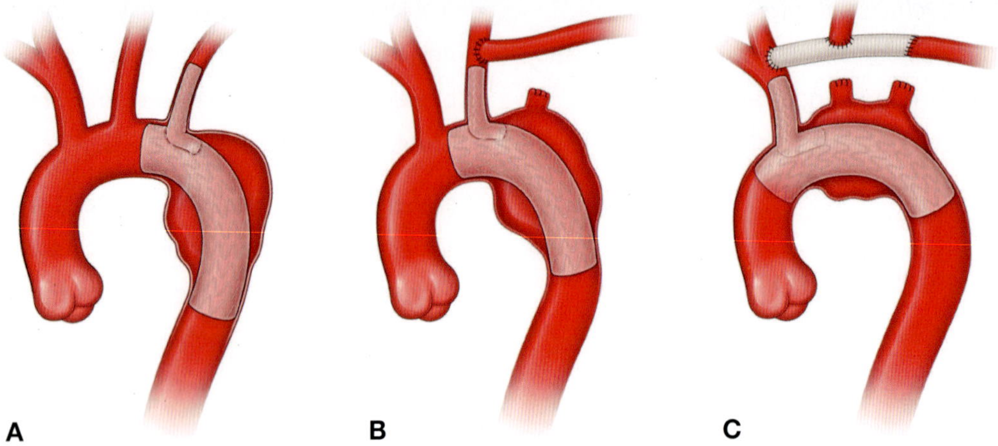

Figure 4-6

Complications

Compared to open repair of thoracic aortic injuries, endovascular repair has been associated with better outcomes and lower mortality in the perioperative period; however, there is a lack of long-term data for comparison. Complications associated with aortic repair include spinal cord injury and acute kidney injury. Specific complications associated with thoracotomy include but are not limited to bleeding, infection, pneumothorax, pleural effusion, shoulder dysfunction, pain, and postthoracotomy pain syndrome. Endovascular complications include graft thrombosis, endoleaks, aneurysm rupture, and aortoesophageal fistula, and therefore, patients must be monitored for many years postoperatively.

CARDIAC TRAUMA

5

Steven R. Allen, MD, FACS
Scott B. Armen, MD, FACS, FCCP, FCCM, COL, MC USAR

TIPS

1. **One must rapidly choose the appropriate incision (median sternotomy vs anterolateral thoracotomy, etc.) for access to the chest based on mechanism of injury, hemodynamic stability, and predicted injury patterns to ensure optimal and expeditious access to the injured organs and blood vessels.**

2. **Penetrating cardiac injuries may be temporarily controlled using a number of methods that include direct finger pressure, a Foley catheter, or surgical staples. Despite these resourceful methods, great care must be taken to prevent converting a controlled injury to one that is uncontrollable and ultimately fatal.**

3. **For penetrating cardiac injuries in proximity to a coronary artery, care must be taken and a U-stitch must be placed under and around the coronary to repair the wound without compromising the blood flow in the distribution of the coronary artery to prevent myocardial ischemia.**

Introduction

Blunt and penetrating cardiac injuries offer a significant challenge to even the most seasoned trauma team due to their high morbidity and mortality. Approximately 25% of all trauma-related deaths are due to injuries of the heart or great vessels. Over 50% of those with penetrating cardiac injuries die before they reach the hospital.

Injuries to the heart and great vessels involve any combination of the anatomic structures that include the great vessels, pericardium, myocardium, and coronary vessels. Published series have demonstrated that the right ventricle and atrium are the most frequently injured, followed by the left ventricle and aorta. The clinical presentation of cardiac and great vessel injuries is dependent on several factors, including mechanism, location, and size of the wound and degree of energy transmitted. Manifestations of these injuries range from asymptomatic changes on electrocardiogram to cardiogenic or hemorrhagic shock, cardiovascular collapse, and death.

The trauma surgeon faced with penetrating injuries to the chest must quickly assess the situation and make multiple decisions based on hemodynamic stability, clinical presentation and exam, as well as mechanism and anatomic location of the wound(s). Rapid decisions to be made include location of the surgical intervention (trauma bay if impending cardiovascular collapse or cardiac arrest are present vs operating room for patients whose clinical situations permit it) and the type of incision based on the predicted injuries. Furthermore, understanding the various repair options, both temporizing and definitive, for cardiac and great vessel injuries is critical. One must also know what resources are immediately available to help with the repair of penetrating cardiac injuries. Knowing when to request the assistance of a fully trained cardiac surgeon and requesting the use of cardiopulmonary bypass for particularly severe or complex injuries are paramount.

This chapter provides an overview of the most useful incisions and repair techniques for penetrating cardiac injuries. It is not a comprehensive review of complex techniques for definitive repair of challenging cardiac injuries as these should be performed under controlled conditions often with the assistance of cardiopulmonary bypass by appropriately trained personnel. However, understanding the techniques that allow access to the cardiac injury and allow for temporary control of life-threatening hemorrhage is of the utmost importance.

Anatomy

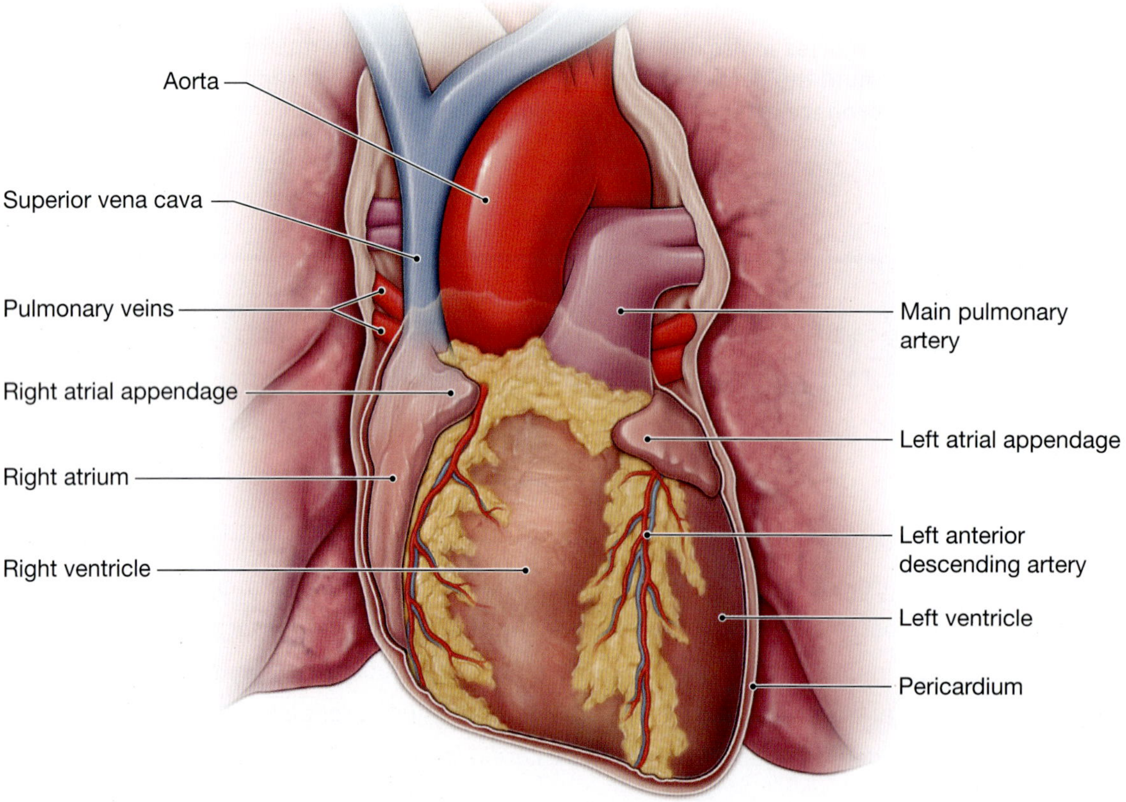

Figure 5-1

5 CARDIAC TRAUMA

TABLE 5-1. American Association for the Surgery of Trauma Organ Injury Scale

Grade	Injury
Grade I	1. Blunt cardiac injury with minor ECG abnormality (nonspecific ST- or T-wave changes, premature atrial or ventricular contractions, or persistent sinus tachycardia) 2. Blunt or penetrating pericardial wound without cardiac injury, tamponade, or cardiac herniation
Grade II	1. Blunt cardiac injury with heart block or ischemic changes without cardiac failure 2. Penetrating tangential cardiac wound, up to but not extending through endocardium, without tamponade
Grade III	1. Blunt cardiac injury with sustained or multifocal ventricular contractions 2. Blunt or penetrating cardiac injury with septal rupture, pulmonary or tricuspid incompetence, papillary muscle dysfunction, or distal coronary artery occlusion without cardiac failure 3. Blunt pericardial laceration with cardiac herniation 4. Blunt cardiac injury with cardiac failure 5. Penetrating tangential myocardial wound, up to but not through endocardium, with tamponade
Grade IV	1. Blunt or penetrating cardiac injury with septal rupture, pulmonary or tricuspid incompetence, papillary muscle dysfunction, or distal coronary artery occlusion producing cardiac failure 2. Blunt or penetrating cardiac injury with aortic or mitral incompetence 3. Blunt or penetrating cardiac injury of the right ventricle, right or left atrium
Grade V	1. Blunt or penetrating cardiac injury with proximal coronary artery occlusion 2. Blunt or penetrating left ventricular perforation 3. Stellate injuries, less than 50% tissue loss of the right ventricle, right or left atrium
Grade VI	1. Blunt avulsion of the heart 2. Penetrating wound producing more than 50% tissue loss of a chamber

Source: Reproduced with permission from Moore EE et al. Organ injury scaling. IV: Thoracic vascular, lung, cardiac, and diaphragm. *J Trauma.* 1994;36(3):299-300.

Incisions

Sternotomy

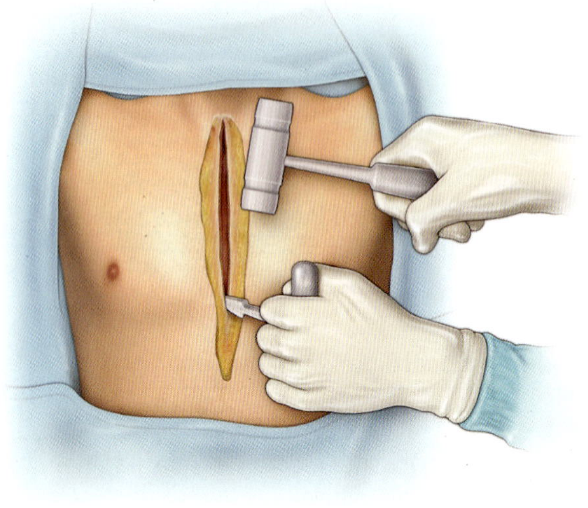

Figure 5-2

Indications: A midline sternotomy is indicated for penetrating injuries to the anterior chest. It allows maximal access to the heart, lungs, middle and distal trachea, and the left mainstem bronchus. Additionally, access to the main pulmonary artery, ascending aorta, and upper mediastinal vessels such as the innominate artery is achieved through this incision. The sternotomy also allows one to extend the incision superiorly over the sternocleidomastoid muscle or over the clavicles to improve access to the carotid or subclavian vessels.

Pitfalls: The sternotomy does not allow access to the posterior mediastinal structures such as esophagus or descending thoracic aorta and impairs access for cross-clamping the descending thoracic aorta for resuscitation purposes.

Technique: Patient is positioned in the supine position with arms tucked to the side. A horizontal roll is placed under the shoulders to help extend the chest and neck. The chest is prepped from the chin to the knees and table to table laterally. One must identify the middle of the sternal notch superiorly and the center of the xiphoid process distally to ensure the incision is carried through the middle of the sternum. One may also palpate the sternal margins along the length of the sternum to ensure to not deviate to one side or the other. A vertical incision is made from the sternal notch to the xiphoid process. Soft tissues are dissected down to the periosteum. One should ensure that the decussation of the pectoralis muscle fibers is separated to the respective sides (occasionally pectoralis muscle fibers cross over midline and the surgeon must take note of this to ensure staying midline on the sternum). The soft tissue superior and deep to the sternal notch, including the interclavicular ligament, is divided with electrocautery, allowing one to bluntly dissect a plane under the superior-most portion of the manubrium. This will help to ensure the innominate vein is out of the way of the saw blade. Similarly, soft tissue overlying the xiphoid process is divided and a straight line is created with electrocautery between the superior- and inferior-most portions. Along this line in the center of the sternum, the sternal periosteum is scored with electrocautery. The anesthesia team should be directed to hold ventilation during the division of the sternum. The sternum is then divided using the sternal saw. Ventilation may be resumed once the sternum is completely divided. It should be noted that one may divide the sternum in the superior to inferior direction or vice versa based on training and the type of saw utilized.

Once the sternum is divided, hemostasis must be obtained from the surrounding soft tissue, the periosteal borders (both outer and inner tables of the sternum and manubrium) using electrocautery, and the marrow of the raw cut surface using bone wax spread into the marrow bed on both sides of the divided sternum.

Left Anterolateral Thoracotomy

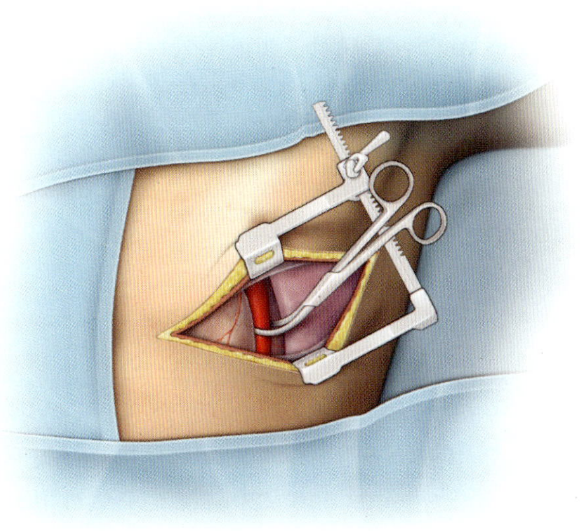

Figure 5-3

Indications: The left anterolateral thoracotomy allows rapid access to the left chest cavity in the event of thoracic trauma and allows resuscitative efforts in the event of prehospital or impending cardiovascular collapse from both blunt and penetrating torso trauma. This incision allows one to directly control bleeding from the heart, lungs, or other thoracic vessels in the field of view; cross-clamp the descending thoracic aorta in an effort to prevent exsanguination (both thoracic and extrathoracic) and improve coronary perfusion; open the pericardium to alleviate the effects of cardiac tamponade; facilitate evacuation of air embolism; and provide internal cardiac massage.

Pitfalls: The left anterolateral thoracotomy offers limited visualization of the heart (apex and anterior surface of the right ventricle) but may provide a challenge for penetrating injuries beyond these areas of the heart to be repaired in a successful manner. Additionally, there is no access to the right chest cavity provided by this incision.

Technique: With the patient in the supine position, the left arm is raised superiorly to remove it from the surgical field. The entire chest is rapidly prepped and draped in a sterile fashion. A large incision is made starting on the right border of the sternum and carried to the left chest along the inframammary fold (approximately the fifth intercostal space). The incision should be curved gently toward the left axilla and extend as low as possible (to the bed) to allow for maximal access to the contents of the left chest. This incision should be made rapidly and must extend through the soft tissue just superficial to the intercostal muscles. The intercostal muscle layers should be carefully penetrated with a Mayo scissors. Once the chest cavity is penetrated, the Mayo scissors are used to divide the intercostal muscles off the superior aspect of the ribs both anteriorly and posteriorly to allow for the chest to be opened. A rib spreader is then inserted with the back end of the rib spreader directed toward the axilla, allowing maximal access to the anterior chest and ensuring it does not preclude extension of the incision should a clamshell thoracotomy need to be performed.

Clamshell Thoracotomy

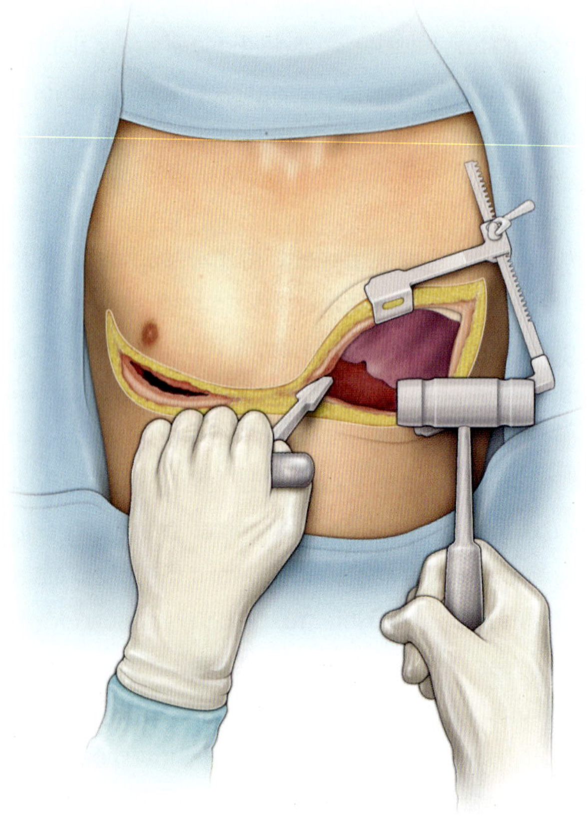

Figure 5-4

Indications: The clamshell thoracotomy is an extension of the left anterolateral thoracotomy across the right side of the chest (addition of a right anterolateral thoracotomy). This is done in order to gain rapid access to the right chest and is usually indicated if blood is returned from placement of a right tube thoracostomy during the initial resuscitative thoracotomy. It may also be utilized to improve access to the mediastinal structures (heart, aorta, main pulmonary artery, superior or inferior vena cavae) once a left anterolateral thoracotomy has been performed and a discrete injury has been identified in any of these mediastinal structures.

Pitfalls: Although the clamshell incision offers an excellent vantage point for many injuries to the chest due to the access of not only the mediastinum but also both pleural cavities, several disadvantages of the clamshell incision are evident. First is the extent of the incision across both sides of the chest. With that comes a significant amount of pain during the patient's recovery. Infectious complications and wound healing issues are also abundant with the clamshell thoracotomy.

Technique: The clamshell thoracotomy is created by extending the left anterolateral thoracotomy across the right chest. The incision is traditionally carried superior to the right nipple at the level of the third intercostal space and extends across in a curvilinear fashion toward the right axilla again as far posterior as possible (limited by the bed). Similar to the left anterolateral thoracotomy, this initial incision must be rapid and nearly full thickness of all soft tissues to the level of the intercostal muscles. The sternum is then transected, and the intercostal muscles are divided off of the rib inferior to the incision. The sternum may be divided in a number of ways. The Lebsche knife is a common instrument used for this purpose. In this method, the blade is struck with a metal mallet to drive the blade into and across the lower one-third of the sternum, dividing it in a horizontal fashion. This will inevitably lead to the division of the bilateral internal mammary arteries, and once the chest is completely opened, the internal mammary arteries should be identified and ligated to control hemorrhage. A rib spreader is then inserted in a similar fashion to the left anterolateral thoracotomy with the back end of the retractor directed toward the axilla.

Trapdoor

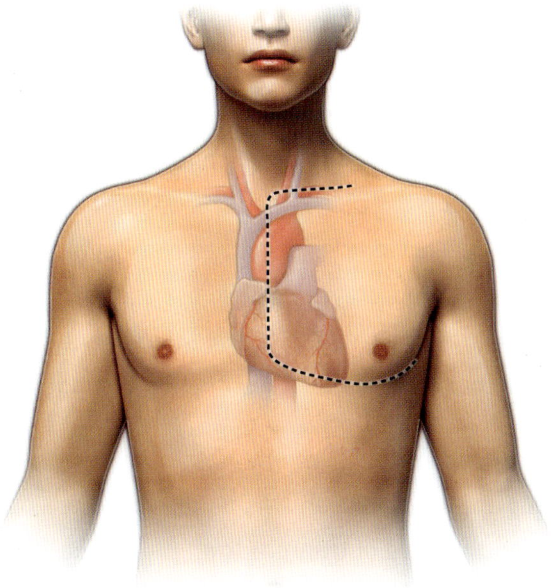

Figure 5-5

Indications: The trapdoor is a combination of an anterolateral thoracotomy, a sternotomy, and a supraclavicular incision with division of the clavicle. While highly morbid, this incision may prove to be lifesaving in the event of a distal great vessel injury or proximal subclavian artery or vein injury. These injuries tend to be difficult to address and repair with the anterolateral thoracotomy because they are superiorly out of reach from that incision alone. Similarly, one may not gain enough access from a sternotomy alone, necessitating the combination of these incisions.

Pitfalls: This incision has been found to be highly morbid due to bleeding complications related to the complex incisions and the muscle (pectoralis muscles) and bones (clavicle and sternum) divided to perform the trapdoor incision. This incision is also associated with significant pain. Pulmonary complications are common due to the structural compromise of the chest wall from the incision but also due to the aforementioned pain preventing adequate coughing, deep breathing, and clearance of secretions.

Technique: The trapdoor incision is typically created once the surgeon realizes that the identified injury is inaccessible through the already created left anterolateral thoracotomy incision as it may be too superior in the chest (left subclavian artery or vein injury). The left anterolateral incision is typically created first as the patient usually is moribund and may initially require a resuscitative thoracotomy (described in detail below). Once the injury is deemed out of reach from the initial incision, a median sternotomy may be connected to the medial aspect of the thoracotomy. A supraclavicular incision with division of the proximal clavicle is also performed. The combination of these incisions allows one to open the chest cavity widely to allow access to the distal great vessels or the proximal brachiocephalic vessels (carotid and subclavian arteries and veins) of the ipsilateral side of the trapdoor incision.

Steps of Resuscitative Thoracotomy

1. Left anterolateral thoracotomy (described above) is performed.
2. Simultaneous to the left anterolateral thoracotomy, a right-sided tube thoracostomy is performed in the standard fashion. This is undertaken to help triage the right chest. Should significant blood be encountered upon insertion of the tube, the left anterolateral incision should be extended across the chest into a clamshell incision (described above).
3. A pericardiotomy should be performed upon entering the chest. The pericardiotomy should

be made with the use of toothed forceps and Metzenbaum scissors. The pericardium is often smooth, tense, slippery, and difficult to grasp. Also, one must take great care not to injure the underlying heart. The pericardiotomy should be extended cranially and caudally anterior to the phrenic nerve. Once the pericardial sac is incised in its entirety, the heart should be carefully eviscerated. This step is undertaken not only to relieve cardiac tamponade but also to allow access to the heart for manual cardiac massage as well as for placement of internal defibrillator paddles.

4. The inferior pulmonary ligament must be incised. Care must be taken to avoid transecting the inferior pulmonary vein. Incising the inferior pulmonary ligament allows for better mobilization of the left lung to allow for improved access to the aorta as well as to allow one to perform a hilar twist of the lung if needed.
5. Next, the aorta should be cross-clamped. This occurs by identifying the aorta along the left lateral aspect of the vertebral column. Because these patients are pulseless, one may request that the airway team place a nasogastric tube down the esophagus to help delineate the esophagus from the aorta, which is posterior to the esophagus. Just proximal to the diaphragm, the parietal pleura overlying the aorta is dissected anteriorly and posteriorly to the aorta. The aortic cross-clamp is then applied across the entire diameter of the aorta. If the parietal pleura is not adequately cleared from the aorta, the cross-clamp will slide off the aorta. The aortic cross-clamp serves several purposes. First, it increases coronary perfusion during diastole with increased afterload. Second, cross-clamping the aorta helps maintain cerebral perfusion, and finally, the supradiaphragmatic cross-clamp helps to control infradiaphragmatic hemorrhage.
6. Life-threatening hemorrhage from the lung must be controlled. This may be accomplished with digital pressure or suture ligation of the bleeding lung or blood vessel, or if bleeding is uncontrollable distal to the hilum, a hilar twist maneuver may be performed to twist the hilar blood supply and eliminate blood flow through the pulmonary and bronchial vessels.
7. Direct cardiac injuries should also be repaired (usually temporarily until definitive repair is possible) with any of the techniques described below to control life-threatening hemorrhage.

Pericardiocentesis

Indications: Pericardiocentesis is utilized to drain fluid (blood in the case of trauma) from the pericardial sac to relieve cardiac tamponade. Cardiac tamponade is usually a result of bleeding into the pericardial sac caused by a penetrating injury to the heart or great vessels or even the pericardium itself. In the setting of cardiac tamponade, blood fills the pericardial sac and restricts filling of the heart (specifically the right and left ventricles). Stroke volume and cardiac output are significantly reduced, which results in cardiovascular collapse if not treated immediately. One may suspect cardiac tamponade based on the classic clinical signs known as Beck's triad, which include jugular venous distension, hypotension, and muffled heart sounds. However, these signs of cardiac tamponade are rarely present, and one must maintain a high level of suspicion for cardiac tamponade based on mechanism, injury trajectory, and hemodynamic instability. Focused assessment sonography for trauma (FAST) should be performed in the pericardial view as a rapid assessment of fluid in the pericardial sac to confirm the diagnosis of hemopericardium.

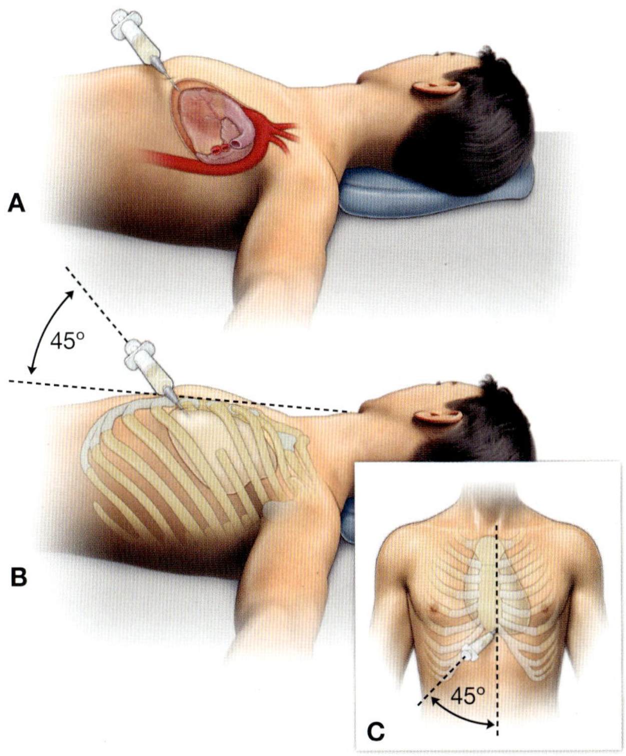

Figure 5-6

Pitfalls: Cardiac tamponade may occur with only a small volume of blood (approximately 200 mL of blood in the acute setting); therefore, one may injure the heart (right ventricle or nearby coronary artery) if the pericardiocentesis needle is passed too deeply. Additionally, a coexisting aortic dissection or myocardial free wall rupture may be worsened by rapid decompression of the cardiac tamponade with return of cardiac filling and rapid increase in cardiac output. However, neither is an absolute contraindication, and pericardiocentesis should be considered in the case of cardiac tamponade in settings in which immediate surgical resources are not available or the patient is profoundly hemodynamically unstable. Finally, pericardiocentesis is a temporizing procedure and should not be considered a definitive treatment for cardiac tamponade.

Techniques: Pericardiocentesis is performed with a needle (2.5-inch angiocath preferred) and syringe. In the urgent or nonemergent setting, lidocaine may be used to minimize patient discomfort. But as often is the case, the patient is too unstable and every second counts; therefore, local anesthetic is forsaken. With the patient in the supine position, the chest and subxiphoid area are prepared and draped in a sterile fashion. The puncture site is located between the xiphoid process and the left costal arch. At this point, the needle is advanced at a 45-degree angle to the skin and inserted 2 cm. One must aspirate continuously during insertion. Once nonclotting blood is aspirated, the needle of the angiocath is withdrawn and the plastic angiocath is left in place within the pericardial sac. With successful aspiration of hemopericardium in the face of cardiac tamponade, systolic blood pressure should improve and central venous pressures should decrease. The advantage of using the angiocath is that it may be left (secured with tape) in place for the short term to prevent cardiac tamponade from reoccurring and to maintain hemodynamic stability.

Pericardial Window

Indications: Similar to pericardiocentesis, the pericardial window may be used to help diagnose injuries to the pericardium, heart, or great vessels. The same clinical signs and symptoms (eg, tachycardia, hypotension, distended neck veins, precordial wound within the "cardiac box") that may indicate possible tamponade may direct one to perform a pericardial window. Additionally, injured patients who may not demonstrate the specific signs and symptoms but have a concerning mechanism or injury trajectory (penetrating injury to the anterior chest) must be considered for pericardial window. Pericardial window has been supplanted by the pericardial view of the FAST exam. However, there are clinical situations where the utility of the FAST is limited and the pericardial window must be performed to rule out cardiac/great vessel injury.

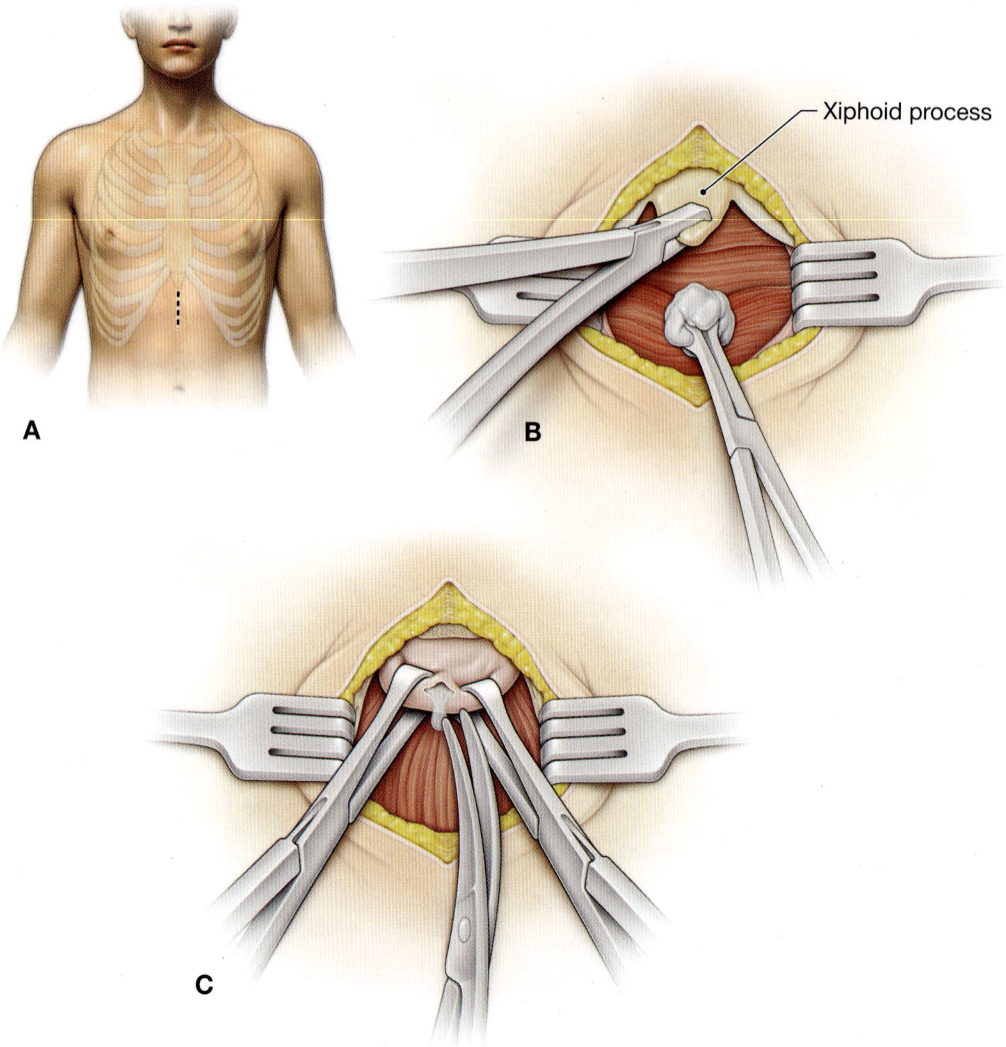

Figure 5-7

Pitfalls: One must be aware of the limitations of the pericardial window. Once the pericardial space is opened, one may encounter clear, serous fluid in the pericardial sac. If insufficient time is allowed for bloody fluid from around the heart to evacuate from the pericardiotomy, then one may obtain a false-negative result that may delay a patient from receiving a potentially life-saving procedure. Conversely, if the pericardium is not meticulously incised and blood from that incision is interpreted as blood from an underlying injury, the pericardial window could be interpreted as a false positive and the patient could be subjected to an unnecessary sternotomy or thoracotomy.

Technique: There are multiple methods to perform a pericardial window. One is the subxiphoid approach, and the other is through the central tendon of the diaphragm. In the subxiphoid approach, a vertical incision is made just inferior to the xiphoid process. The soft tissues are dissected at an angle in the cephalad direction under the xiphoid process. The fibrous pericardial sac is identified and grasped with Allis clamps and firmly retracted downward toward the surgeon. The pericardial sac is then incised with Metzenbaum scissors. Once the pericardiotomy is completed, the nature of the fluid is inspected. The pericardial sac and the fluid contents are then observed for at least 10 beats of the heart to ensure that the fluid does not change in color, consistency, or volume.

The other technique is a transabdominal approach in which the abdominal cavity is entered. The central tendon of the diaphragm is identified and grasped with Allis clamps and pulled down into the operative field. The central tendon of the diaphragm is then carefully incised with Metzenbaum scissors down to the pericardial sac. Once the pericardium is identified, it is grasped and incised in a similar fashion to the subxiphoid technique. The heart must be allowed to beat least 10 times to monitor the quality of the fluid in the pericardial sac to ensure that blood is not encountered.

Open Cardiac Massage and Use of Internal Defibrillation Paddles

Indications: Open cardiac massage must be rapidly instituted upon entering the pericardial sac during the resuscitative thoracotomy or sternotomy when the heart is found to be in asystole, poorly contracting, or fibrillating (while the defibrillation paddles are being set up and charged for imminent defibrillation). Internal defibrillation is attempted when the heart is discovered to be in fibrillation on visualization of the heart.

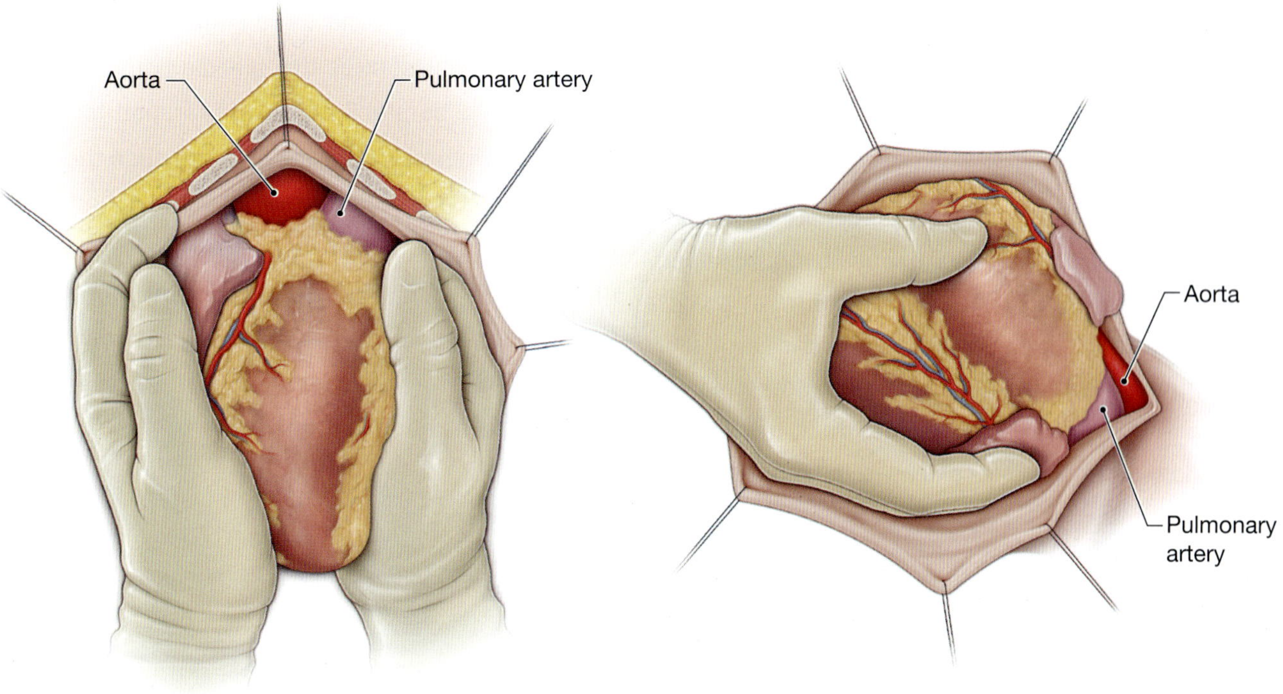

Figure 5-8

Pitfalls: Open cardiac massage offers its own risks. If proper technique is not followed, one may inadvertently perforate the heart with a thumb or finger. Additionally, the heart should be fully eviscerated from the pericardial sac to allow for proper placement of the hands on either side of the heart to allow for the most effective cardiac compressions.

Technique: Proper technique for open cardiac massage is critical to ensure optimal massage and prevent injury to the heart. One hand must be placed behind the heart, while the other hand is placed over the anterior surface of the heart. The hands must be positioned so that the fingers and thumbs are straight and compress the heart in a clapping motion in a way that sequentially compresses the heart from the apex up toward the aorta. This motion should be repetitive, and as time progresses with ongoing massage, one must be cognizant of proper form because it is easy to curl the fingers or thumbs in a way that may perforate the heart muscle.

Upon identification of cardiac fibrillation, internal defibrillation is utilized with internal defibrillation paddles. The exact type may vary by institution. However, the overall procedure of the paddles is similar across models. One paddle is placed on the posterior aspect of the heart near the apex, while the other paddle is placed on the anterior surface of the heart more toward the right atrium. Gentle pressure is used to hold the heart between the paddles. The defibrillator is charged by another team member. The initial defibrillation should occur at 10 J (joules), increasing by 10 J with each subsequent defibrillation attempt to a maximum energy recommended of 50 J. Internal defibrillation may be attempted serially as long as the heart is noted to be fibrillating. No additional defibrillation attempts should occur in the face of an organized cardiac rhythm.

Hemorrhage Control for Penetrating Cardiac Wounds

Multiple methods may be employed to help control hemorrhage from a penetrating cardiac injury. Bleeding may be controlled from the heart using digital control with a finger, a Foley catheter may be inserted into the wound, and surgical staples may be used to temporarily close the wound and staunch bleeding. Each method is described in more detail below.

Digital Control: In the face of a small wound of the right ventricle, often gently placing a finger over the wound may adequately control the bleeding and allow for the patient to be stabilized in preparation for definitive repair. One must be careful to not push the finger deeper into the wound as to make the wound larger and often uncontrollable. Additionally, not all wounds are amenable to this method because they may be too large to simply control with digital pressure. This must be assessed and recognized rapidly to prevent what may be a devastating iatrogenic injury.

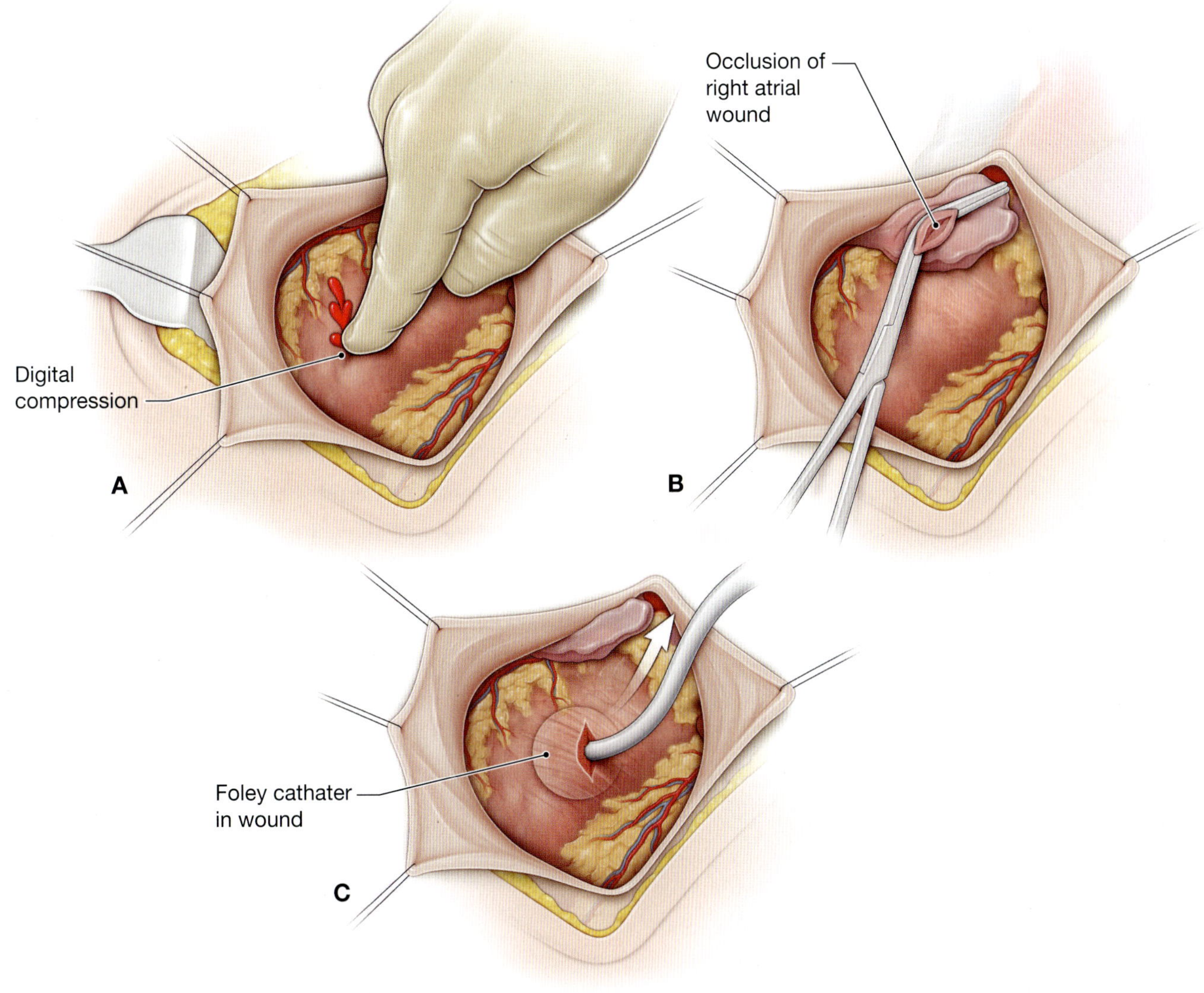

Figure 5-9

Foley Catheter: Larger penetrating cardiac injuries may be temporarily controlled with the insertion of a Foley catheter into the wound and gently inflating the balloon on the catheter. The Foley catheter is then pulled very gently to seal the balloon to the inner wall of the heart. Great caution must be taken when attempting this method. The inflation of the balloon may injure the chamber of the heart in which it is inserted. Additionally, even the lightest traction on the heart may inadvertently tear the heart open, turning a potentially salvageable situation into an uncontrolled and mortal injury.

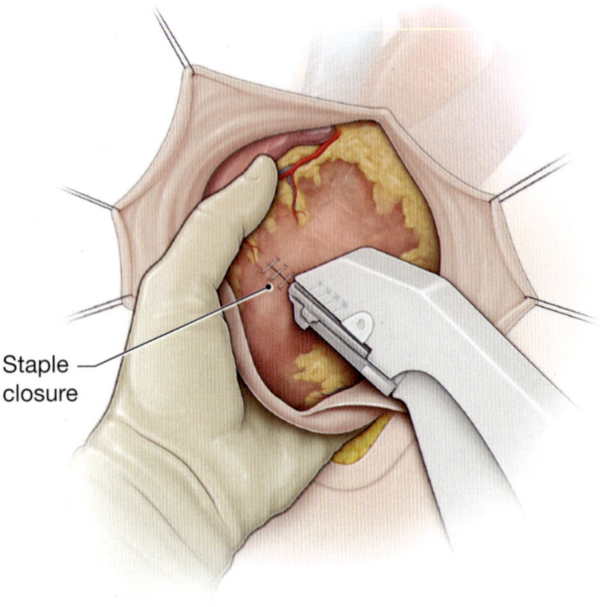

Figure 5-10

Surgical Staples: Often, linear lacerations on the heart (stab wounds) may not be amenable to the other methods previously described. In the face of hemorrhage, the linear nature of these wounds may be better suited for temporary control with surgical staples. In this case, the stapling device is used to approximate the edges of the lacerated heart. Caution must be used with this method as well because the right atrium and ventricle may be very thin and friable and may tear very easily. For this reason, staples may lacerate the already injured heart muscle, making a wound larger and more difficult to control.

No matter the method selected to control hemorrhage of a penetrating cardiac injury, one must take great care to ensure that the wound is not exacerbated and rendered uncontrollable.

Penetrating Wound in Close Proximity to a Coronary Artery

Indications: Penetrating wounds in close proximity to a coronary artery require an understanding of the coronary anatomy of the heart and appropriate identification so that the coronary artery is not inadvertently ligated in the repair of the cardiac injury. This may be difficult to recognize given that the heart can be covered in epicardial fat in the region of the coronary arteries or the coronary arteries may actually be intramuscular. Because of these anatomical challenges, one must be cognizant of the coronary anatomy and typical course of the various coronaries, especially the right main, left main, and left anterior descending coronary arteries.

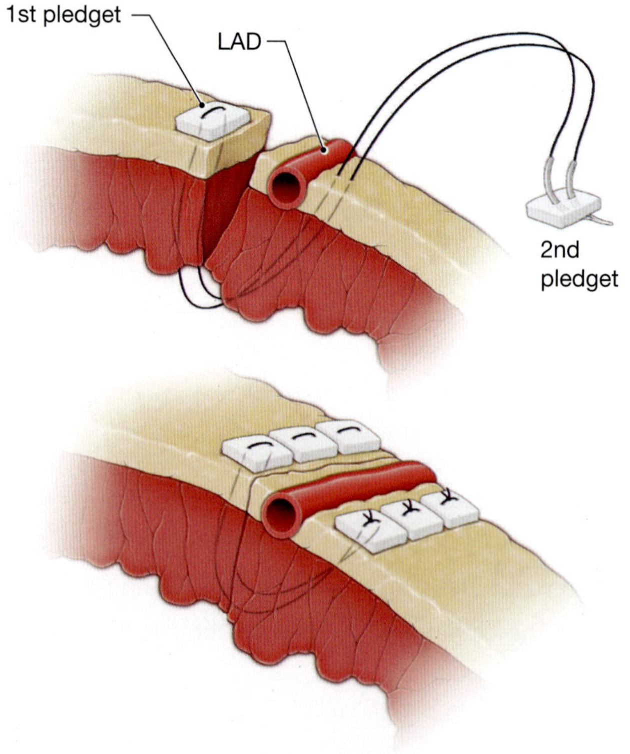

Figure 5-11

Pitfalls: Penetrating injuries in close proximity to the coronary arteries present a technical challenge to the surgeon. Not only must the surgeon identify the close proximity, but one must also use meticulous technique in repairing the injury. If the penetrating injury is repaired in a manner that results in ligation of the coronary artery, the heart will become ischemic. Depending on the vascular distribution of the ligated coronary artery, this may result in massive cardiac ischemia with subsequent patient demise.

Technique: To repair a penetrating injury in close proximity to a coronary artery, one must first identify the injury as such. Once the injury is noted to be in close proximity to a coronary artery, the injury is repaired using a U-stitch consisting of a pledgeted 4-0 Prolene suture. The U-stitch is positioned so that the suture traverses under the coronary and the pledgets are positioned on either side of the injury on one side and the coronary artery on the other side. Once this suture is placed and tied down and the wound is noted to be adequately repaired, one must watch the electrocardiogram on the monitor to identify ST changes concerning for coronary ischemia. If arrhythmias or ST changes are noted, the suture must be removed and repositioned either deeper or wider on the wall of the heart to avoid the coronary artery and its branches and thus minimize the risk of myocardial ischemia.

Coronary Artery Laceration

Indications: Penetrating cardiac injuries may result in lacerations to the coronary arteries. In the face of a coronary artery injury, the surgeon must first identify the injury and determine if the laceration involves the proximal or distal segment of the coronary artery and decide whether the associated myocardial distribution warrants coronary artery bypass versus simple ligation of the injured vessel.

Pitfalls: Lacerations of the coronary arteries may result in devastating myocardial ischemia. One must understand the vascular distribution of each of the main coronary arteries to appropriately judge the extent of the myocardial ischemia should one decide to simply ligate the injured vessel instead of performing a bypass graft. Massive myocardial ischemia (ie, left anterior descending artery distribution) may lead to significant and unrecoverable myocardial ischemia.

Technique: The technique one selects to repair a lacerated coronary artery depends on the location of the laceration. Distal injuries may be amenable to simple suture ligation, leading to a very small but survivable area of myocardial ischemia, whereas more proximal injuries will require a more complex repair often requiring cardiopulmonary bypass and a coronary artery bypass graft.

Distal Injury: A coronary artery injury to the distal most segment of the artery may simply be ligated. This may be accomplished using a 6-0 Prolene suture ligature. Both the proximal and distal ends of the artery must be ligated to effectively control hemorrhage. The concomitant cardiac muscle injury must also be repaired usually with the previously described U-stitch to avoid additional injury to the more proximal segment of the injured coronary artery.

Proximal Injury: A proximal coronary artery injury offers a very difficult and dire circumstance that will likely require cardiopulmonary bypass and a formal coronary bypass graft. The trauma surgery team must remember to appropriately prepare the patient in the typical trauma fashion (chin to knees and table to table). Preparing and draping the thighs into the field allows adequate access should the saphenous vein need to be harvested for a vascular conduit. If a proximal or mid-coronary artery laceration is identified, one should solicit assistance in the rapid harvest of the greater saphenous vein in order to perform a reversed saphenous bypass.

Simultaneous to the harvest of vein conduit, the surgeon must call for assistance from an appropriately trained cardiac surgeon. The patient must undergo rapid arterial and venous cannulation, either centrally (aorta and right atrium) or peripherally (femoral artery and vein), for the institution of cardiopulmonary bypass (CPB) (described below). Hemorrhage control may be obtained with suture ligation of the bleeding coronary artery. Once on CPB and based on the hemodynamic status of the patient, there are various conduits that may be used to restore coronary arterial flow. One may perform a bypass graft using the vein conduit to the distal segment of the lacerated artery. If the patient is hemodynamically stable, one may also rapidly harvest the left internal mammary artery (LIMA) in the standard fashion and perform a bypass graft of the LIMA to the distal segment of the lacerated artery. The distal anastomosis is typically completed with 7-0 Prolene sutures, whereas the proximal anastomosis to the aorta (as used with vein grafts) is performed with 6-0 Prolene sutures.

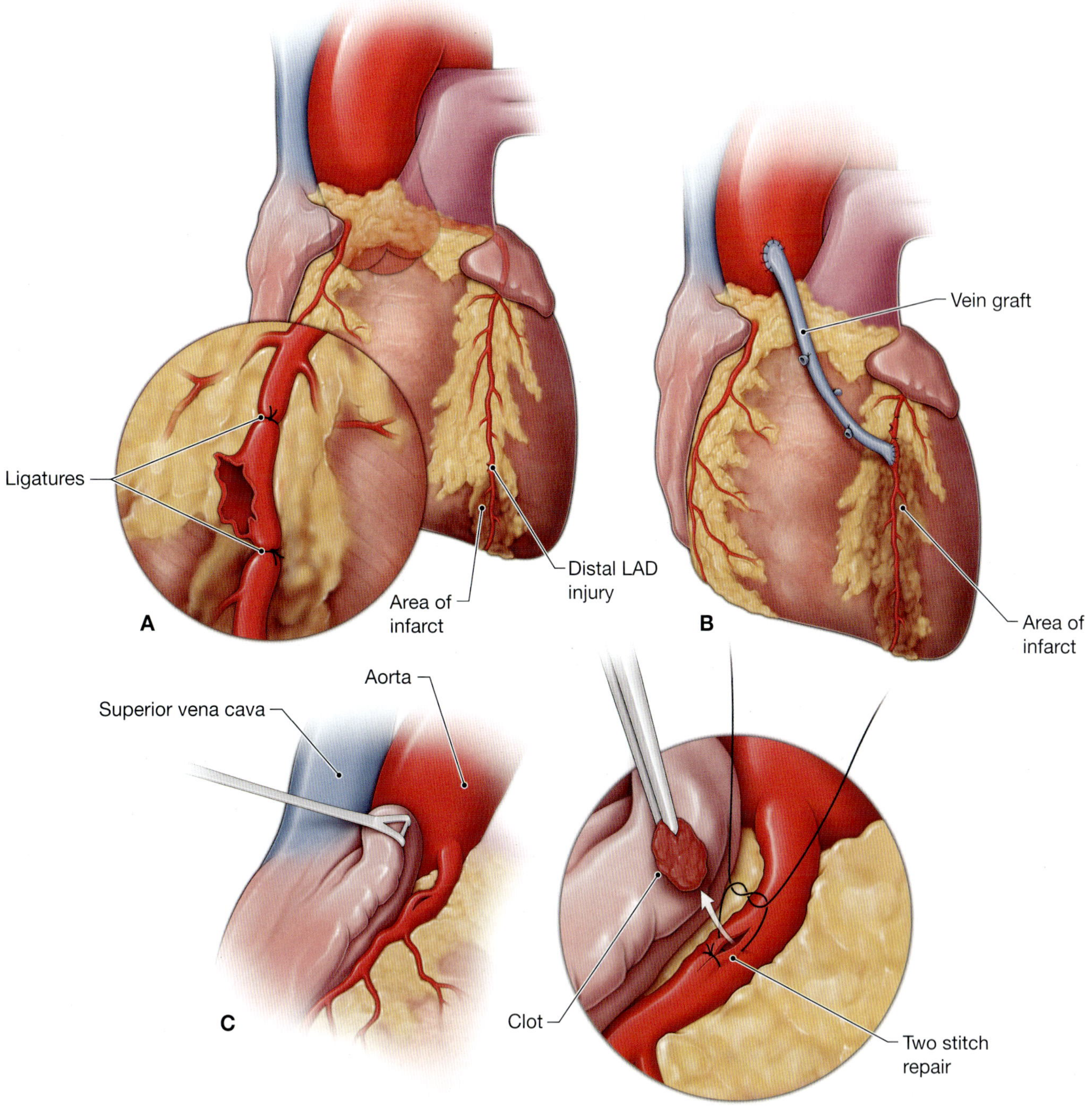
Ligatures
Area of infarct
Distal LAD injury
A
Vein graft
B
Area of infarct
Aorta
Superior vena cava
C
Clot
Two stitch repair

Figure 5-12

Cardiopulmonary Bypass in Trauma

Indications: The use of CPB in trauma, specifically for penetrating cardiac injuries, is widely debated due to the varied survival benefit published in the literature. Indications for the use of CPB in those with penetrating injuries to the heart include hemodynamic support in the face of cardiovascular collapse and to facilitate the repair of injuries that are not amenable to simple repair, with examples being wounds to the posterior surface of the heart, multichamber cardiac injuries, injuries to one or more of the cardiac valves, and coronary artery injuries

Pitfalls: Improved survival through the use of CPB in trauma is strongly debated; therefore, it is unclear whether patients actually benefit. This may be related to the dire circumstances surrounding a penetrating injury to the heart and the overall poor physiologic condition of the patient upon arrival to the hospital. Aside from the questionable benefit of CPB, CPB brings with it its own set of complications that include a significant inflammatory response with widespread systemic effects such as renal dysfunction, coagulopathy, thrombocytopenia, and stroke. Furthermore, trauma patients may have multiple sites of bleeding in addition to the cardiac injury. Thus, the need for full-dose heparinization certainly puts the patient at risk for significant bleeding complications from concurrent injuries (eg, associated open wounds, solid organ injuries, concomitant intracranial hemorrhage).

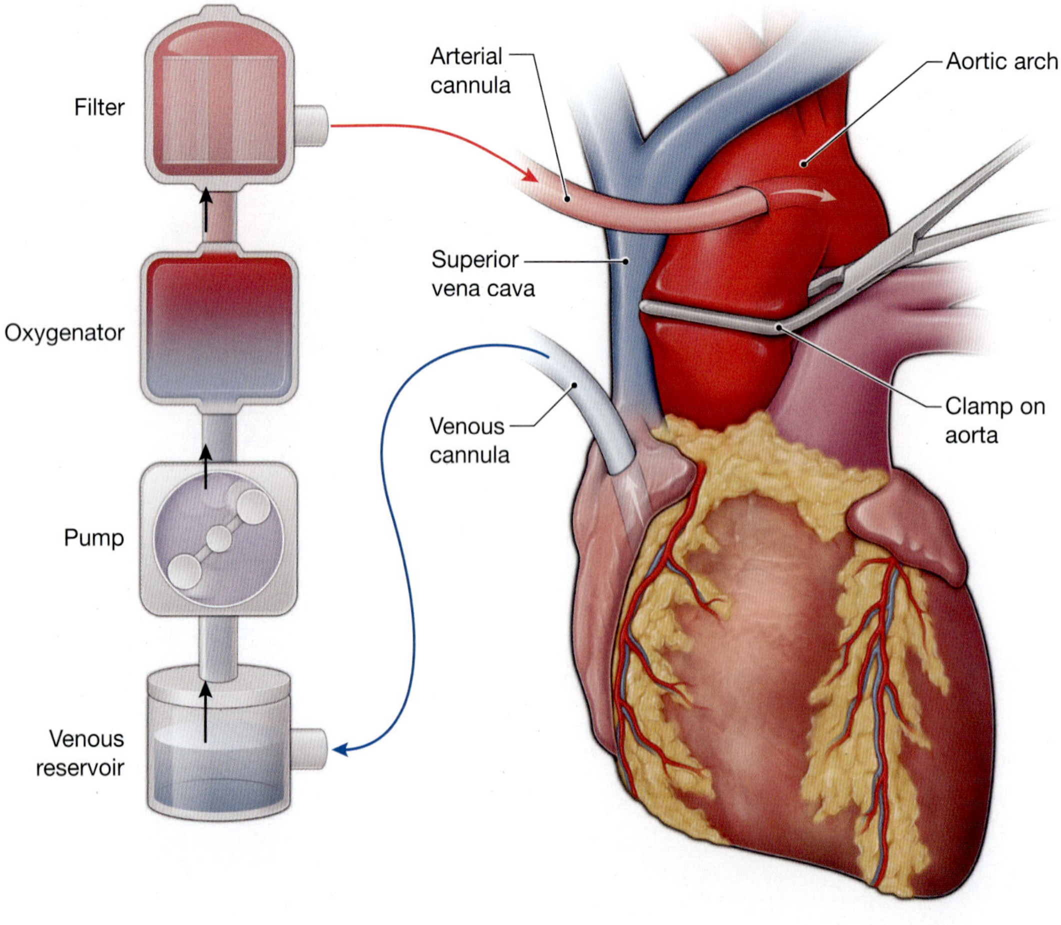

Figure 5-13

Technique: To initiate CPB, one must obtain both arterial and venous access. This may be done centrally via the aorta and right atrium or peripherally via the common femoral artery and femoral vein. Once arterial and venous access is obtained and the CPB machine is set up and primed, the cannulas are connected via tubing to the CPB pump. It is critical that the arterial cannula is free of any bubbles when connecting to the tubing to prevent air emboli. This is not critical when connecting the venous cannula. One must fully heparinize the patient as well using 300 units/kg of heparin intravenously. Upon obtaining an activated clotting time >400 seconds, one may "go on bypass" safely. The pump is initiated, and blood is drained from the large venous cannula. Upon full CPB support, the heart is stopped with a dose of cardioplegia (beyond the scope of this chapter), and ventilation is ceased by turning off the ventilator.

Once on CPB, to repair an intracardiac injury (multichamber, valvular, or septal injuries), the aorta must be cross-clamped. At this time, cardioplegia solution must be administered to stop the heart and protect the myocardium. The cardioplegia solution is instilled via a separate antegrade cardioplegia cannula that is placed in the aorta, proximal to the aortic cross-clamp. A retrograde cardioplegia cannula may be placed in the right atrium and the balloon settled in the coronary sinus. With CPB at full flow and the heart stopped with appropriate myocardial protection strategies, one may undertake the necessary repairs of the heart such as valve repair, closure of septal defects, or coronary artery bypass, especially to the posterior aspect of the heart where the heart would not otherwise tolerate being twisted and positioned to reach the injured vessel.

Chest Wall Closure

Indications: Chest wall closure is dependent on the type of incision that is undertaken to gain access to the injury. One must work hard to close the chest as rapidly as possible, with every attempt made to close the chest at the completion of the index operation. However, this is not always possible due to severe hemodynamic instability in which the chest may be left open temporarily in a damage-control fashion. Chest wall closure for each of the incisions is described below.

Pitfalls: Chest wall closure must be meticulous to prevent any one of the many associated complications. The most common complications include wound infection with associated osteomyelitis and mediastinitis. Other complications include sternal instability and dehiscence, wound/soft tissue dehiscence, exposure of the underlying sternum and wires, retained hemothorax from poorly positioned or nonfunctioning chest tubes, and pneumothorax again from nonfunctioning chest tubes or from inappropriate technique upon removing the chest tube.

Techniques: Techniques for each type of incision are described below.

Sternotomy—The sternum is approximated with a series of wires placed horizontally along the length of the sternum. Prior to definitive closure of the sternum, chest tubes are placed in the pleural spaces (if violated) and mediastinum to drain fluid and blood from these spaces to prevent pleural effusions and cardiac tamponade, respectively. These are secured with zero silk sutures, and a Pleur-evac® system is used to accumulate the drainage.

The sternum is then closed in any number of ways. For patients with thin body habitus, one may use "single wires" that contain a single wire attached to a large cutting needle. For larger patients, "double wires" are preferred. Double wires are made up of a wire that is doubled on itself with both ends attached to the large cutting needle. The wires are carefully driven through the body of the sternum. While one must follow the curve of the needle, one must first drive the needle through both tables of the sternum in a very straight direction either from above or below depending on which side of the sternum is being approached. Once through both tables of the sternum, one must follow the curve of the needle to bring the wire into its appropriate position. The wire is twisted off of each needle.

Most methods use three wires in the manubrium, with one immediately distal to the angle of Louis and the additional wires placed equally down the body of the sternum. Once all wires are placed, the wires are crossed (again, there are many ways to secure the wires in closing the sternum), pulled upward, and then pulled together to reapproximate the cut edges of the sternum. Once the sternum is reapproximated, the wires are twisted together and cut. Care must be taken in the final tightening of each wire to prevent breaking the wires. The wires are then bent down into the sternum and soft tissues to prevent them from protruding through the wound and causing the patient significant pain. The fascial layer of muscle and soft tissue immediately over the sternum is then closed using 0 vicryl suture to cover the sternum and wires in their entirety. The additional soft tissue is closed in layers with 2-0 vicryl, and the skin may be closed with surgical staples or using a running subcuticular suture depending on the acuity of the clinical situation.

Left Anterolateral Thoracotomy—The left anterolateral thoracotomy may also be closed in a manner that prevents lung herniation and stabilizes any fractured ribs that occurred either as a result of the injury or from performing the procedure itself.

Multiple chest tubes are typically placed in the left pleural space prior to definitive closure of the chest cavity. The chest tubes are placed such that one runs along the posterior chest wall into the apical position. An anterior tube is positioned along the anterior chest wall, while a curved chest tube is positioned over the dome of the diaphragm. These tubes exit the chest wall several centimeters inferior to the thoracotomy incision. One must take care to ensure that they exit the skin in a lateral to anterolateral position on the chest wall to prevent patient discomfort should they be placed too far posteriorly.

The ribs may be approximated in a variety of ways. One may simply place heavy (#1 or #2) permanent sutures in a figure-of-eight fashion around the superior and inferior ribs and reapproximate the ribs to restore anatomy. Care must be taken to not cinch the ribs too tightly to one another. An alternative technique involves drilling intermittent holes in the inferior rib and then using the same heavy suture material as previously described. The upper rib is encircled while the suture is placed through each of the holes in the rib. Again, these sutures are tied down to simply restore anatomy. Once the ribs are reapproximated, then the overlying serratus anterior muscle is reapproximated in a single layer using 0 vicryl suture. If the latissimus muscle was divided, it should also be repaired in a similar fashion. These muscles must be reapproximated with the overlying fascia included during each pass of the needle. The soft tissue and skin are then closed in layers.

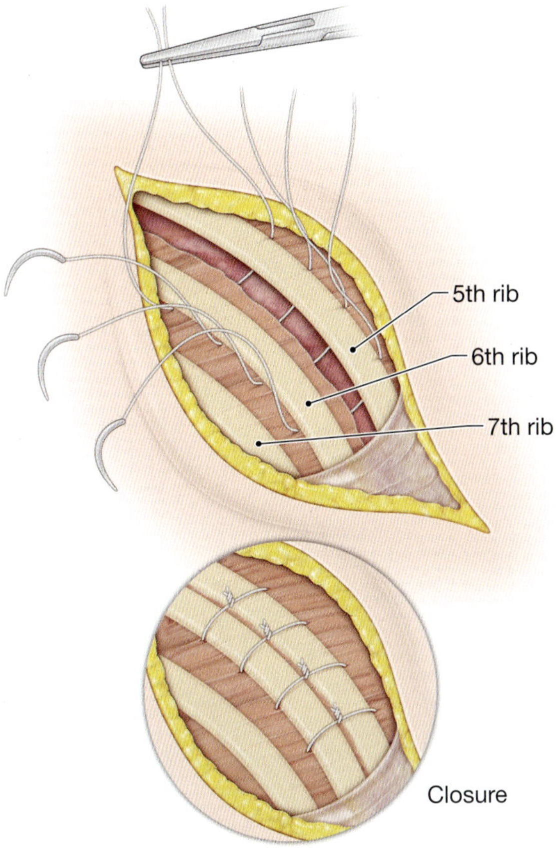

Figure 5-14

Clamshell Thoracotomy—The clamshell is closed in a similar fashion to the left anterolateral thoracotomy. Chest tubes are placed in each chest cavity as described above. Each chest cavity is also closed in a similar fashion. The challenge with closure of the clamshell is reapproximation of the lowest portion of the sternum that is often transected during the creation of the clamshell thoracotomy. The proximal sternum may be approximated to the short distal segment of sternum using wires. This may be accomplished by placing a wire in a figure-of-eight fashion or by placing two wires in a simple interrupted fashion as described previously for sternotomy closure. The blood supply to the short distal segment of sternum is often tenuous and may lead to sternal wound complications and impaired healing. The soft tissue and skin are again closed in multiple layers as previously described.

Trapdoor Incision—The trapdoor incision is highly morbid and difficult to adequately close given the combination of incisions. Closure should be initiated by approximating the sternum with closure of the sternotomy using wires as described above. Once the sternum is completely reapproximated, the clavicle may be plated or simply reapproximated with a cerclage stitch to help stabilize the bone. Finally, the thoracotomy aspect of the incision is closed separately. This may be performed using any of the preferred techniques described above depending on surgeon comfort and experience. Once the sternum and clavicle are reapproximated and the anatomy of the ribs from the thoracotomy is restored, one must reapproximate the incised muscle fascia of the pectoralis muscle as well as the serratus muscle from the thoracotomy. The overlying soft tissue and skin are closed in separate layers as previously described to ensure adequate tissue coverage over any wires, plates, and other hardware that may have been placed during the definitive closure.

6 LUNG TRAUMA

Renaldo Williams, MD
Geoffrey A. Anderson, MD, MPH
Ali Salim, MD

TIPS

1. **Patients with pulmonary injuries will often have associated serious injuries, including cardiac and intra-abdominal injuries, that may need to be addressed first or in conjunction with thoracic injuries.**

2. **Ninety percent of blunt chest trauma is managed nonoperatively, with chest tube insertion being the likely intervention. Patients sustaining severe penetrating injuries with hemodynamic collapse or significant blood loss are more likely to require operative intervention.**

3. **There is almost no role for anatomic resections in trauma; preserve as much lung parenchyma as possible with resections.**

Introduction

Thoracic injuries sustained secondary to trauma represent 20% to 25% of all trauma deaths. The true incidence of pulmonary injuries secondary to trauma remains unknown but is significant.

Most chest trauma injuries, whether penetrating or blunt in etiology, can be managed with nonoperative management. Five percent of chest injuries involve severe penetrating pulmonary injuries with hemodynamic compromise and/or significant amount of blood loss that cannot be managed with chest tube insertion alone and will require operative intervention. If the patient is hemodynamically stable, this may allow time for computed tomography imaging that may assist with diagnosis and operative planning. Understanding thoracic anatomy is key to achieving a successful outcome with low morbidity.

The mortality rate for traumatic thoracic injuries ranges from 10% to 60% depending on several risk factors including, but not limited to, mechanism of the injury, location of the injury, associated extrathoracic injuries, prehospital transport time, presence of hemodynamic collapse, and need for multiple procedures.

Anatomy

The thorax (or chest) is composed of the chest cavity and chest wall (Figure 6-1). It contains the major organs: the heart and the lung. Other major internal structures that are housed here include the trachea, the esophagus, and major blood vessels such as the aorta, vena cavae, and pulmonary arteries and their branches (Figure 6-2).

The thoracic skeleton is composed of the ribs and the sternum. The ribs are numbered 1-12 on either side. The true ribs (1-7) connect to the sternum proper. False ribs (8-10) are connected to the proceeding ribs by cartilage. Floating ribs (11 and 12) do not have anterior attachments to the sternum.

There are important anatomical landmarks that help us describe the chest location and are particularly useful in thoracic injury. The nipple line of the male patient roughly estimates the location of the fourth intercostal space. The inframammary crease line in the female patient corresponds to the fourth intercostal space. These are useful when deciding chest tube insertion sites and incisions. Additionally, the midclavicular line roughly correlates to the nipple line in a vertical plane and can be utilized in identifying injuries associated with "the cardiac box." The "cardiac box" is a term referring to the space that has the sternal notch, costal margins, and midclavicular lines as boundaries and is associated with increased risk of cardiac injury.

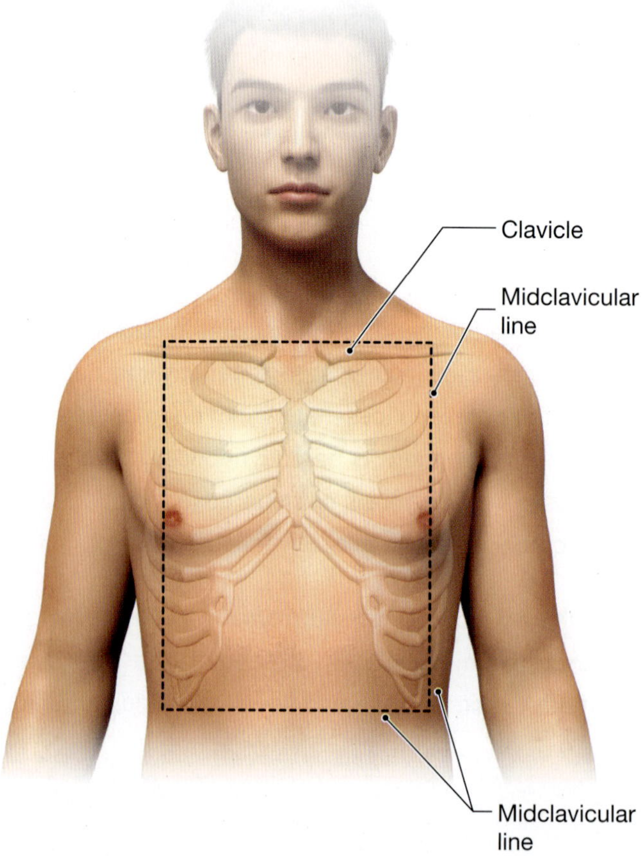

Figure 6-1

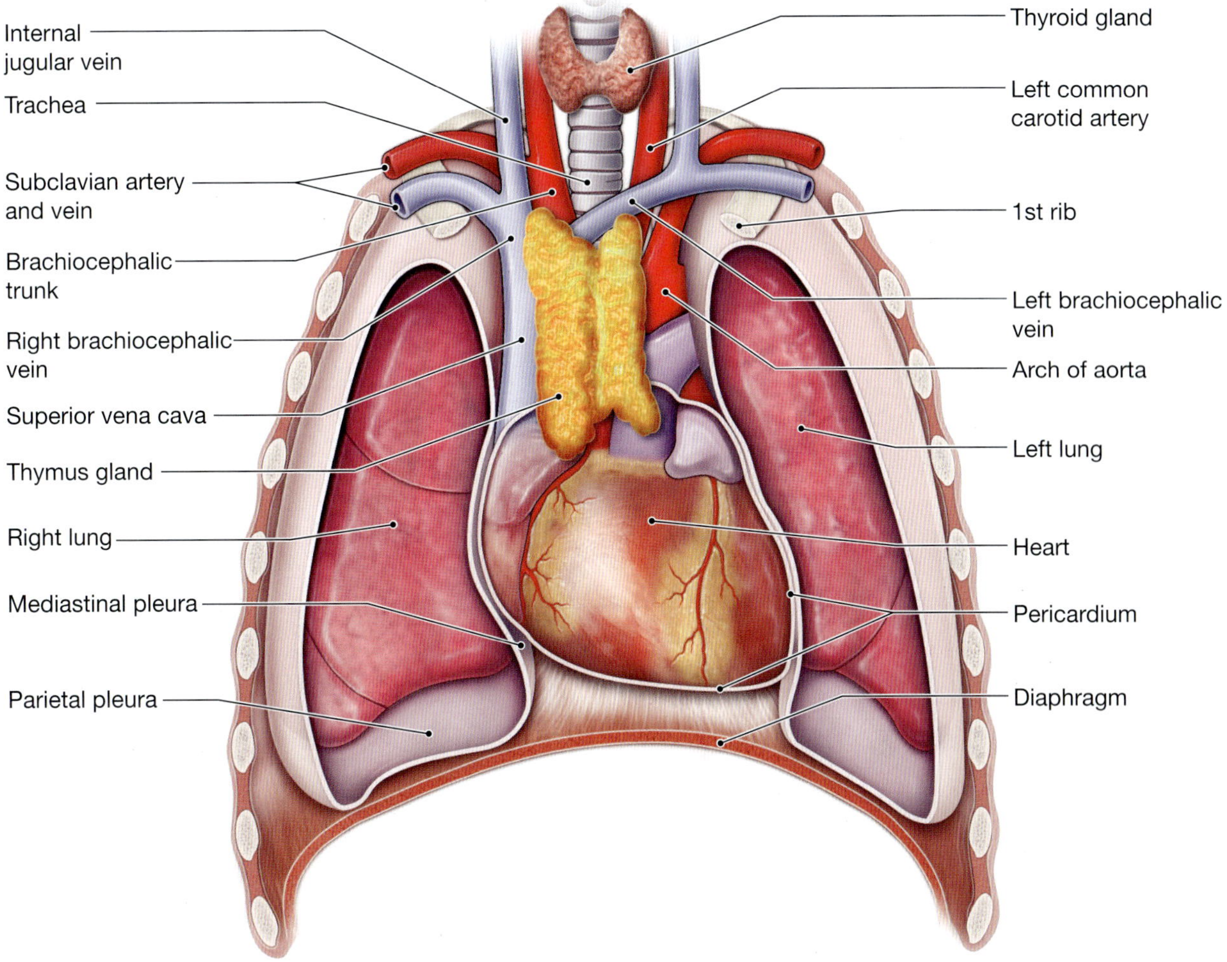

Figure 6-2

American Association for the Surgery of Trauma Organ Injury Scale

The American Association for the Surgery of Trauma (AAST) has developed a grading system (Table 6-1) that helps standardize language when addressing the severity of thoracic injuries. The grading system alone does not dictate the intervention needed. The vital signs, condition of the patient, and the grading system together help the physician develop an appropriate treatment plan for the trauma patient.

6 LUNG TRAUMA

TABLE 6-1. Organ Injury Scale

Grade	AAST Injury Scale - Lung
I Contusion Unilateral, <1 lobe	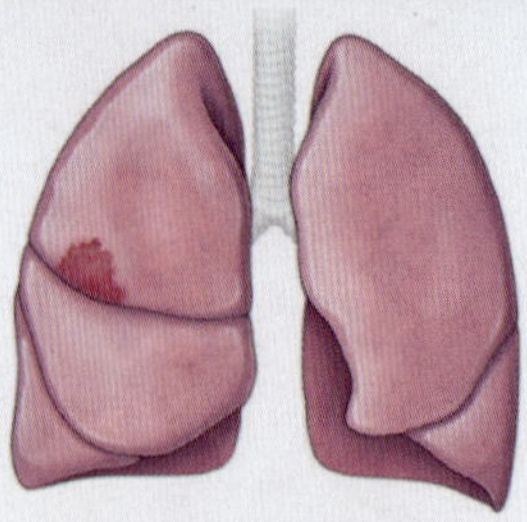
II Contusion Unilateral, > 1 lobe	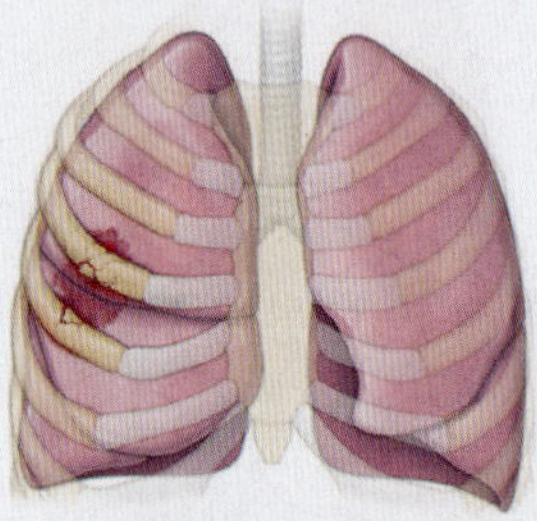
III Hematoma Nonexpanding intraparenchymal	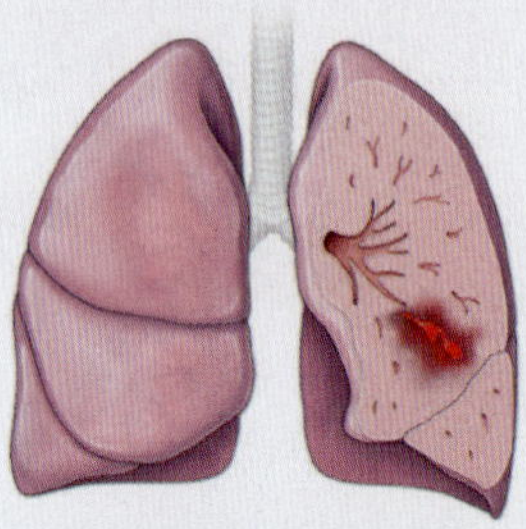
IV Vascular Primary branch intrapulmonary vessel disruption	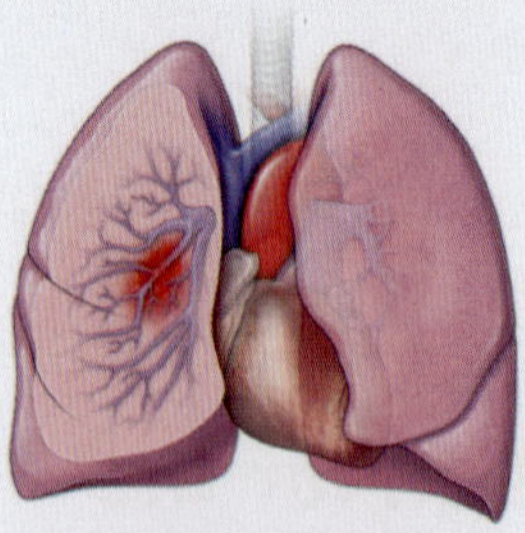
V Hilar vessel disruption	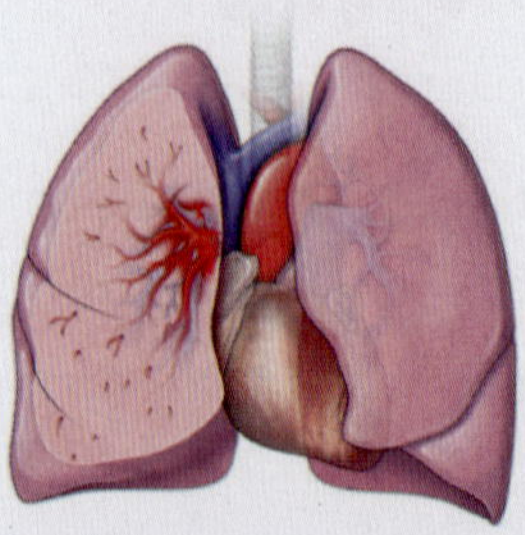

Source: Adapted with permission from Moore EE, Malangoni MA, Cogbill TH, et al. Organ injury scaling. IV: Thoracic vascular, lung, cardiac, and diaphragm. *J Trauma.* 1994;36(3):299-300.

Operative Steps

Patient Positioning

Patient positioning will depend on the location of the injury and the patient's hemodynamics. If the patient is hemodynamically unstable, then the patient should be placed in a supine position with a bump underneath the patient to allow for positioning a thoracotomy incision. In the supine position, this will allow for quick conversion to sternotomy if needed. A patient needing a posterolateral thoracotomy will need to have appropriate hemodynamics before placing them in lateral decubitus position; this is rarely done acutely in trauma. Anesthesia will start with a single-lumen endotracheal tube and convert to a double-lumen endotracheal tube if single-lung ventilation is needed. Low tidal volume ventilation is utilized to prevent air embolism during resection.

Equipment

These procedures require additional equipment that may not be included in the standard tray. Some of these additional items include a Finochietto retractor (Figure 6-3) (or two of these if clamshell is needed), Duval forceps (Figure 6-4), Allison lung retractor, sternal saw, Lebsche knife, rib shears, and a vascular tray. The Finochietto retractor will be utilized with the thoracotomy or median sternotomy incision to allow for exposure. It is important to make sure to place the retractor side with the crank toward the bed to allow for additional exposure and keep it from being pulled on during the procedure. The sternal saw, rib shears, and Lebsche knife are used when cutting through the sternum and/or ribs to access the chest cavity. The sternal saw should be checked to make sure the blade is appropriately positioned before use. The Lebsche knife (Figure 6-5) has a mallet that comes with it

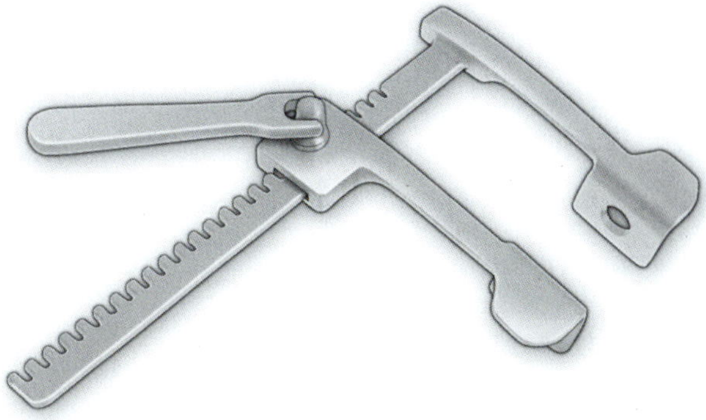

Figure 6-3. Finochietto retractor.

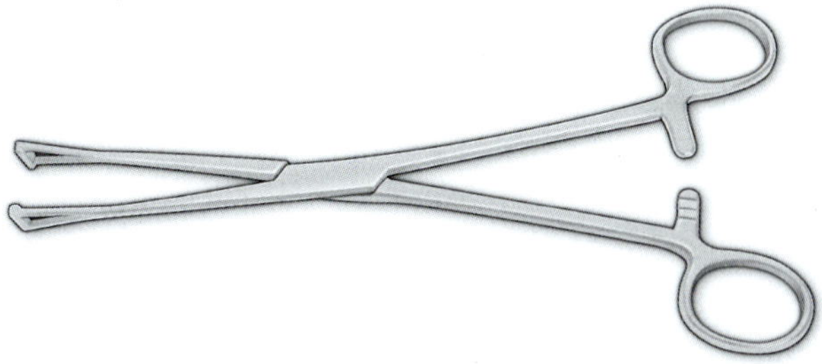

Figure 6-4. Duval lung clamp.

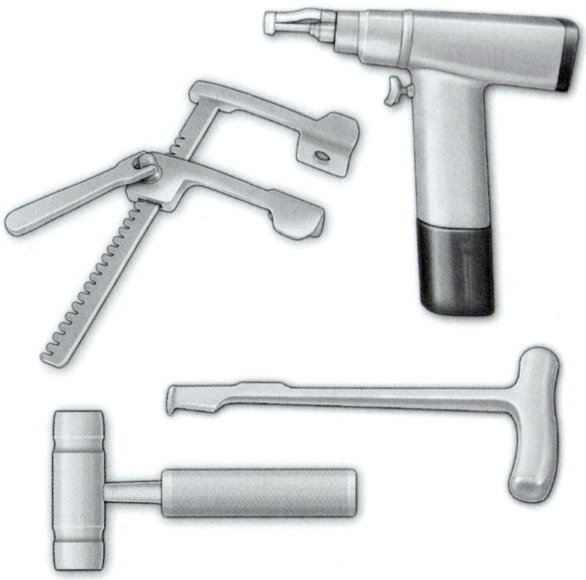

Figure 6-5. Lebsche knife.

that is utilized in quickly cutting the sternum to allow for access. A vascular tray should be on hand to help deal with the major vessel injuries that may be encountered. Making sure these instruments, along with Prolene sutures, are available should be done before proceeding with vascular repair.

Procedural Steps

Chest Entry

1. Anterolateral thoracotomy: The first step will be to enter the chest through a thoracotomy incision. The most common will be the anterolateral thoracotomy incision (Figure 6-6) due to ease of access if the patient is hemodynamically unstable or if access is also needed to enter the abdominal cavity. It may be extended to the contralateral hemithorax if a concomitant injury is found. The incision begins at the lateral border of the sternum at the fourth or fifth intercostal space and extends laterally to the latissimus dorsi and curves into the axilla (Figure 6-7). It is carried through skin, subcutaneous tissue, pectoralis major and minor muscles anteriorly and the serratus posteriorly, and then finally through the intercostal muscles.

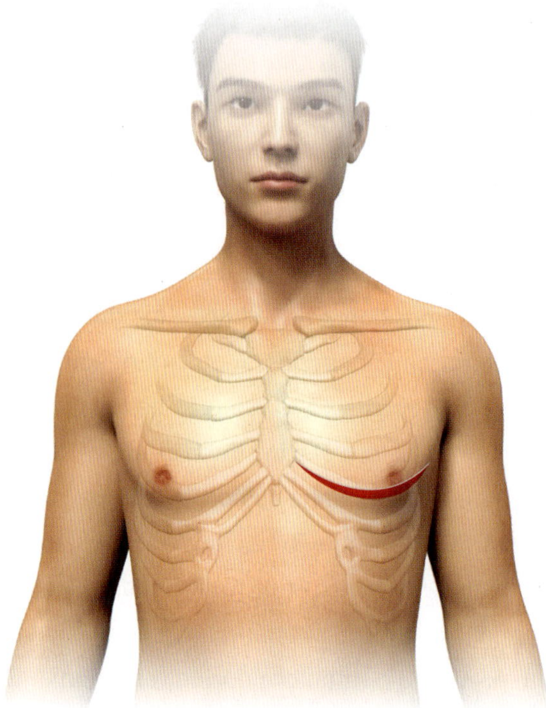

Figure 6-6. Thoracotomy incision.

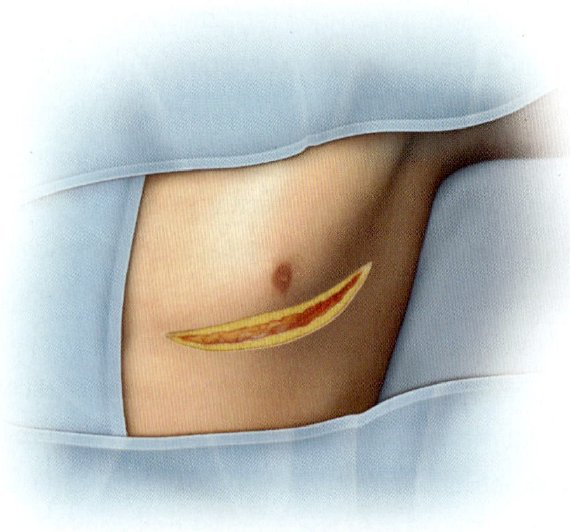

Figure 6-7. Anterolateral thoracotomy incision.

When dividing the intercostal muscles, it is important to be as close as possible to the superior border of the rib to avoid the neurovascular bundle (Figure 6-8). Before pleural entry, anesthesia should be asked to hold ventilation if possible. The pleura is entered and a Finochietto retractor is used to separate the ribs slowly and expose the structures of the thoracic cavity. (Note the position of the Finochietto in Figure 6-9.)

2. Clamshell thoracotomy: To improve exposure, the original thoracotomy incision can be extended to the contralateral intercostal space by utilizing the Lebsche knife to cross the sternum horizontally (Figures 6-10 and 6-11).

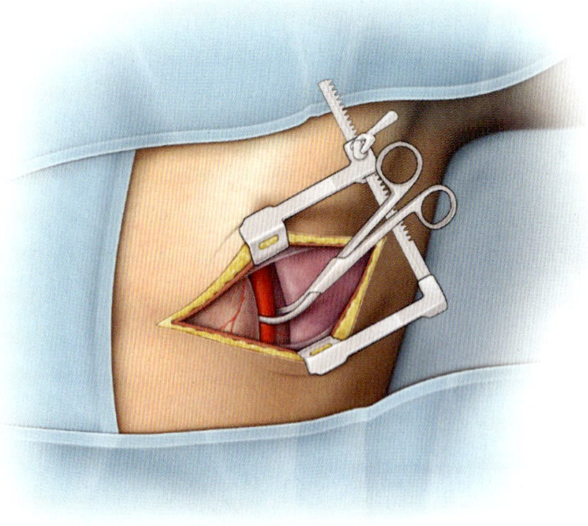

Figure 6-9

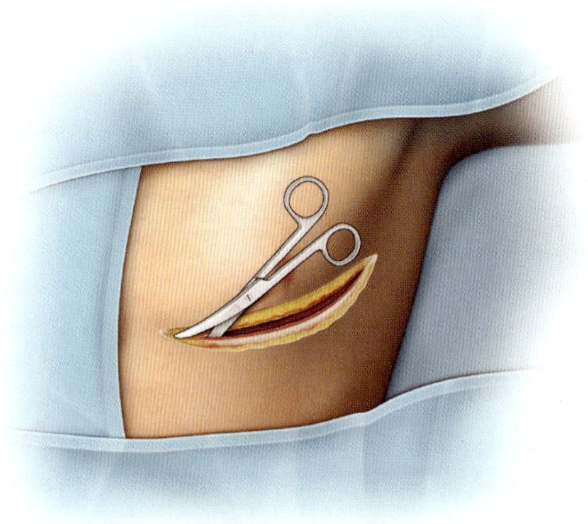

Figure 6-8

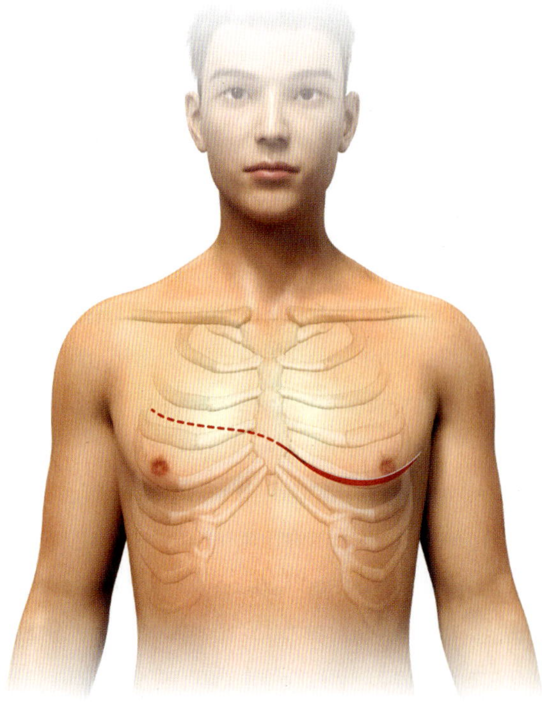

Figure 6-10. Clamshell thoracotomy.

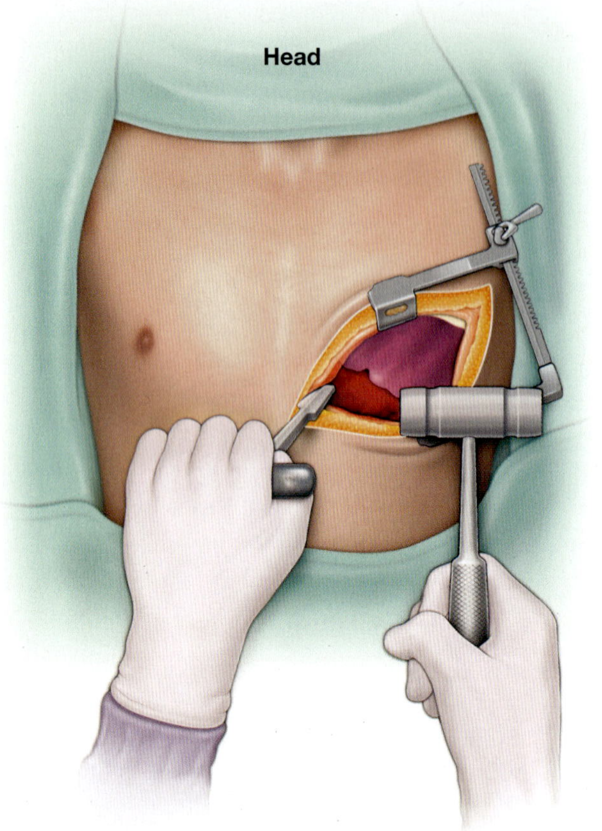

Figure 6-11. Lebsche knife used to extend the contralateral intercostal space.

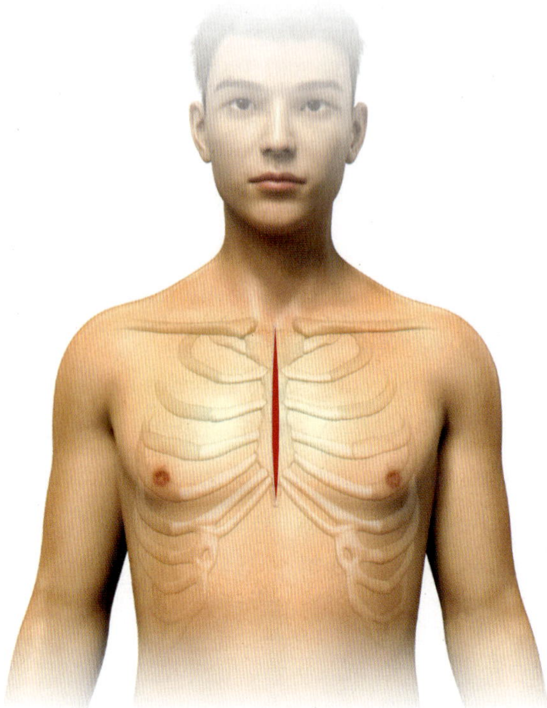

Figure 6-12. Median sternotomy.

3. The median sternotomy (Figure 6-12) may need to be utilized for very proximal lung injuries and hilar injuries near the mediastinum. First, a vertical incision is made from the sternal notch to the xiphoid. Utilizing cautery, the incision is carried through the subcutaneous tissue to the bone. Next, blunt dissection is used superiorly at the sternal notch (Figure 6-13) to sweep down the innominate artery and left innominate vein that could be right underneath and to divide the robust interclavicular ligament. At the xiphoid process, cautery may be utilized to incise the inferior ligament that is identified. Occasionally, the xiphoid process must be removed.

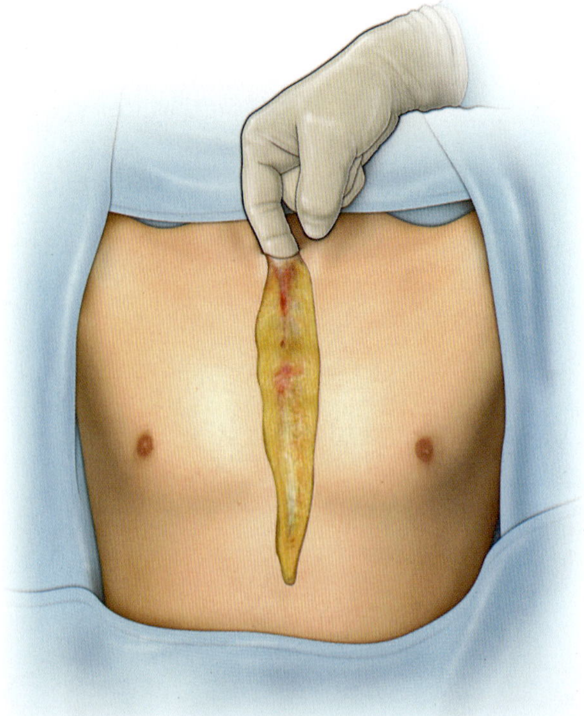

Figure 6-13. Blunt dissection at the sternal notch.

Next, a sternal saw is used in cutting through the sternum in a vertical fashion, allowing accessing to the heart and mediastinal structures. Mark the sternum with cautery first to ensure that the sternum is divided at its center (Figures 6-14 and 6-15).

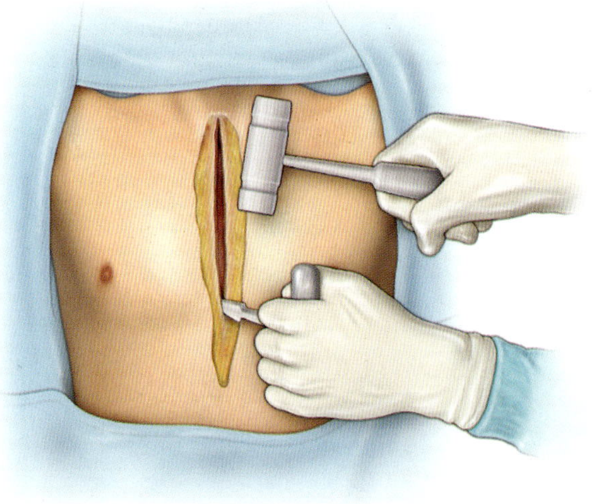

Figure 6-14

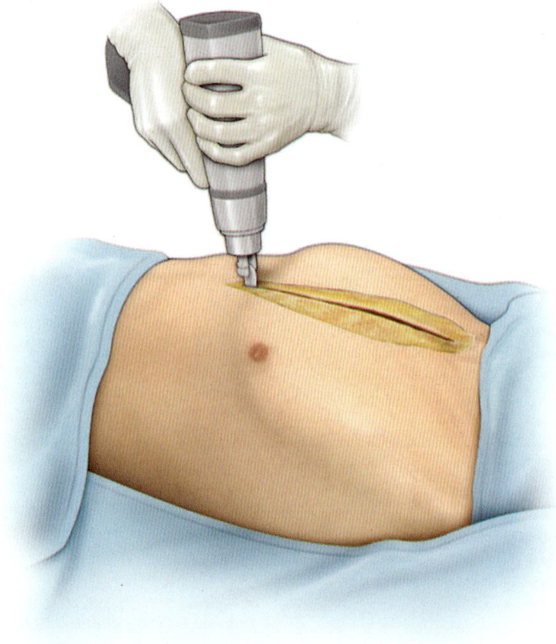

Figure 6-15

4. Pneumorrhaphy: This is utilized in small, peripheral lung repairs only. Never suture the entrance and exit wound due to the risk of air embolism. Once the retractor is in place to expose the structures in the chest cavity, the lung should be stabilized using Duval forceps or other suitable forceps. This exposes the injured tissue and allows for the approximation of bronchi and ligation of vessels (Figure 6-16). Vessels should be ligated with 3-0 or 4-0 nonabsorbable suture. Bronchi should be closed with absorbable sutures such as 3-0 PDS.

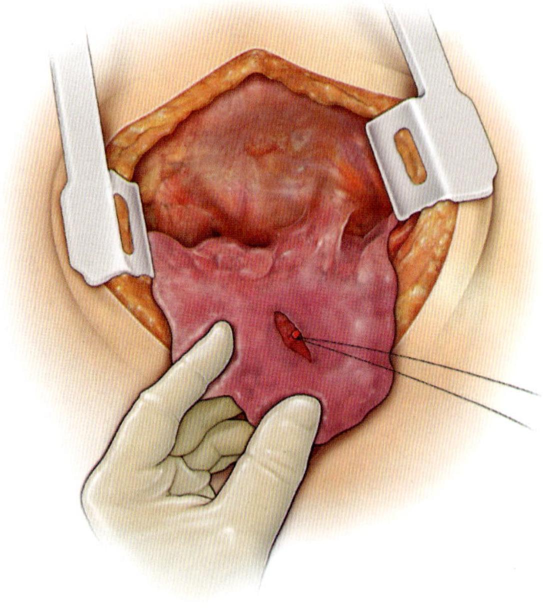

Figure 6-16. Pneumorrhaphy.

5. Tractotomy: This is used for deep wounds from penetrating injury without hilar injury. After stabilization with Duval forceps (Figures 6-17 and 6-18), the entrance and exit wounds for the penetrating injury are identified. Next, a GIA stapler is placed through the entry site and used to staple the tissue. This will allow for identification of bleeding vessels and injured bronchi that will need to be separately ligated using suture. The lung tissue can be reapproximated with a running suture. Air leak test is performed, and additional repairs are made. Tissue sealants may be used in this setting. Chest tubes are placed, and the incision is closed.

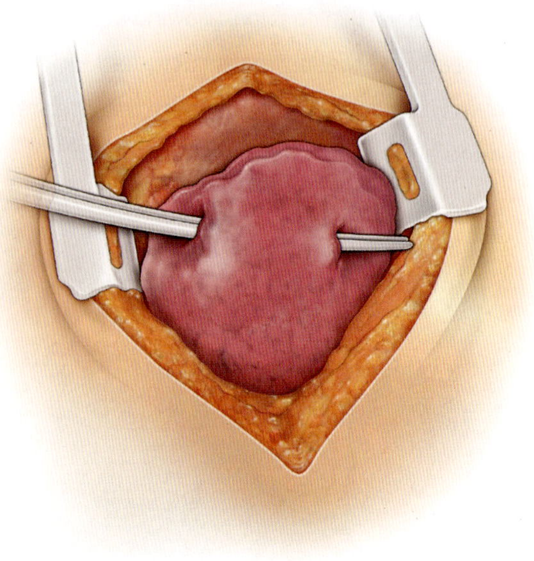

Figure 6-17

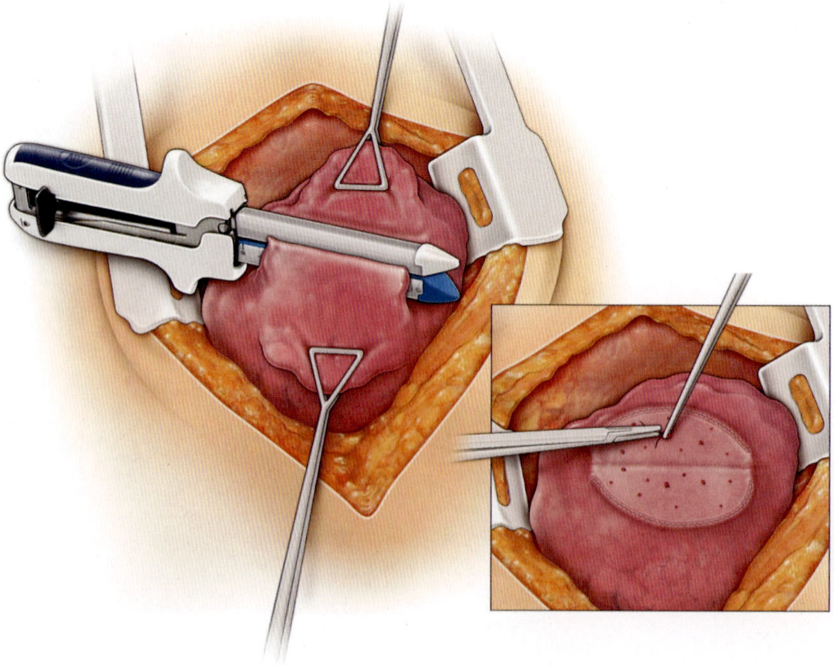

Figure 6-18

6. Wedge resection: For peripheral injuries or small injuries requiring resection, wedge resection may be used. The lung tissue to be divided will be grasped with Duval forceps (Figure 6-19). Next, the GIA stapler will be placed across the lung tissue including the injured portion of the lung (Figure 6-20). This may take a couple of staple loads. After completion of the staple fires, the staple lines should be inspected for hemostasis and addressed. The staple line will be immersed under saline and positive pressure to test for air leak. Any air leak identified can be oversewn with absorbable suture. After placing chest tubes, the incision can be closed.

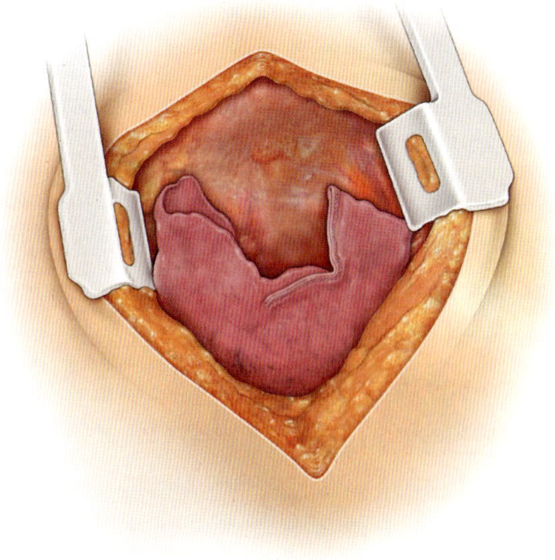

Figure 6-20

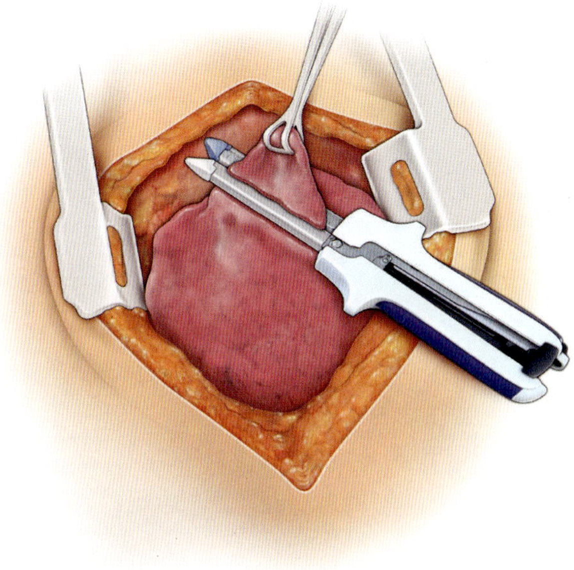

Figure 6-19. Lung tissue grasped with Duval forceps.

7. Lobectomy: Lobectomy is rarely undertaken and best utilized when there is a need for resection of major portions of devitalized lung parenchyma or control of major air leaks or hemorrhage. The vast majority of the time, a nonanatomic resection can be performed. The first step should be gaining control of major bleeding with digital control or vascular clamp. Next, dividing the inferior pulmonary ligament will allow for greater exposure of the lower poles. Major hilar vessels should be identified, and then lobar vessels should be noted and controlled. These vessels may be ligated with nonabsorbable sutures or using a vascular stapler. The major bronchi corresponding to the appropriate segment or lobe should be transected utilizing a TA stapler. Stay sutures placed before the transection will help to prevent retraction of the tissue once the transection is complete. The suture and staple lines should be assessed with a leak test. They should be immersed under saline, and

the anesthesiologist will provide positive pressure. Additional sutures and staples may be needed for any leaks identified. Any stumps may be covered with a pericardial, pleural, diaphragmatic, or intercostal muscle flap if time permits. After lobectomy, the remaining lobes are secured to the thoracic wall to prevent torsion. Torsion can occur easily after these cases, and failure to recognize can result in tissue necrosis. Next, chest tubes are placed, and the incision is closed.

8. Pneumonectomy: This procedure is rarely performed. Anesthesia should be in close communication when undertaking a pneumonectomy. The fluid management strategy will change dramatically once the lung has been resected and the hemorrhage has stopped. If it is undertaken when the patient is exsanguinating, the pulmonary hilum should be encircled quickly and digitally to provide enough compression to the hilar structures to allow anesthesia to catch up with the resuscitation of the patient. An aortic cross-clamp is placed across the hilum a few centimeters from the mediastinal pleura. Depending on the side, the phrenic and vagus nerves with accompanying branches should be identified and preserved (Figures 6-21 and 6-22).
9. If the hemorrhage is stopped, intrapericardial control of the pulmonary vasculature will not be needed. If the hemorrhage continues, there may be bleeding from a location that is more proximal. This is quite difficult to address. Additional cardiothoracic expertise may be needed including

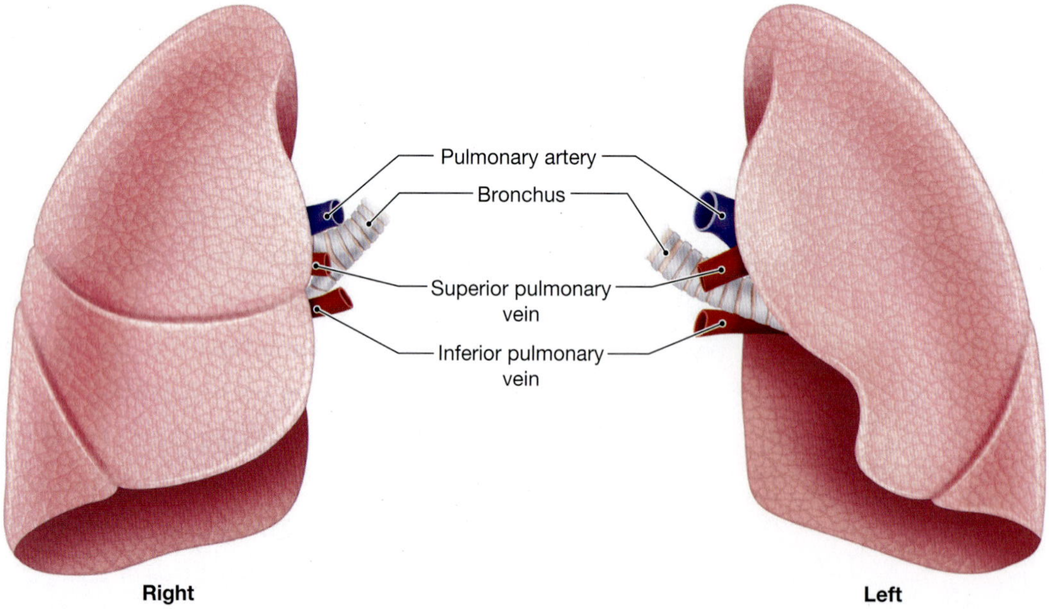

Figure 6-21

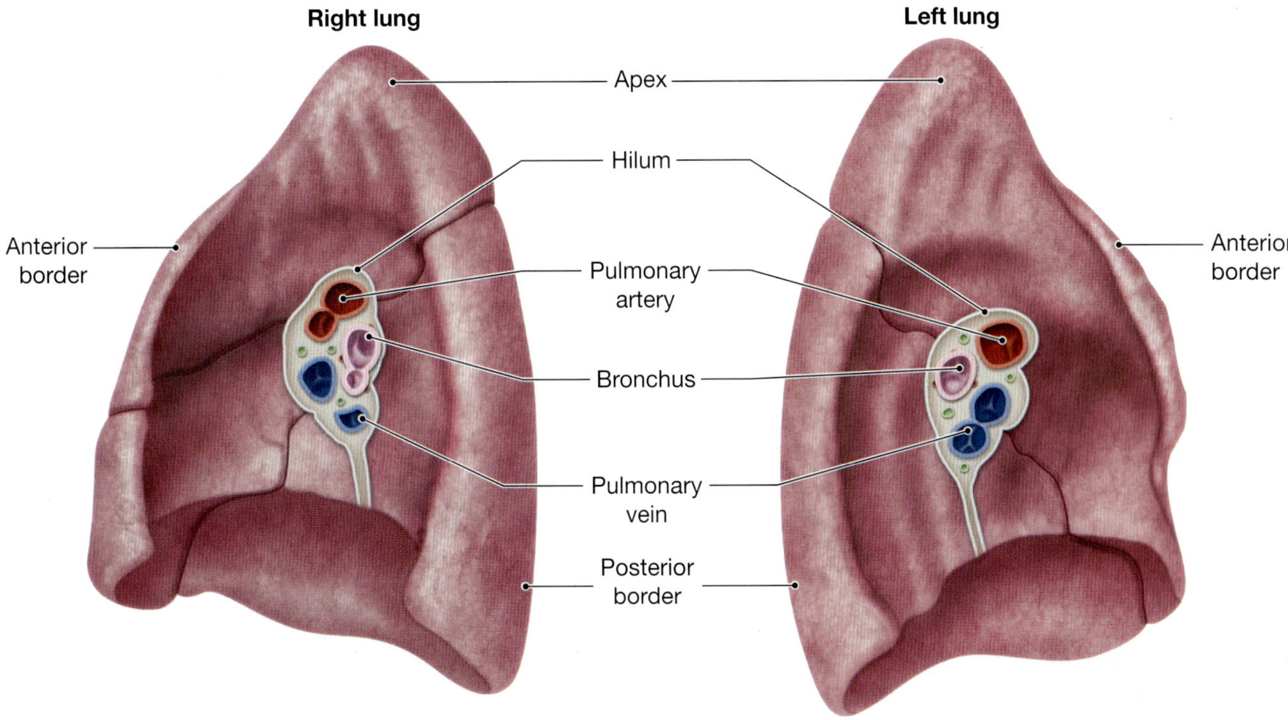

Figure 6-22

placing the patient on cardiopulmonary bypass. If the bleeding has subsided after cross-clamp of the hilum, a TA-90 may be placed across the pulmonary hilum to transect the pulmonary artery, veins, and main bronchus in one maneuver. Alternatively, TA-45 and TA-30 staplers including vascular loads may be utilized if the vessels and bronchus have been individually isolated. A chest tube(s) should be placed at the end of the procedure (Figure 6-23).

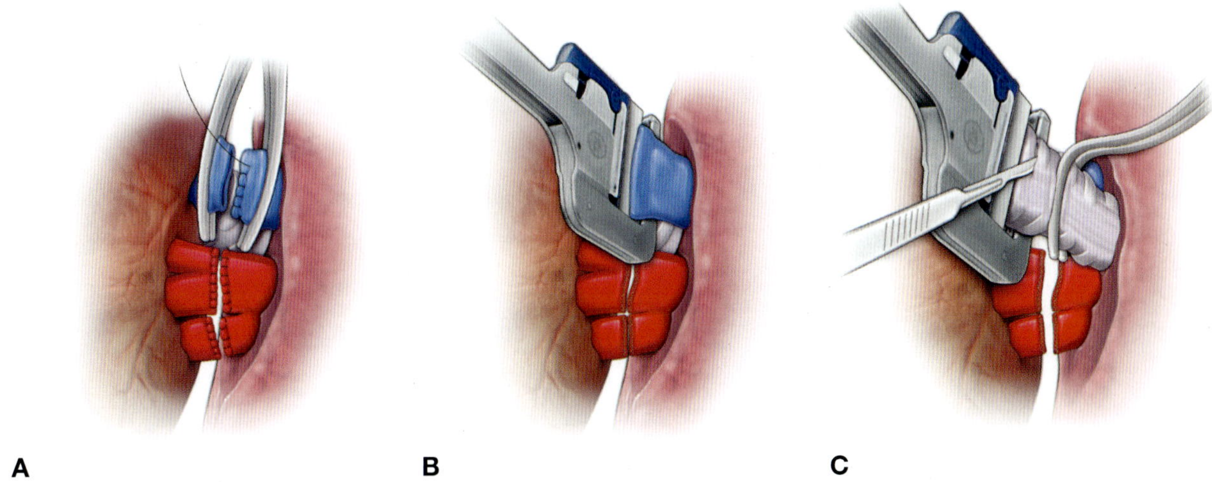

Figure 6-23. A. Division of pulmonary vessels using clamp and sew technique. B. Division of pulmonary vessels using TA stapler. C. Division of main bronchus using TA stapler.

10. Closure: The thoracotomy incisions should be closed in multiple layers using an absorbable suture. The ribs should reapproximated with #0 or #1 Vicryl sutures. The sutures should be placed in a figure-of-eight fashion and not include neurovascular bundles on the inferior border of the rib. The muscle layer groups of the pectorals and serratus anterior and latissimus dorsi should be closed individually using 2-0 Vicryl sutures. The subcutaneous layer is closed with 3-0 Vicryl sutures, and the skin is closed with staples. Sternotomy incision will be closed in layers. The sternum will be reapproximated with sternal wires (made from different types of metallic alloys). They can be closed in interrupted figure-of-eight fashion or interrupted simple stitches. The subcutaneous layer is closed with Vicryl sutures, and the skin is closed with Monocryl sutures or staples (Figures 6-24 and 6-25).

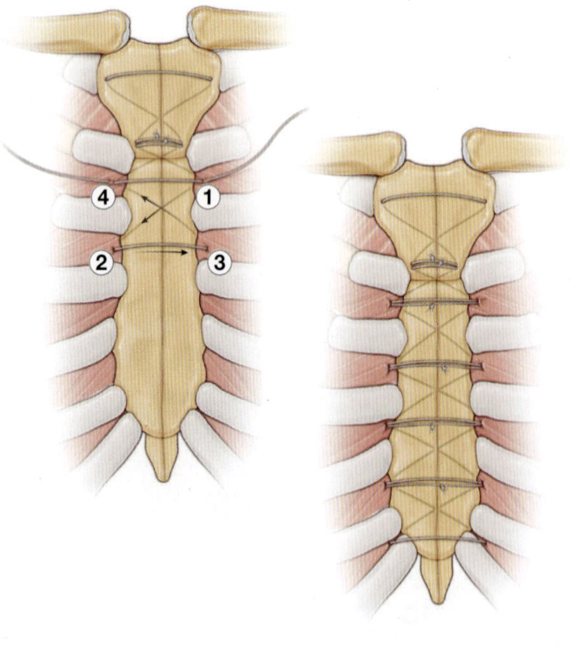

Figure 6-24

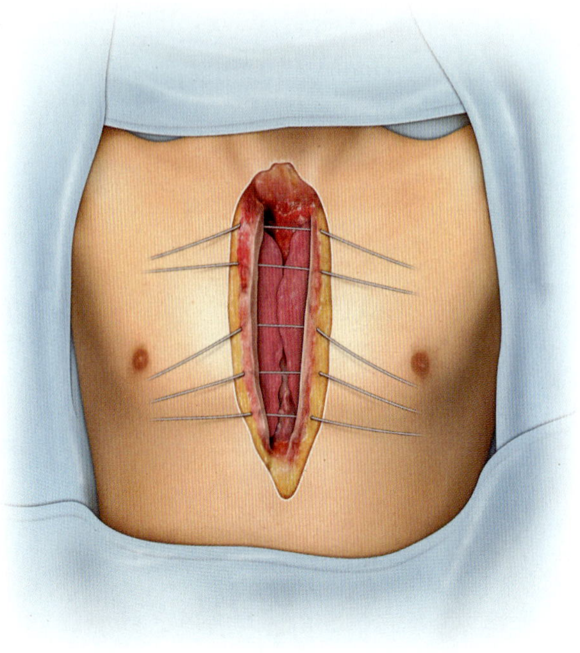

Figure 6-25

Complications

Morbidity is common after suffering lung trauma. There are several complications that can arise including pulmonary contusion, pneumothorax, hemothorax, pneumonia, empyema, lung abscess, air embolism, heart failure, and pulmonary hypertension. Some other technical complications from intervention include lung torsion, bronchopleural fistulas, hemorrhage, and bronchial stump leaks. The type of complication will direct the course of treatment options available. Major postoperative hemorrhage, empyema, and large air leaks secondary to major stump blowouts may require the patient to return to the operative theater for surgical intervention.

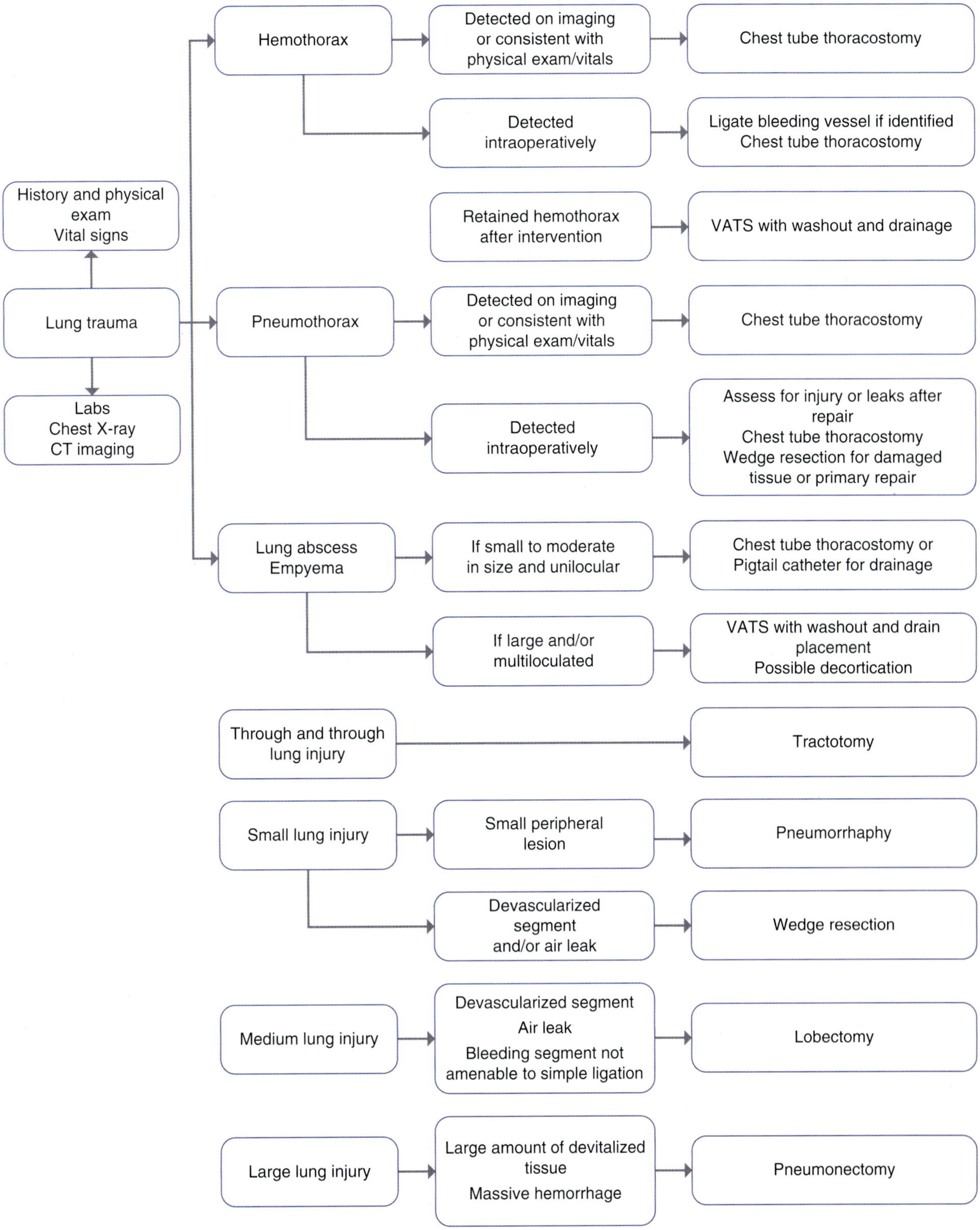
History and physical exam
Vital signs
Lung trauma
Labs
Chest X-ray
CT imaging
Hemothorax
Detected on imaging or consistent with physical exam/vitals
Chest tube thoracostomy
Detected intraoperatively
Ligate bleeding vessel if identified
Chest tube thoracostomy
Retained hemothorax after intervention
VATS with washout and drainage
Pneumothorax
Detected on imaging or consistent with physical exam/vitals
Chest tube thoracostomy
Detected intraoperatively
Assess for injury or leaks after repair
Chest tube thoracostomy
Wedge resection for damaged tissue or primary repair
Lung abscess
Empyema
If small to moderate in size and unilocular
Chest tube thoracostomy or Pigtail catheter for drainage
If large and/or multiloculated
VATS with washout and drain placement
Possible decortication
Through and through lung injury
Tractotomy
Small lung injury
Small peripheral lesion
Pneumorrhaphy
Devascularized segment and/or air leak
Wedge resection
Medium lung injury
Devascularized segment
Air leak
Bleeding segment not amenable to simple ligation
Lobectomy
Large lung injury
Large amount of devitalized tissue
Massive hemorrhage
Pneumonectomy

Figure 6-26

7

AIRWAY INJURIES

Daniel Lim, DO, FACS
Adam Peton, DO
Dale A. Dangleben, MD, FACS

TIPS

1. Avoid placing a tracheostomy through the tracheal injury; ideally, these should be distal to the injury.
2. Use absorbable monofilament sutures.
3. Conserve as much healthy trachea as possible.
4. Always have separate tracheal and esophageal suture lines.
5. Avoid searching for the recurrent laryngeal nerve.
6. Keep neck in flexion postoperatively (may have to suture chin to chest).

Introduction

Laryngotracheal Injury is a rare entity accounting for 1 in ever 30,000 emergency room visits in the United States. It is the second most common cause of death in patients with head and neck trauma after intracranial injury. Only 0.5% of multiple trauma patients will have reported injury to the airway at any level. Blunt trauma is by far the most common cause of tracheal injury. The predominant mechanism, accounting for greater than 50% of cases, is motor vehicle collision. This usually occurs when the driver's extended neck hits the windshield, dashboard, or steering wheel. Other mechanisms of blunt injury occur during sports and hanging or strangulation. Penetrating injuries are much less common and are due to stabs or gunshot wounds. Iatrogenic injuries are extremely uncommon and may occur during procedures such as tracheostomy, emergent intubation, or bronchoscopy. Symptoms can include, but are not limited to, dyspnea, hoarseness, neck pain, and dysphagia.

Regardless of the extent of injuries, a protected airway is paramount in all trauma patients. At times, a surgical airway is mandated, and there are several ways in which this can be established. The standard of care for emergent surgical airways remains cricothyroidotomy. However, in the nonemergent situation, there exists other forms of establishing a surgical airway, which are described in detail below.

Anatomy

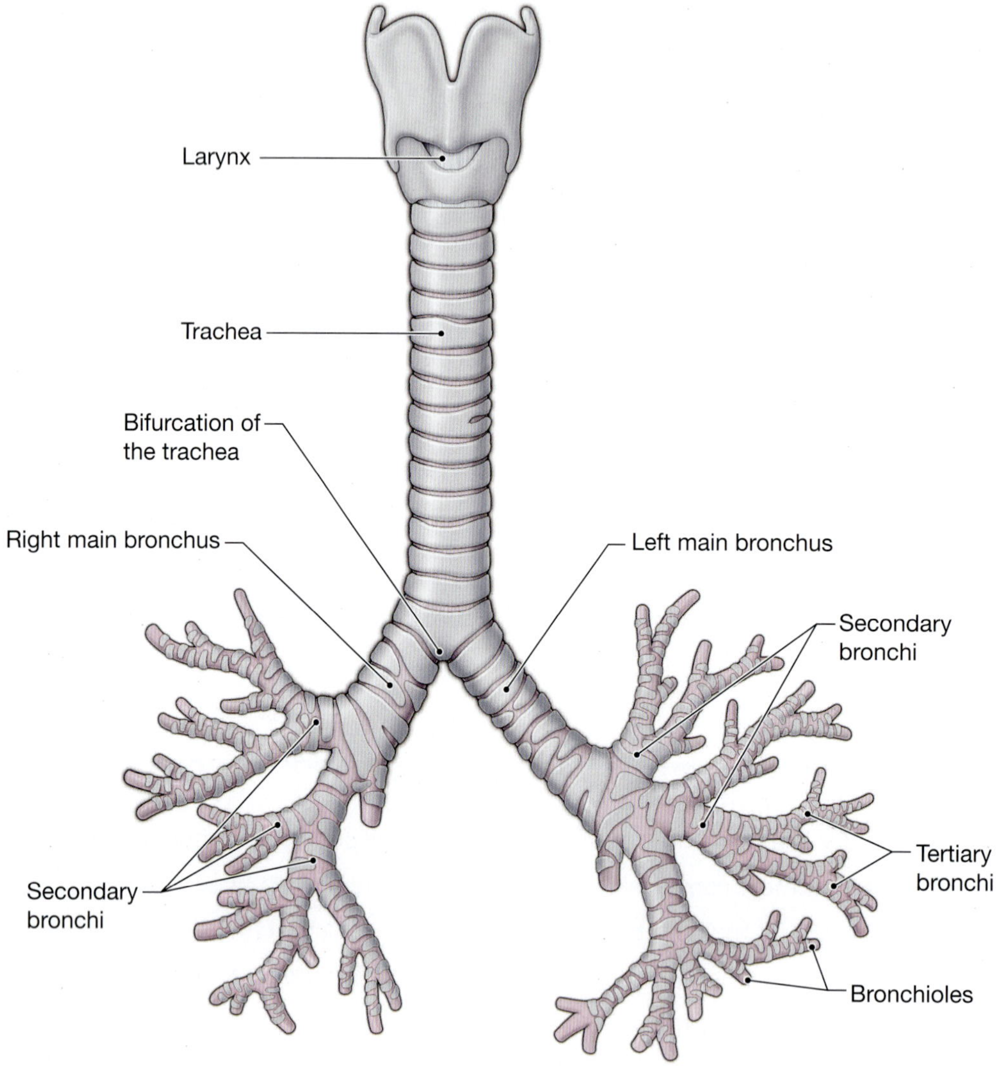

Figure 7-1

A system known as the Schaefer classification system has been widely used and accepted by the American Academy of Otolaryngology–Head and Neck Surgery to help characterize laryngotracheal injury and assist with treatment decisions based on severity. The classification system is divided into five groups, each representing a different level of injury severity (Table 7-1).

TABLE 7-1. Schaefer Classification System

Severity		Number of Patients (%)
Grade 1	Minor endolaryngeal hematoma without detectable fracture	7 (33.33)
Grade 2	Edema, hematoma, minor mucosal disruption without exposed cartilage, nondisplaced fractures	7 (33.33)
Grade 3	Massive edema, mucosal disruption, exposed cartilage, focal fold immobility, displaced fracture	1 (4.76)
Grade 4	Group 3 with two or more fracture lines or massive trauma to laryngeal mucosa	3 (14.2)
Grade 5	Complete laryngotracheal separation	3 (14.2)

Management of Laryngotracheal Injuries

After establishing a secure airway, the injury is identified, classified, and managed either operatively or nonoperatively. The ultimate goal of repair should consider reestablishing phonation, protection from aspiration, ventilation, and deglutition. The management of the injury is dependent upon the anatomy involved. For example, if the injury involves the hyoid bone, it is common that the hyoid bone injury is managed nonoperatively. When the injury involves thyroid cartilage that is nondisplaced, then supportive management is warranted. If it is displaced, then open surgical reduction is warranted. If the injury involved the cricoid cartilage that is nondisplaced, supportive management and observation are appropriate, whereas if it is displaced, then operative repair is mandated. When tracheal transection is diagnosed, this can be repaired in an open fashion with an end-to-end anastomosis using interrupted absorbable sutures. If there is a mixed-type injury involving the esophagus, a primary-type repair can be undertaken with an interposition flap. (See Chapter 10, Esophagus.)

Surgical Options for Airway Management

Cricothyroidotomy: Open and Percutaneous Techniques

Knowledge of the anatomy is very important, especially the landmarks, when performing these procedures.

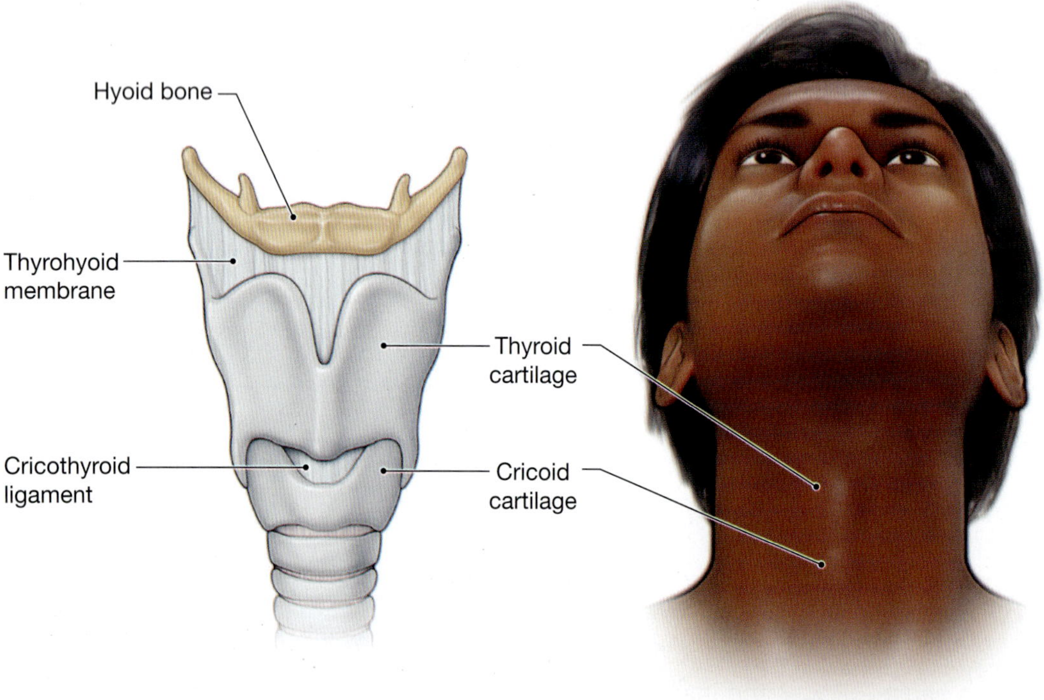

Figure 7-2

Open: Create a 4-cm vertical, midline incision through the skin. At the superior border of the cricoid cartilage, perform a 2-cm transverse incision of the cricothyroid membrane. Immediately, insert the tracheal hook and retract the tissues in a cephalad direction. Then, insert a trousseau dilator with the tips closed, and once inserted, dilate in a cephalad to caudad direction. Gently insert the endotracheal or tracheostomy tube through the dilated trachea opening and inflate the cuff. Ensure proper tube position before removing the tracheal hook and dilator.

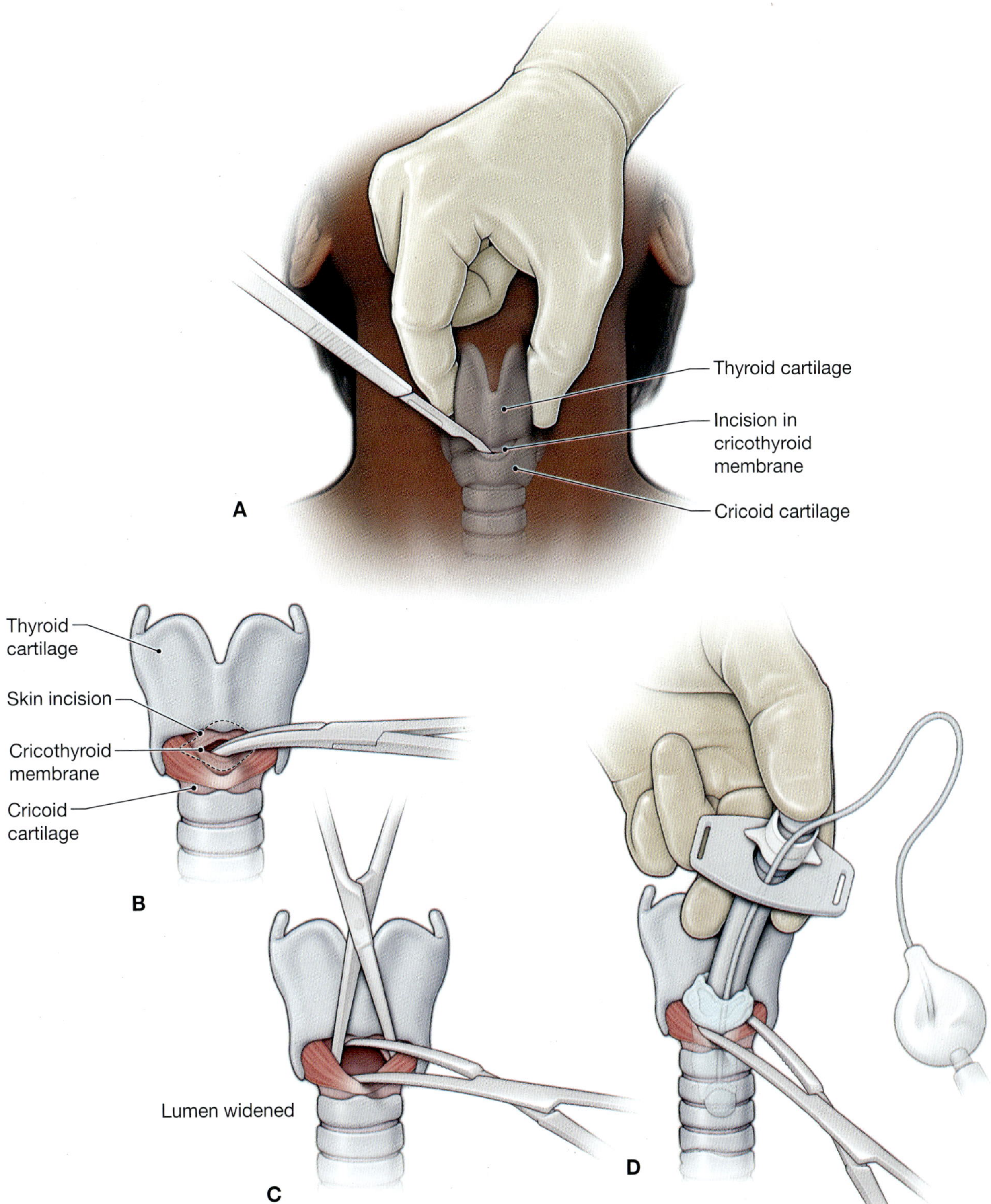
Thyroid cartilage
Incision in cricothyroid membrane
Cricoid cartilage
A
Thyroid cartilage
Skin incision
Cricothyroid membrane
Cricoid cartilage
B
Lumen widened
C
D

Figure 7-3 A-D

Percutaneous There are a few percutaneous cricothyroidotomy kits. Be familiar with the kit at your institution.

Proceed by inserting an 18-gauge needle with fluid-filled syringe into the inferior portion of the cricothyroid membrane. Slowly advance the needle in a slightly caudad angle while continuously aspirating; the needle is within the trachea when air is aspirated. Advance the catheter into the trachea and insert the guidewire through the catheter. Remove the catheter, leaving the guidewire in the trachea. Make an incision along the guidewire through the skin and the cricothyroid membrane. Place the dilator into the airway catheter and advance the loaded dilator/airway catheter over the wire into the trachea. Remove the dilator and confirm the proper placement of the airway catheter by $EtCO_2$. Secure the airway catheter with sutures.

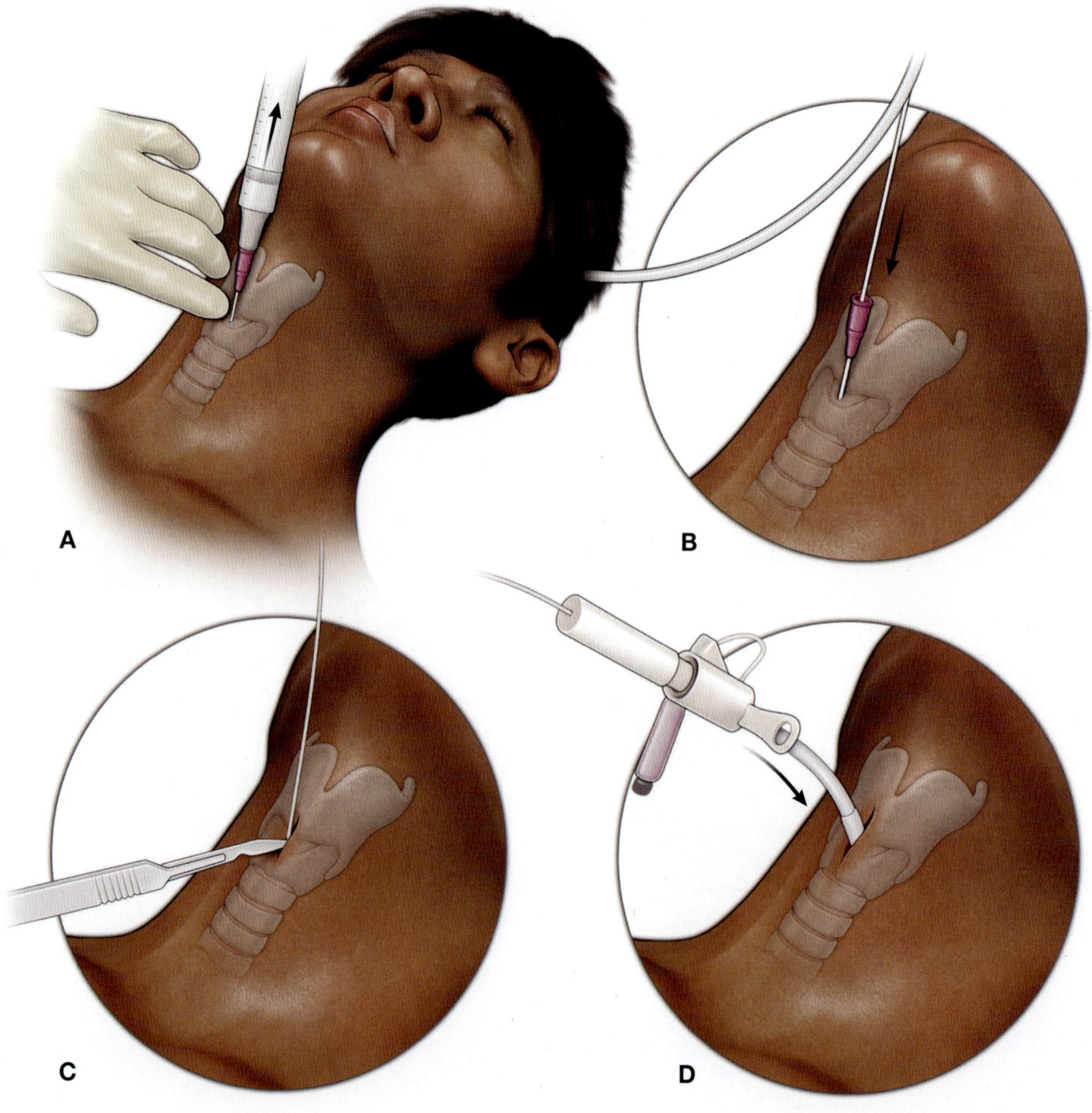

Figure 7-4 A-D

Tracheostomy: Open and Percutaneous Techniques

Percutaneous: This is preferably done under bronchoscopic visualization. Always inspect the patient's neck and palpate the anatomic landmarks. Make a 2-cm midline incision approximately two fingerbreadths above the sternal notch. If the bronchoscope is being utilized and there is an endotracheal tube, pull the tube to about 18 cm at the lip. Using the hemostat, spread gently into the pretracheal space. Then, insert the 18-gauge needle catheter between the tracheal rings. Slowly advance the needle slightly in a caudad angle. When the needle is within the trachea, either on direct bronchoscope visualization or when air is aspirated, the guidewire can be inserted through the catheter. Remove the catheter, leaving the guidewire within the trachea. Pass the serial dilation system over the wire and into the trachea. Place the appropriate dilator into the tracheostomy and then advance the tracheostomy tube into the trachea. Remove the dilation system, inflate the balloon, and confirm correct intratracheal position of the tube. Connect mechanical ventilation and suture the tracheostomy tube to the skin.

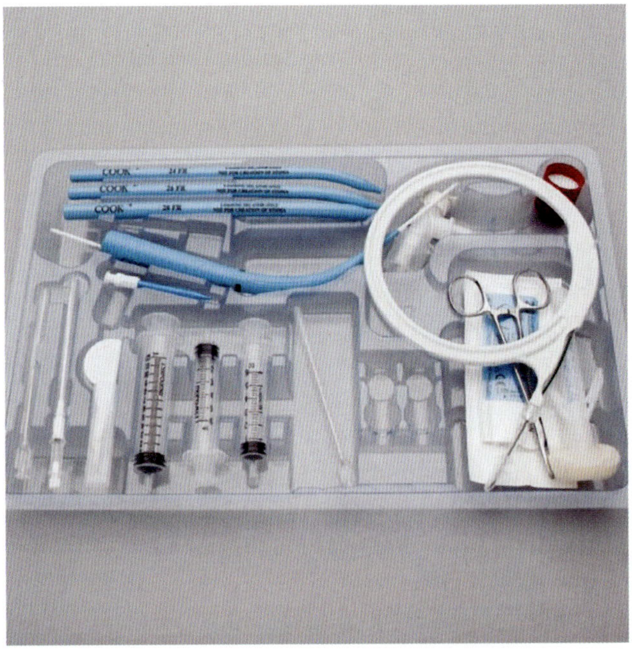

Figure 7-5. Percutaneous tracheostomy kit.

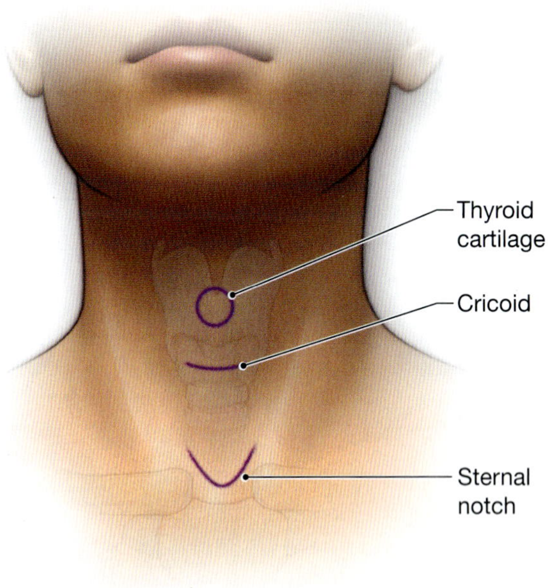

Figure 7-6. Relevant anatomy for percutaneous tracheostomy.

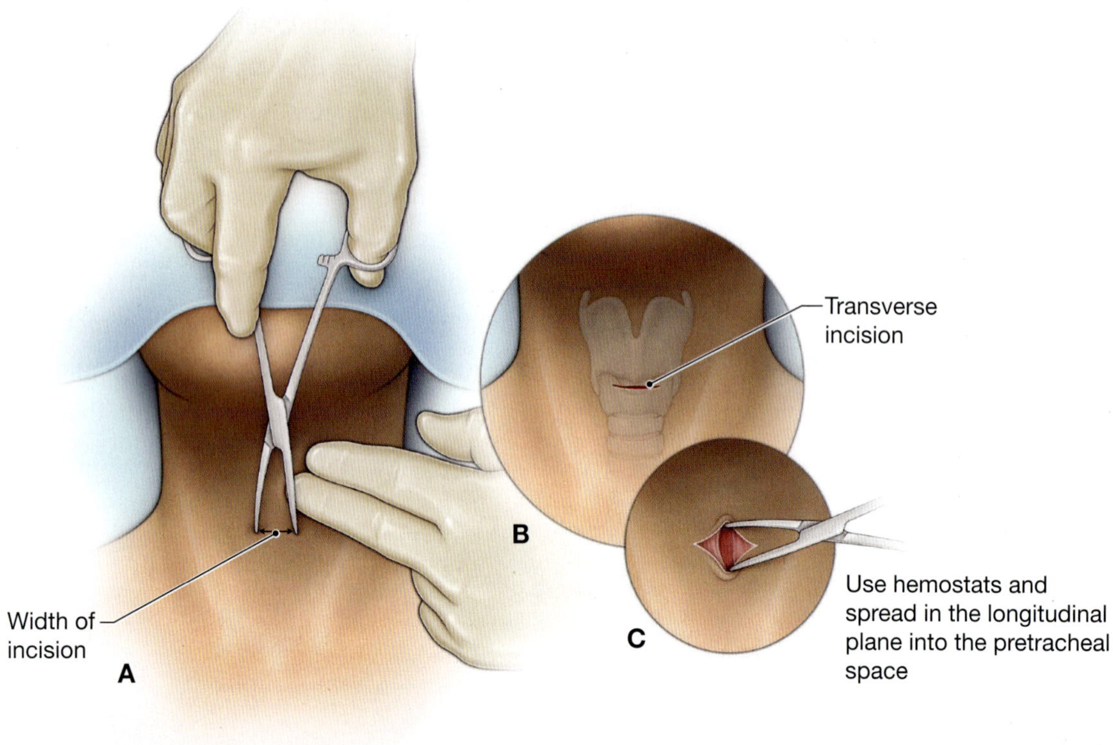
Transverse
incision
B
Use hemostats and
spread in the longitudinal
plane into the pretracheal
space
C
Width of
incision
A

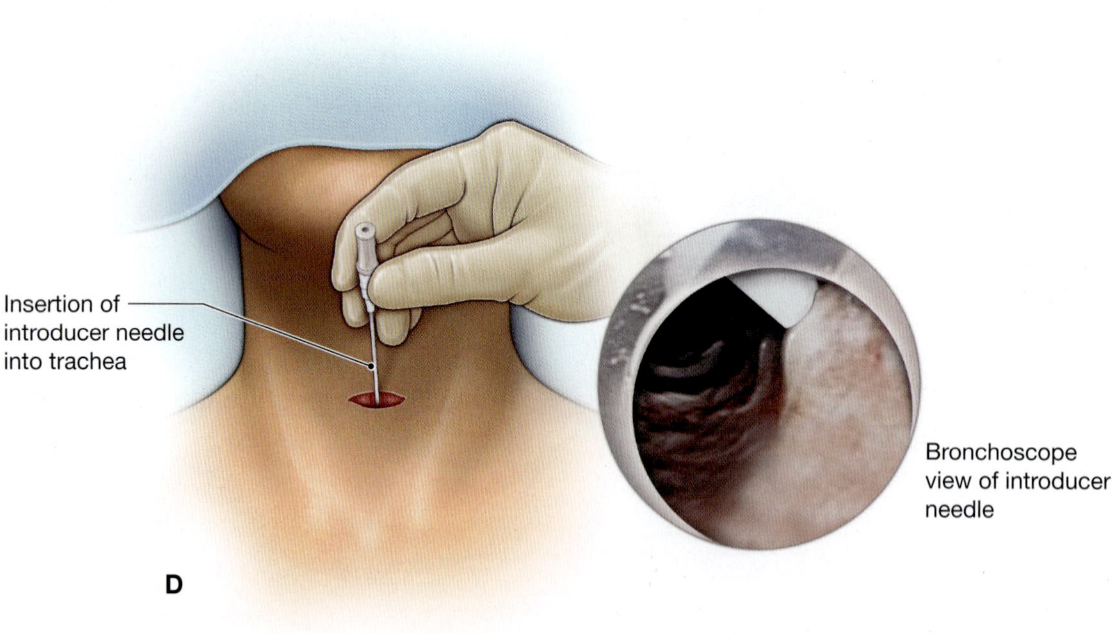
Insertion of
introducer needle
into trachea
Bronchoscope
view of introducer
needle
D

Figure 7-7 A-D

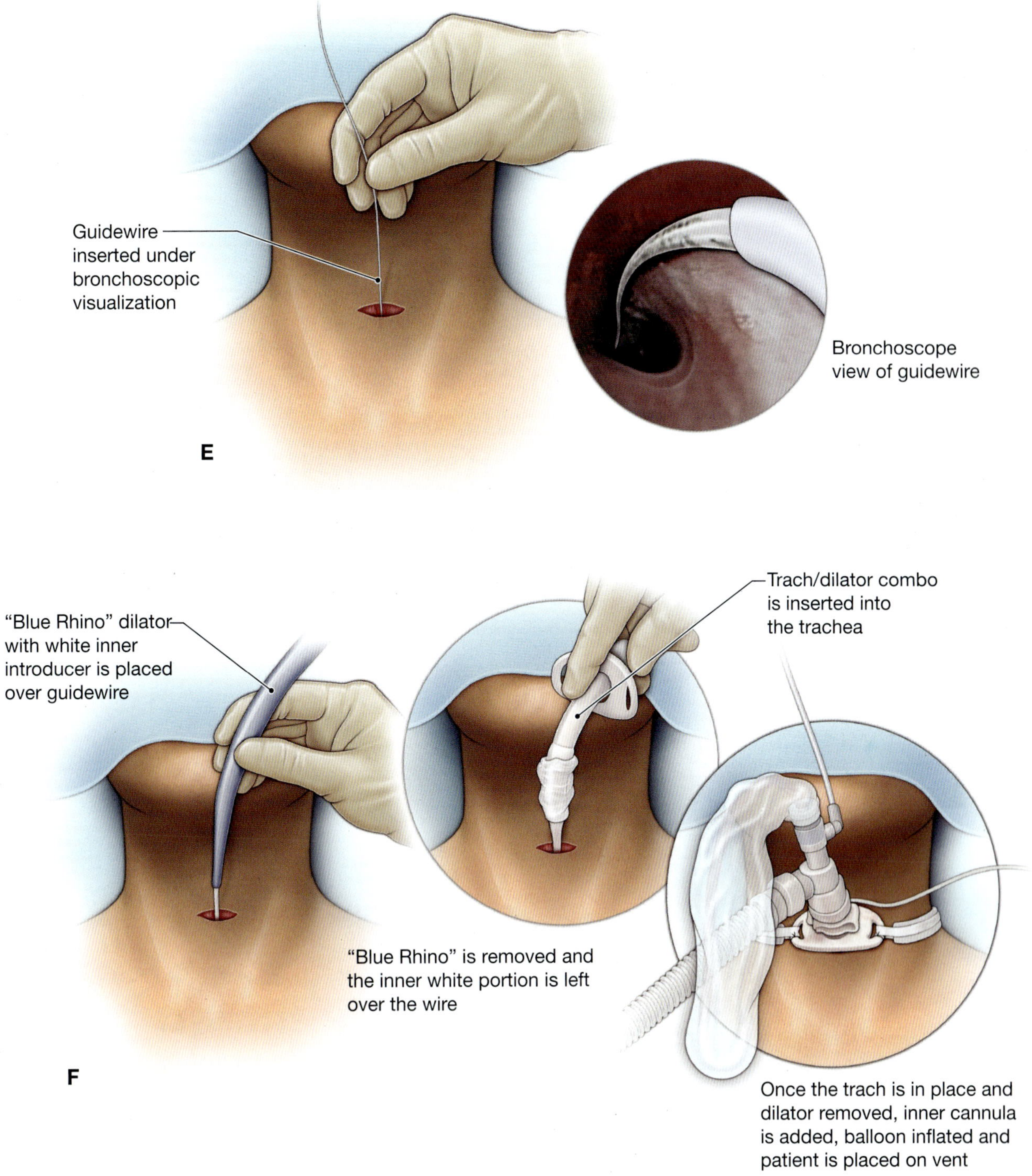
Guidewire inserted under bronchoscopic visualization
Bronchoscope view of guidewire
E
"Blue Rhino" dilator with white inner introducer is placed over guidewire
Trach/dilator combo is inserted into the trachea
"Blue Rhino" is removed and the inner white portion is left over the wire
F
Once the trach is in place and dilator removed, inner cannula is added, balloon inflated and patient is placed on vent

Figure 7-7 E, F

Open Tracheostomy

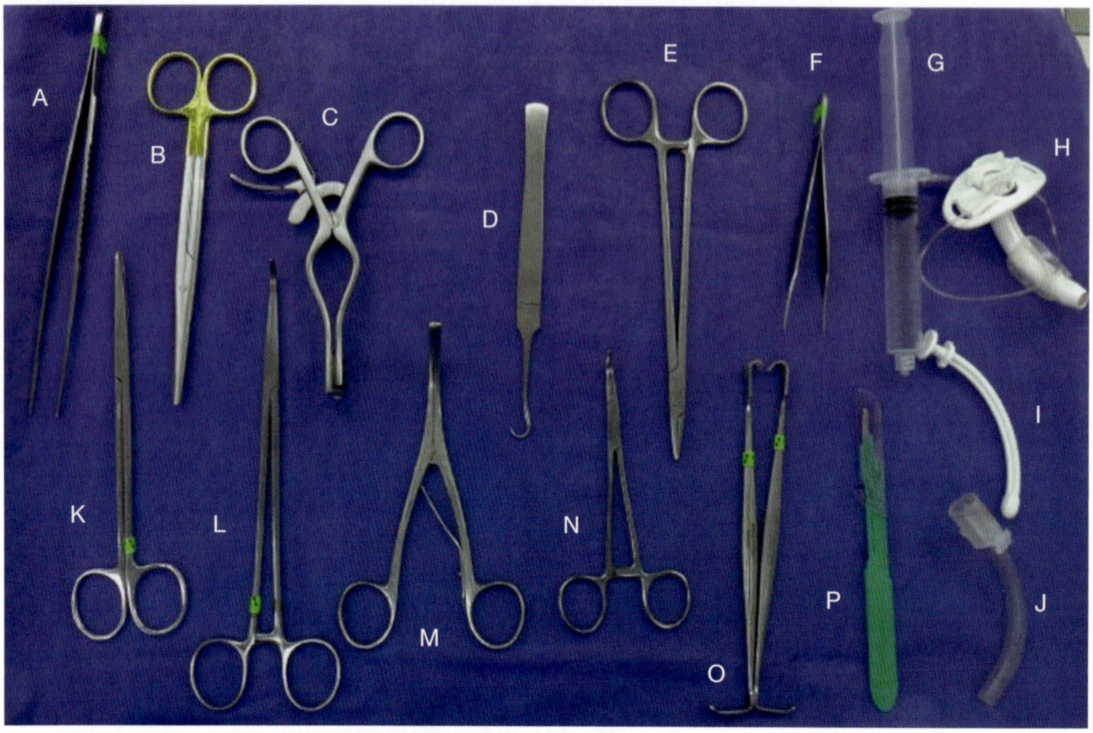

Figure 7-8. Instruments for open tracheostomy.

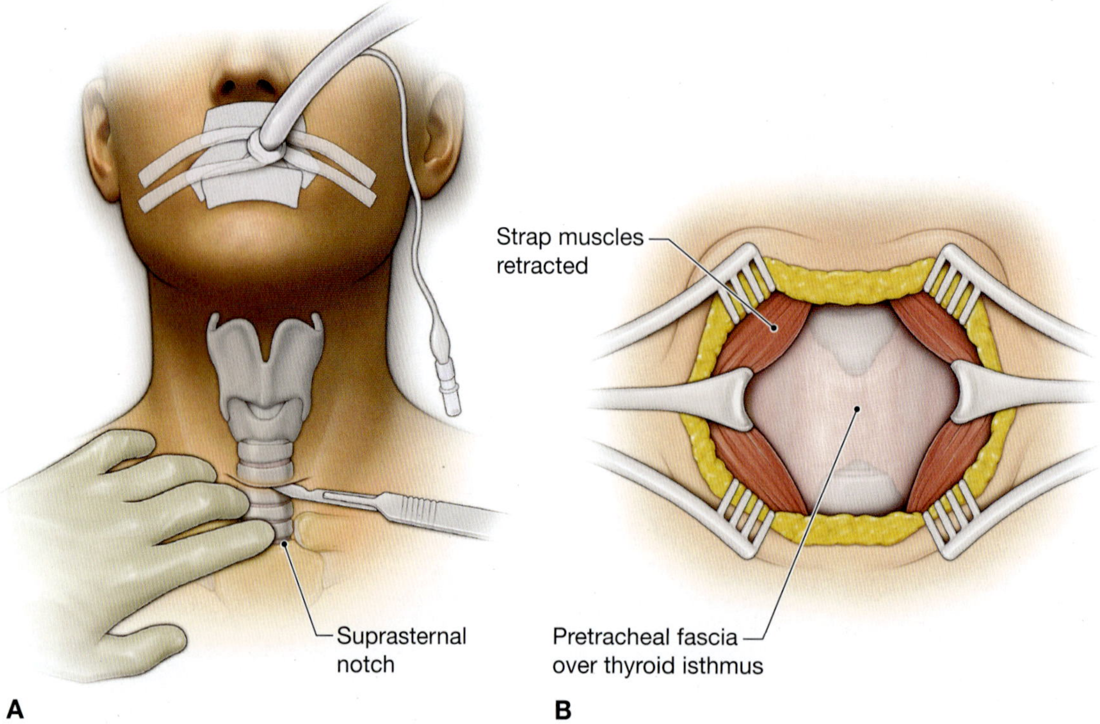

Figure 7-9 A, B

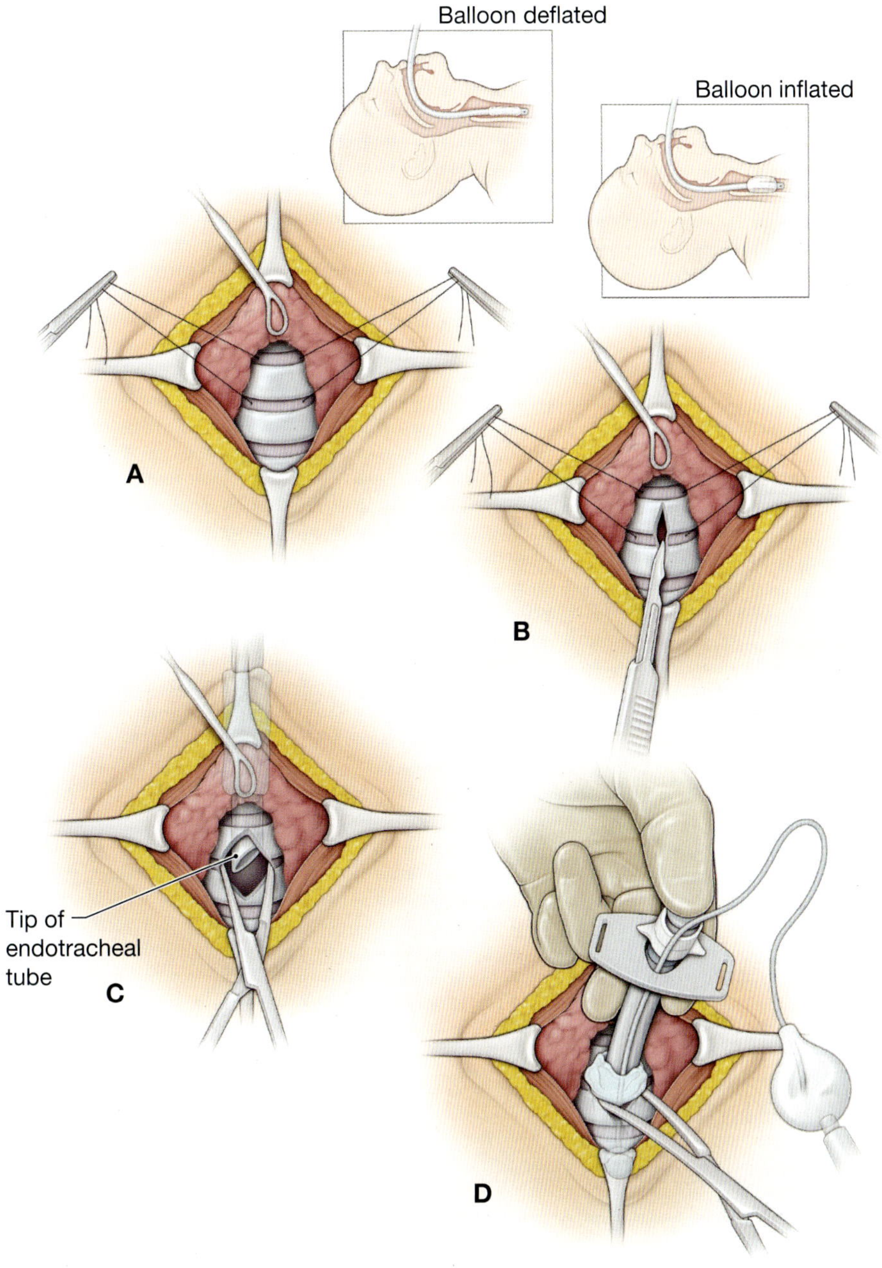

Figure 7-10 A-D

Place neck in extended position if not contraindicated. Make 4-cm midline skin incision approximately two fingerbreadths above the sternal notch. Extend if necessary. Dissection is carried down midline through subcutaneous tissues and platysma muscle. Identify strap muscles and divide vertically midline. Divide the tracheal isthmus. Expose the trachea via blunt dissection. The tracheal hook is then placed beneath the cricoid cartilage to stabilize and elevate the trachea. Create a tracheotomy window between the second and third and third and fourth tracheal rings. Insert the tracheostomy tube tip into the trachea in the axis perpendicular to the trachea, and turn it parallel to the axis once it has entered the trachea. Inflate the balloon and confirm correct intratracheal position of the tube. Place a trach tie. Connect mechanical ventilation and suture the tracheostomy tube to the skin.

Simple Tracheal Laceration

Repair simple tracheal lacerations using absorbable monofilament suture to reduce the chance of anastomotic granulations. Ensure that the suture incorporates the cartilage and the tracheal mucosa. For simple anterior penetration wounds, do not miss a posterior wall injury.

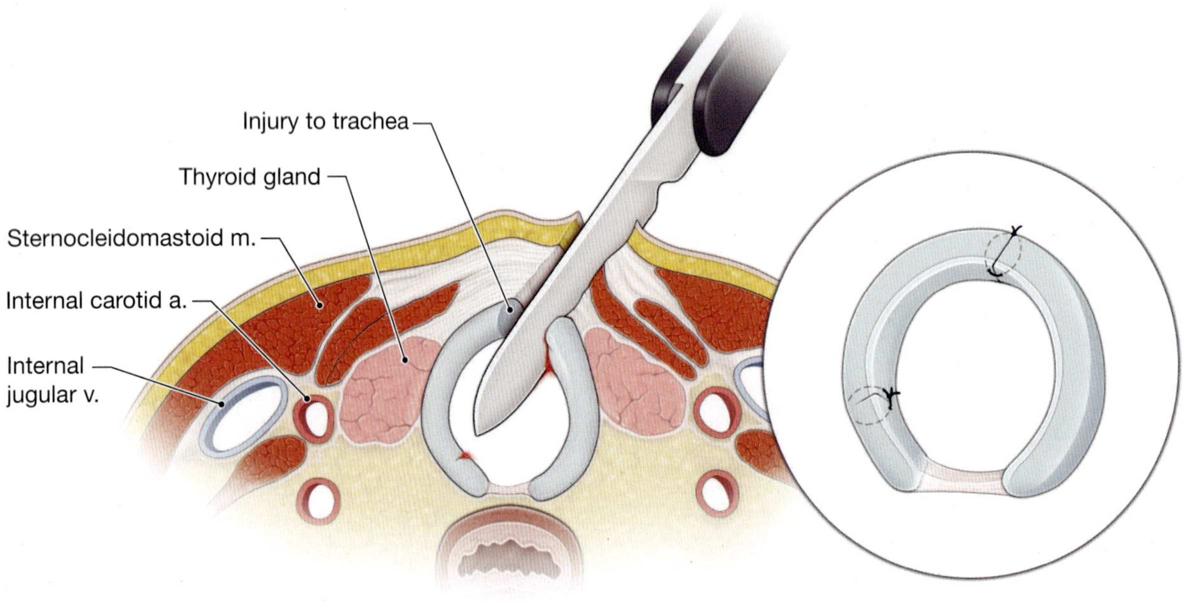

Figure 7-11

Complex Tracheal Injury

This may include loss of or devitalized tissue that may require extensive surgery. Do not hesitate to consult your thoracic or otolaryngology colleagues. These injuries may require tracheal ring resection and flap rotation. Intubation from above and guiding the tube below the injury should be attempted. If the injury is just below the sternal notch, an upper hemisternotomy will be needed for better exposure.

A short segment tracheal resection may be required. Obtain orotracheal intubation and place a pillow under the patient to allow for some neck extension at the start of the case. Once devitalized tissue is debrided and a good tissue margin is obtained circumferentially, mobilize the trachea to decrease suture line tension. Pay attention to the endotracheal tube while ventilation is being maintained. Prior to suturing, remove or deflate the pillow to allow some neck flexion. The trachea is approximated with 3-0 absorbable sutures in an interrupted fashion. The sutures should be 4 mm apart and 5 mm back from the tracheal edge. All knots must be tied outside the tracheal lumen. Place sutures from posterior to lateral, adjust the tracheal tube, and then place the anterior sutures. It is important to note that a tracheostomy is not required. Also, muscle coverage of the anastomosis is relatively indicated. In situations of extreme instability where definitive repair cannot be performed, continue ventilation with endotracheal intubation with a cuffed tube below the level of the injury.

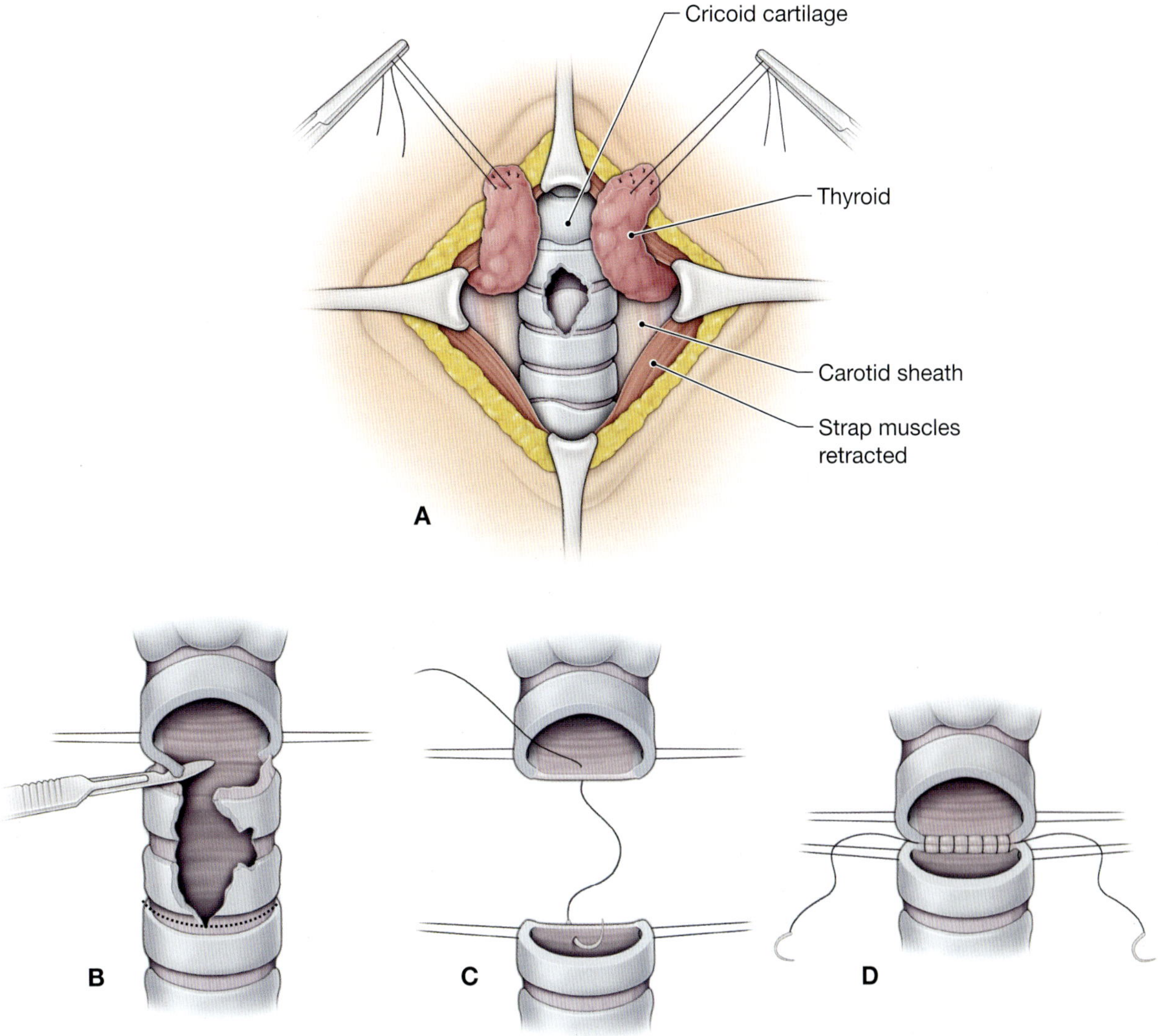

Figure 7-12 A-D

8 SURGICAL STABILIZATION OF RIB FRACTURES

Stephen Stopenski, MD
Sebastian D. Schubl, MD, FACS, FSIS

TIPS

1. **Operative planning with careful review of preoperative computed tomography is crucial for successful stabilization.**
2. **Multiple commercially available plating systems exist, but the basic principles remain constant.**
3. **Video-assisted thoracoscopic surgery (VATS) is an adjunct to clear the pleural space and administer subpleural local anesthesia. Alternatively, VATS can be used to placed intrathoracic plates.**

Introduction

Rib fractures are common injuries following blunt thoracic trauma, being diagnosed in 10% to 20% of all trauma patients. They are a harbinger of trauma severity; 90% will have other associated injuries, and 50% will require an operation or admission to the hospital including the intensive care unit, particularly among elderly patients.

Previously, nonoperative management with multimodal pain control and pulmonary hygiene was used to treat most rib fractures. However, severe pain with chest wall instability can lead to poor respiratory effort, resulting in infection, sepsis, and mortality. Each additional rib fractured correlates to an increased risk of pneumonia and death. Therefore, surgical stabilization of rib fractures (SSRF) has proven to be an effective alternative to treat rib fractures. With the availability of commercially available systems and success of prospective trials, indications for SSRF have expanded (Table 8-1) and an algorithmic approach (Figure 8-1) to the treatment of multiple rib fractures is recommended. The reduction and immobilization of fractured ribs reduce pain, prevent nonunion, and improve pulmonary function.

Surgical planning starts with a thorough understanding of the fracture pattern, for which high-resolution computed tomography (CT) is an indispensable resource. Rib fractures can broadly be divided into three zones: anterior, lateral, and posterior. Once patients are stable and other life-threating injuries are addressed, early fixation within 72 hours is recommended to optimize outcomes.

TABLE 8-1. Indications and Contraindications for Surgical Stabilization of Rib Fractures (SSRF)
Indications
1. Chest wall instability
Flail segment (≥3 consecutive ribs fractured in ≥2 places)
Three bicortically displaced ribs
Paradoxical chest wall motion (flail chest)
2. Three or more displaced rib fractures with 2 or more pulmonary derangements
Respiratory rate >20
Incentive spirometer <50% predicted
Numerical pain score >5/10
Poor cough
3. Ventilated patients with failure to wean
4. Failure of nonoperative management
5. Undergoing thoracic surgery for separate indication ("on the way out")
6. Chronic pain or malunion
Contraindications
1. Hemodynamic instability
2. Severe traumatic brain injury
3. Unstable spine injury
4. Acute myocardial infarction

SURGICAL STABILIZATION OF RIB FRACTURES

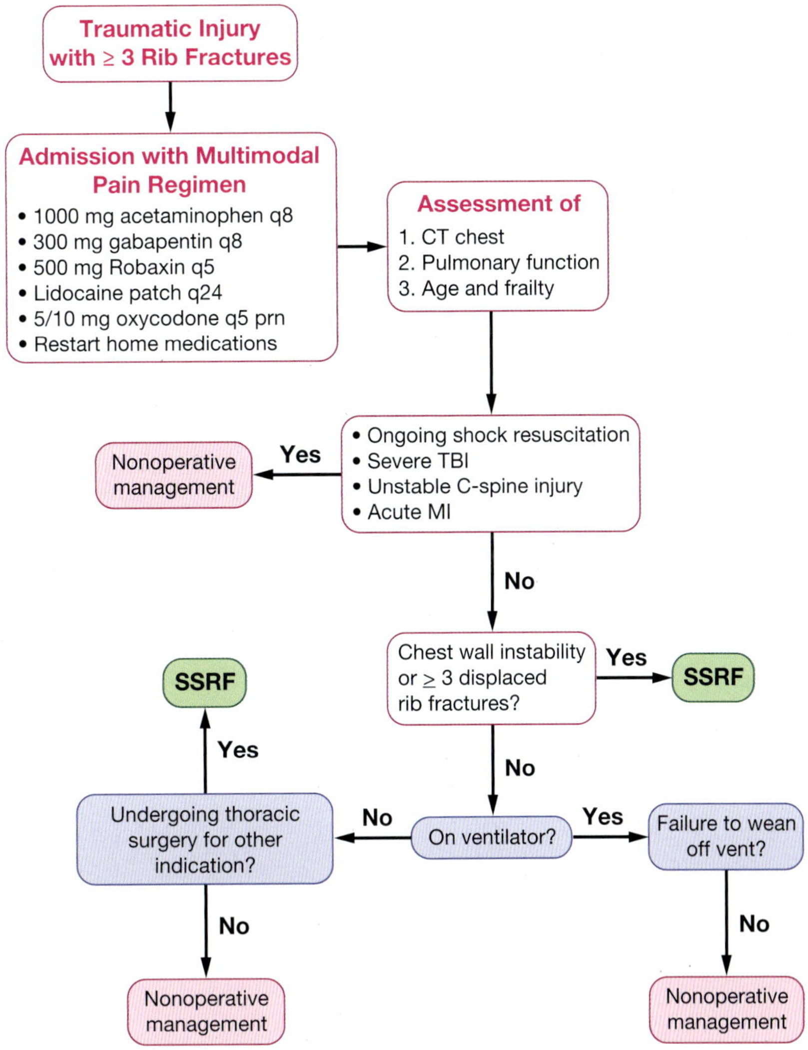

Figure 8-1. Algorithm for management of multiple rib fractures.

Anatomy

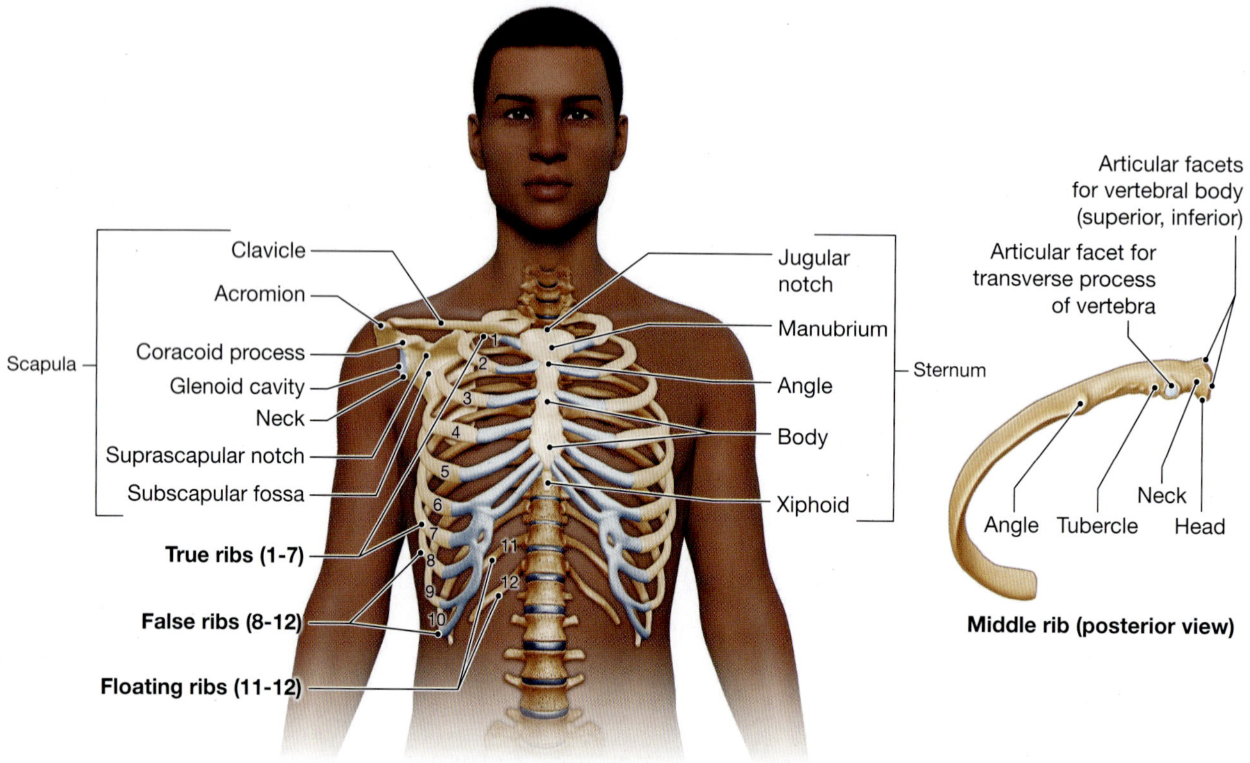

Figure 8-2

TABLE 8-2. American Association for the Surgery of Trauma (AAST) Injury Scale: Chest Wall

Grade	AAST Injury Scale - Chest Wall
I	Fracture: < 3 ribs, closed, no-displaced Nondisplaced clavicle, closed
II	Fracture: ≥ 3 adjacent ribs, closed Open or displaced clavicle Nondisplaced sternum, closed Scapular body, open or closed 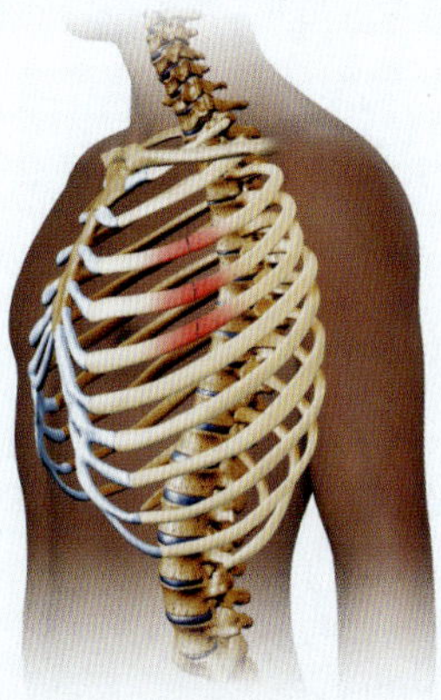
III	Fracture: Unilateral flail segment (< 3 ribs) Open or displaced sternum Flail sternum 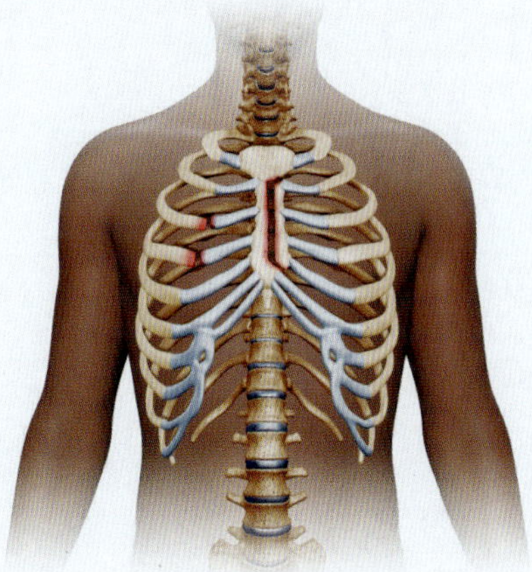
IV	Fracture: Unilateral flail chest (≥ 3 ribs)
V	Fracture: Bilateral flail chest (≥ 3 ribs) 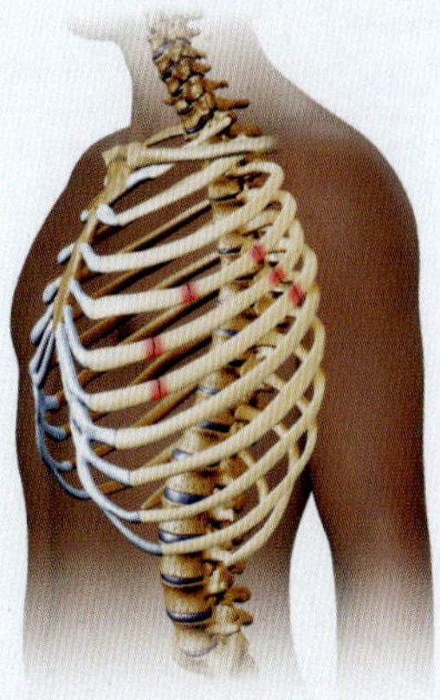

Source: Adapted with permission from Moore EE, Cogbill TH, Jurkovich GJ, et al. Organ injury scaling. III: Chest wall, abdominal vascular, ureter, bladder, and urethra. *J Trauma.* 1992;33(3):337-339, Table 1.

Alternative to American Association for the Surgery of Trauma (AAST) Grade: Nomenclature for Multiple Rib Fractures

	Alternative to AAST grade - Nomenclature for multiple rib fractures
1	Fracture displacement is categorized as nondisplaced (≥90% cortical contact), offset (cortical contact but <90%, and displaced (noncortical contact) 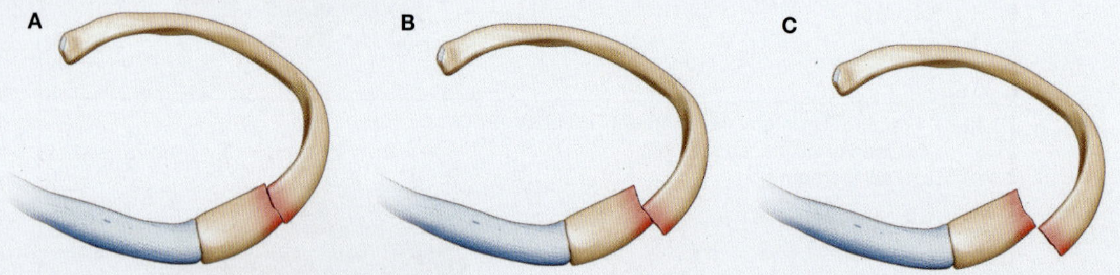
2	Individual fractures can be characterized as simple, wedge, or complex 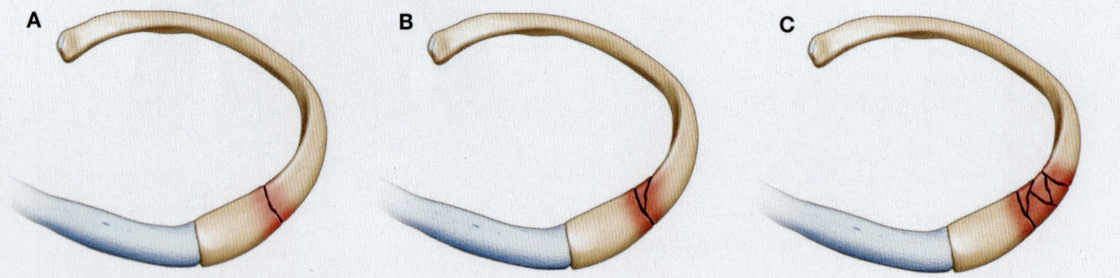
3	Fractures of neighboring ribs are defined as in series
4	Fracture location is based off the anterior and posterior axillary lines and are categorized as anterior, lateral, and posterior

Figure 8-3

Operative Steps

1. Anterior fractures: position and incision
   For fractures anterior to the anterior axillary line, patients are positioned supine with arm abducted 90 degrees or suspended using a candy cane stirrup. Bilateral anterior fractures can be repaired without repositioning. An inframammary incision is used. Muscle-sparing techniques should be used by dividing inferior to the pectoralis muscles to enter the subpectoral plane.

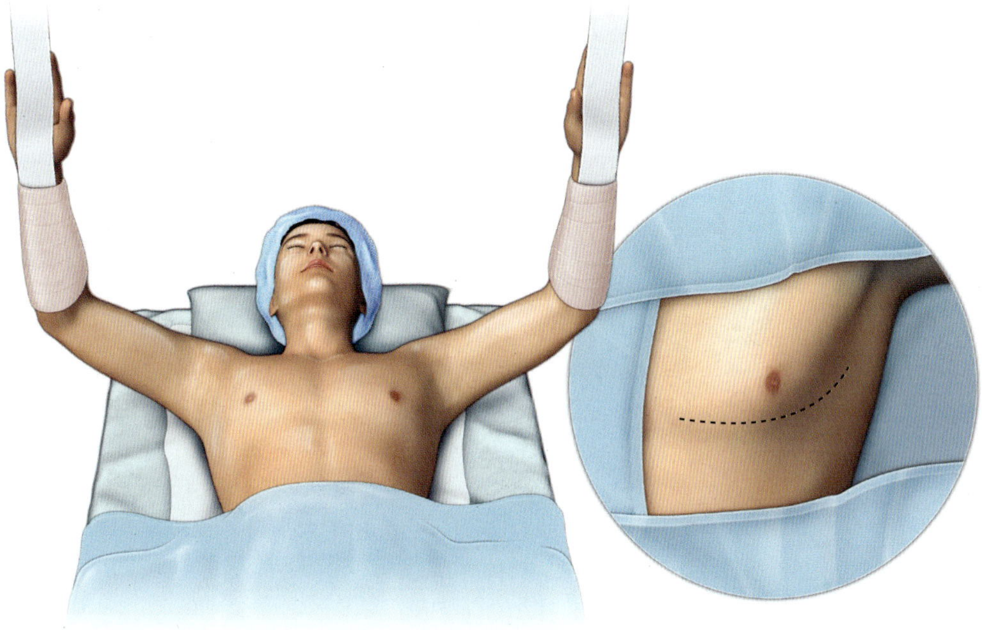

Figure 8-4

2. Lateral fractures: position and incision
   Patients are positioned in lateral decubitus with an axillary roll. Hips should be secured with a strap or band and the arms appropriately padded to avoid brachial plexus injuries. Patients with bilateral fractures are positioned for unilateral SSRF and then either flipped for the contralateral side or have a subsequent operation. The specific incision is tailored to the fracture pattern in a "line of best fit" to the fractures, usually as a vertical axillary or lateral incision. Lateral fractures of three to five levels can be accessed via a longitudinal incision in the mid-axillary line.

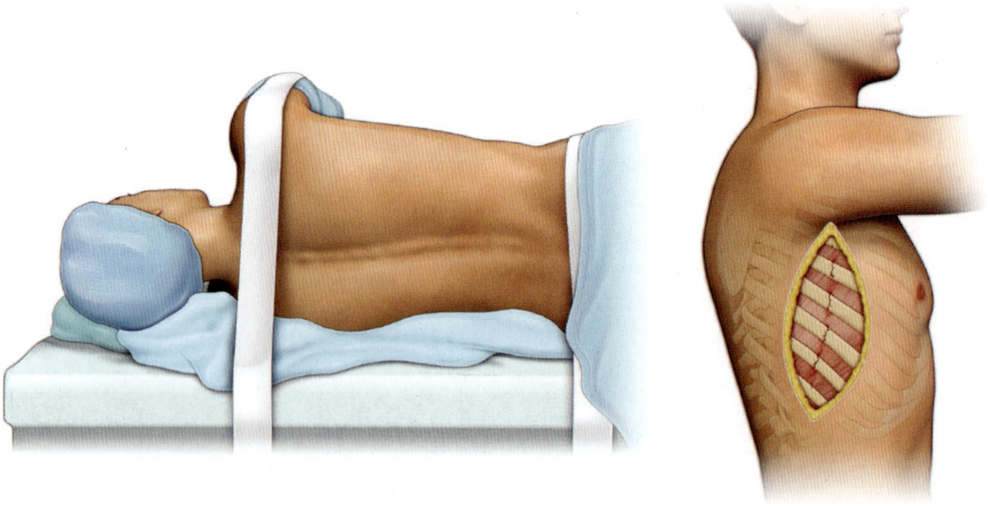

Figure 8-5

3. Posterior fractures: position and incision
   Patients are best positioned prone with their ipsilateral arm outstretched about 10 cm lower than the bed to help mobilize the scapula. A subscapular incision is created over the triangle of auscultation. Flaps are raised under the trapezius and latissimus dorsi until the infrascapular space is accessed. Additional splitting of the serratus anterior may be necessary for exposure. This approach gives excellent visualization of the posterior and lateral chest wall.

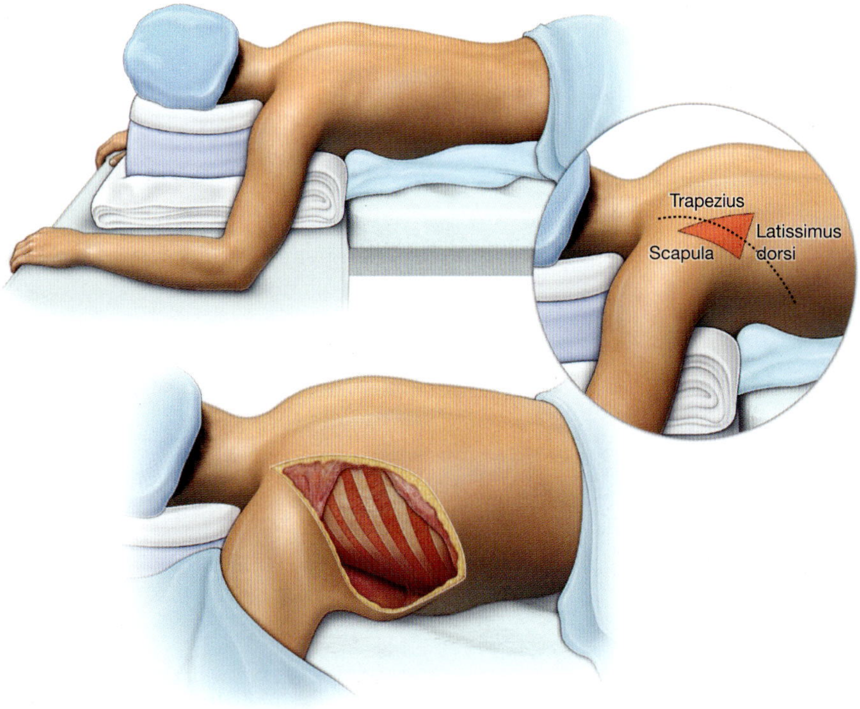

Figure 8-6

4. Rib exposure and reduction
   There are multiple commercial systems available, but the basic principles remain constant. The fractured fragments are exposed 3-5 cm on either side of the fracture line. A penetrating towel clamp, or similar instrument, is used to reduce and align the fracture, while ensuring "bone-to-bone" contact. Although most systems come precontoured, additional bending may be necessary to allow the plates to sit flush with the rib.

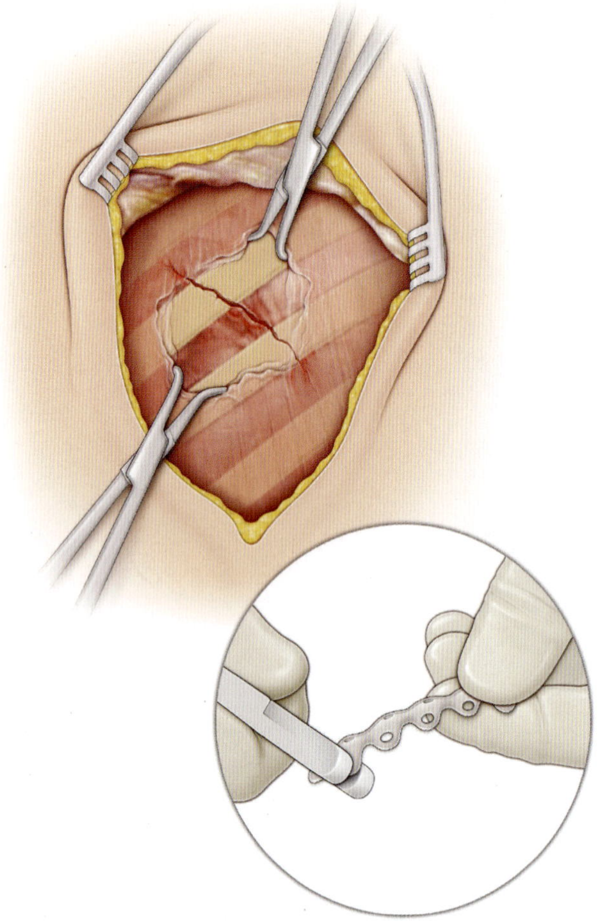

Figure 8-7

5. Rib fixation
   Depending on the system, fixation can be uni- or bicortical. In the case of bicortical fixation, screw length is determined by rib measurement. Drill holes should always be at a right angle into a portion of the rib with intact cortices. Plates should be positioned on the upper two-thirds of the rib to minimize risk of injury to the neurovascular bundle. We recommend three screws on either side of the fracture line. The two most distal screws relative to the fracture line are placed first for partial fixation; this allows for manipulation of the plate into optimal position before placing the rest of the screws and removing the clamps.

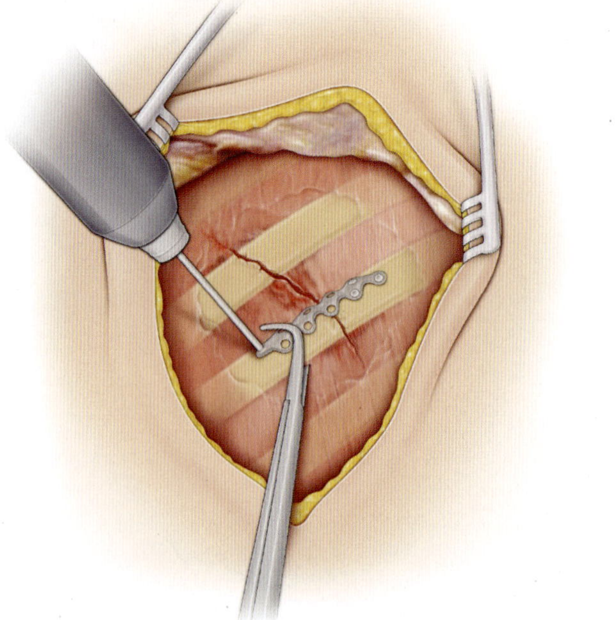

Figure 8-8

6. Video-assisted thoracoscopic surgery (VATS)
Following extrathoracic rib plating, we choose an alternative site for thoracoscopy port placement. This allows for evacuation of any hemothorax, inspection of the lung, insertion of thoracostomy tube, and administration of subpleural intercostal nerve block with liposomal bupivacaine.

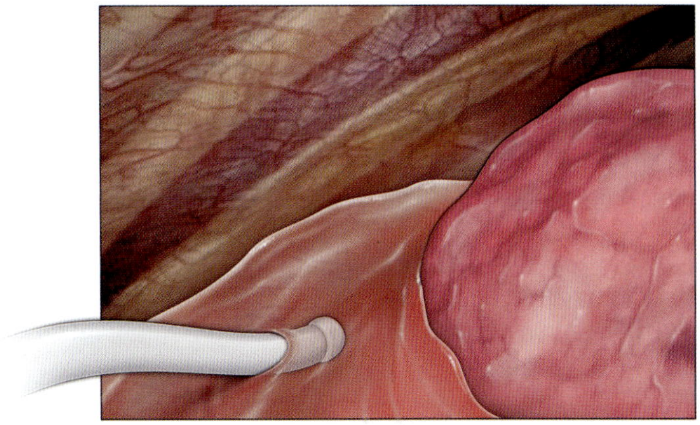

Figure 8-9

7. Intrathoracic SSRF
The RibFix Advantage (Zimmer Biomet, Jacksonville, FL) is currently the only commercially available intrathoracic plating system. Patients are positioned in the lateral decubitus. After flexible bronchoscopy, they undergo double-lumen endotracheal intubation for single-lung ventilation. A 5-mm trocar is placed anterior at the ninth intercostal space for thoracoscopy. One additional 12-mm utility port is placed based on the fracture location. The rib fractures are identified intrathoracically, and an open mini-incision is made over the fracture line. Osteotomies are drilled on either side of the fracture line. Using guide tubes and wires, plates are placed intrathoracically with extrathoracic locking screws.

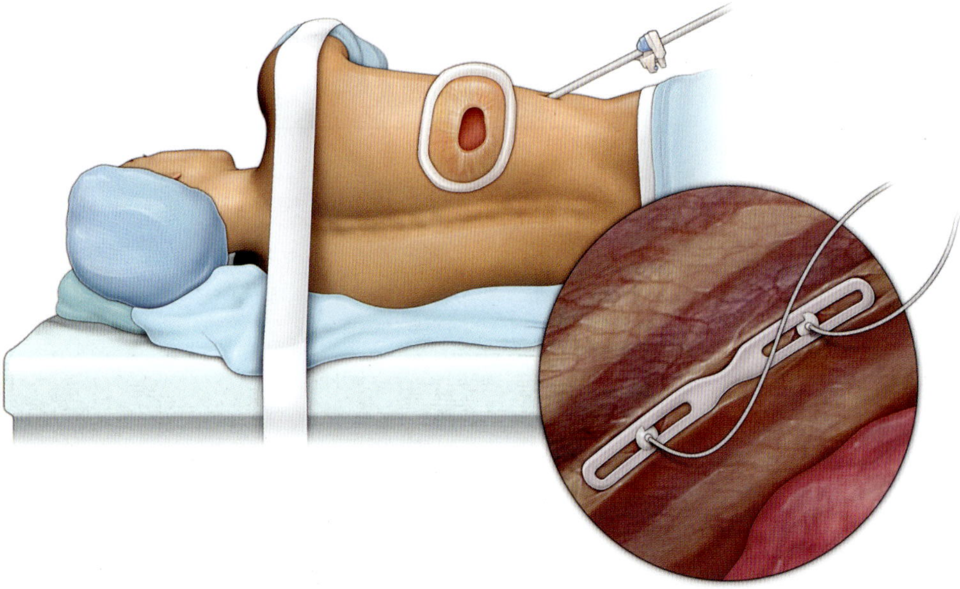

Figure 8-10

Complications

Overall, complications from SSRF are rare. Given the variety of different systems available and lack of head-to-head comparisons, the rates of hardware failure and wound infection vary. The most commonly utilized systems use a low-profile malleable titanium plate with locking screws. Hardware failure can occur from either loosening and migration of hardware or fracturing of the titanium plate. Retrospective data suggest the incidence of hardware failure is around 3%; however, 40% of patients are asymptomatic. Only half of patients will require explantation of hardware, and 10% will require additional SSRF.

Hardware infection is always a concern with the implantation of a foreign material. When infection occurs, treatment typically mandates removal of any foreign body and temporary external fixation to decrease the bacterial load and allow for bony union. Unfortunately, hardware removal after SSRF leads to malunion, chronic pain, and compromised respiratory mechanics. Therefore, treatment of infection after SSRF incorporates an algorithm to minimize hardware removal and promote bony union. In most circumstances, infection can be adequately controlled with drainage, local wound care, and antibiotics. Negative-pressure wound therapy and placement of antibiotic beads have also been effective methods to combat bacterial load.

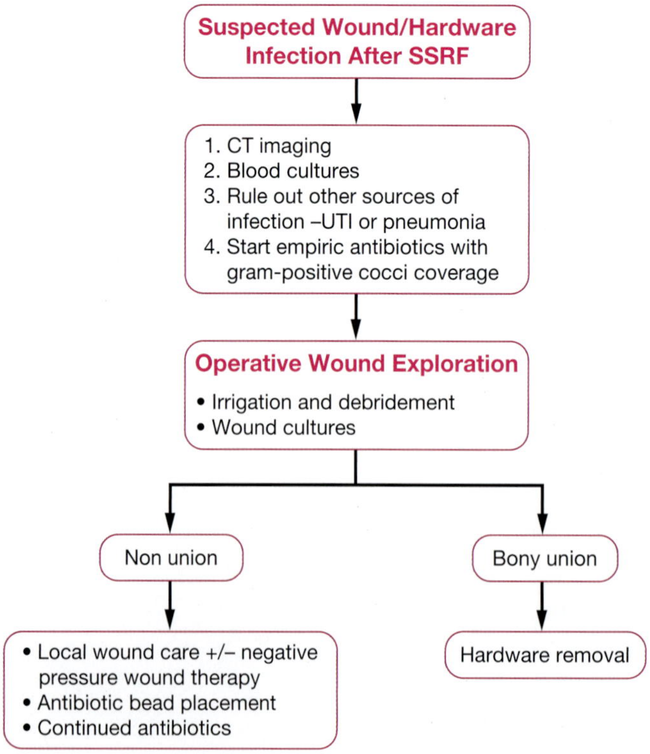

Figure 8-11

CERVICAL ESOPHAGEAL TRAUMA

9

Michael J. Collins, MD

TIPS

1. The myotomy may need to be extended to fully expose extent of mucosal defect.
2. A vascularized muscle flap is ideal to buttress repair.
3. Combining endoscopy and contrast esophagram approaches 100% accuracy for diagnosis.
4. Cervical esophageal injury is best approached via a left neck incision.

Introduction

Traumatic esophageal injuries are rare, with penetrating injuries accounting for 99% of injuries. The predominant mechanism of injury is gunshot wounds in 70% to 80% of cases followed by stab injuries in 15% to 20%. Esophageal injuries due to blunt trauma are exceedingly rare. Although uncommon, these injuries cause significant morbidity and mortality due to delay in diagnosis, complications from esophageal perforation, and associated injuries.

The signs and symptoms of early esophageal injury can be vague and nonspecific. Therefore, a high index of suspicion is critical to avoid delays in establishing an accurate diagnosis. Patients with an injury pattern or transcervical trajectory suggestive of injury should be evaluated for esophageal injury. Physical exam findings are nonspecific, although cervical injuries may present with subcutaneous emphysema, saliva or food particles in the wound, neck hematoma, and cervical tenderness and stiffness (though pain is less severe). In stable patients, a computed tomography (CT) angiogram of the neck should be performed, and although identifying esophageal injury is uncommon, this is helpful in finding associated injuries as well as extraluminal air and fluid in the periesophageal area. CT evidence of cervical esophageal injury should prompt cervical exploration, particularly in the presence of signs or symptoms consistent with injury. This area is easily accessed surgically, with low morbidity, and open exploration allows direct evaluation and repair of the esophagus. This avoids the cost and delays in intervention associated with multiple additional diagnostic studies. In contrast, if clinical suspicion is low, abnormal CT findings may then be further investigated by esophagoscopy and/or esophagography. Combining these two modalities approaches 100% accuracy.

Operative exploration is best accomplished through a left neck incision along the anterior border of the sternocleidomastoid muscle or a transverse collar incision if bilateral exploration is warranted. Principles of surgery include encircling a Penrose drain around the esophagus, debriding nonviable or necrotic tissue, exposing the entire mucosal defect with a longitudinal esophagomyotomy, and performing primary repair using autogenous tissue reinforcement whenever possible.

Early diagnosis and repair, identification of concomitant injuries, and consideration of damage control procedures are imperative to reduce the incidence of mortality, which was found to be 19% in the largest series.

Anatomy

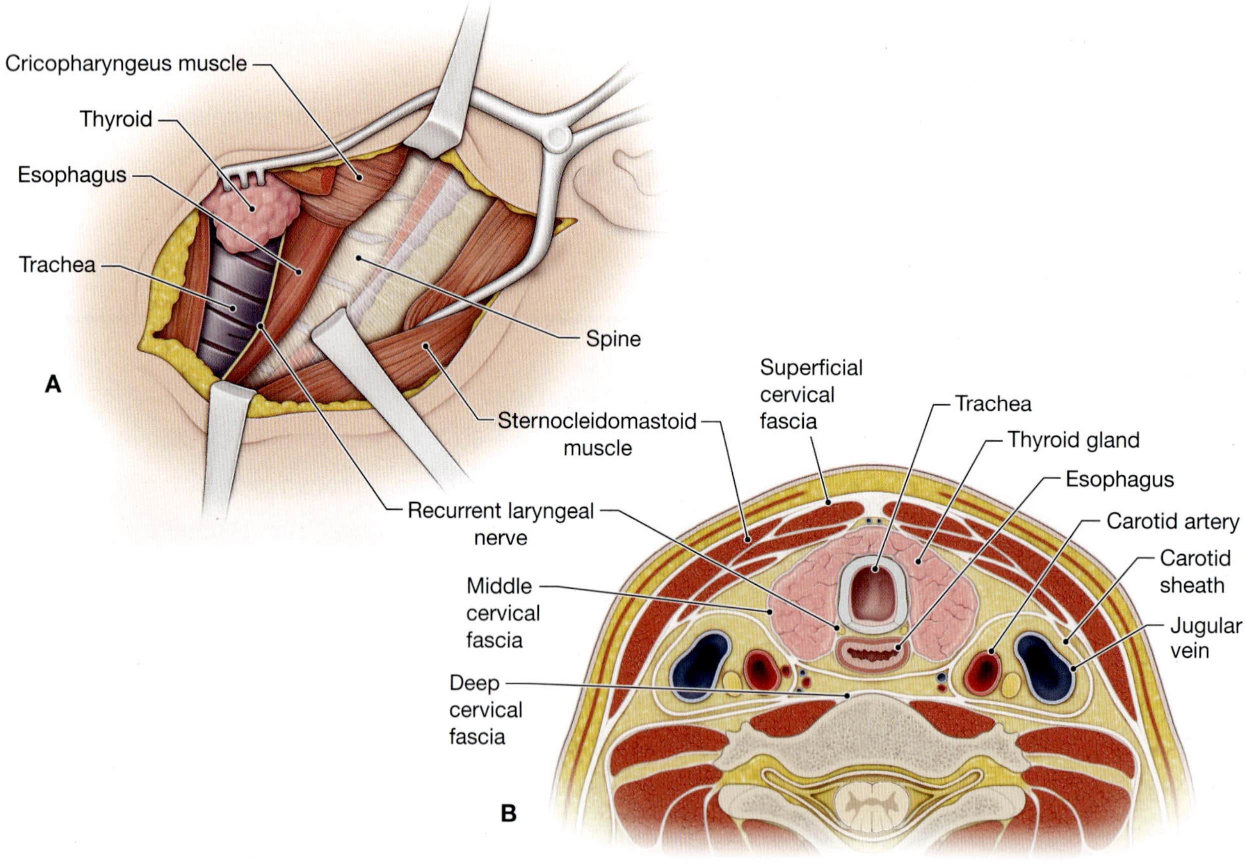

Figure 9-1

American Association for the Surgery of Trauma (AAST) Grades
Grade 1: contusion, hematoma, or partial-thickness laceration
Grade 2: laceration <50% circumference
Grade 3: laceration >50% circumference
Grade 4: segmental loss or devascularization <2 cm
Grade 5: segmental loss or devascularization >2 cm

Operative Steps

A. Exposure to the cervical esophagus is made via a neck incision along the anterior border of the left sternocleidomastoid muscle from the level of the cricoid cartilage to the sternal notch. A transverse collar incision may be used if bilateral exploration is necessary. Dissection carried down until anterior border of SCM is exposed and retracted inferolaterally.

B. The omohyoid muscle will often need to be divided and this is best done laterally so that the muscle may be used as a pedicled flap after repair. Further exposure may be obtained by dividing the sternal head of the SCM as well.

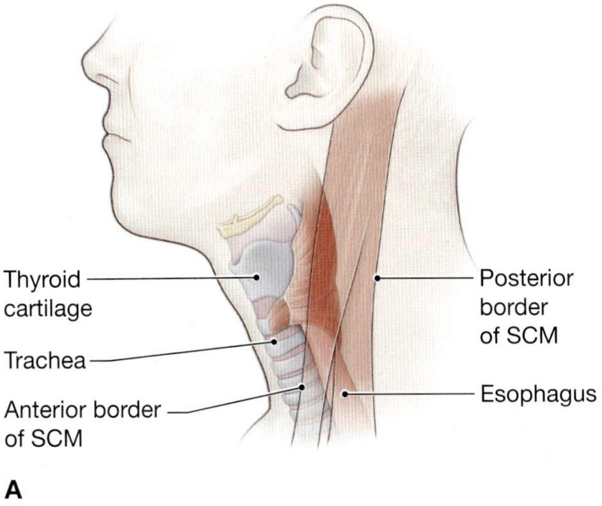

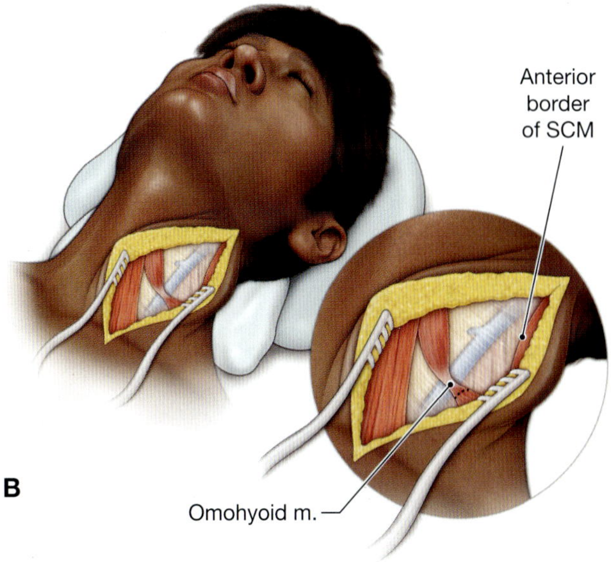

Figure 9-2 A, B

C. Deep cervical fascia incised medial to internal jugular vein. The left lobe of the thyroid is retracted anteriorly and medially. The inferior thyroid artery is ligated and divided. Recurrent laryngeal nerve is identified in tracheoesophageal groove. Care must be taken to avoid superior retraction of the laryngotracheal complex which can cause stretch injuries to the recurrent nerve.

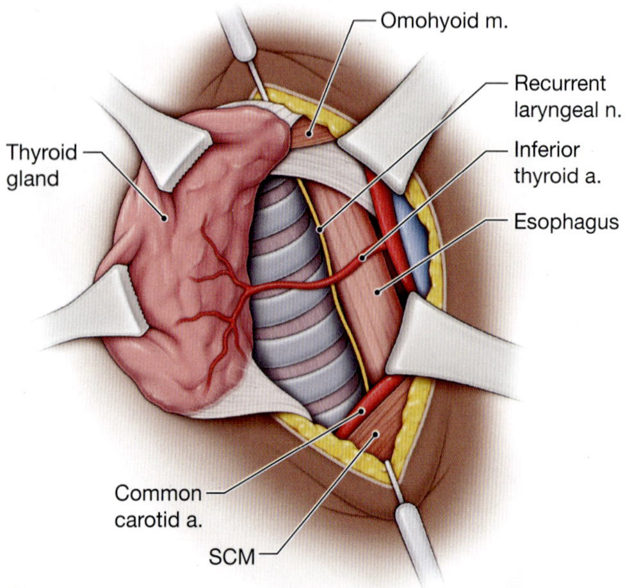

C

D. Blunt finger dissection technique is used to gain access to the prevertebral space, taking care to avoid injury to the recurrent laryngeal nerve in the tracheoesophageal groove. (Alternatively, the prevertebral space can be approached behind the carotid sheath). Once the subfascial plane is entered, dissection with a right angle clamp, the tip of which hugs the muscular layer of the esophagus, is performed starting posteriorly and proceeding anteriorly, working first behind and then anterior to the esophagus, developing a circumferential plane around the esophagus. Using a right angle clamp, the esophagus is dissected circumferentially and a 1" penrose drain is passed around the esophagus. Using this drain, the esophagus is gently retracted laterally and superiorly, and a combination of sharp and blunt (finger/peanut) dissection performed starting superiorly and proceeding inferiorly towards the thoracic inlet to gradually mobilize and dissect the esophagus from the surrounding soft tissues. Care must be taken to avoid injury to the posterior tracheal wall while doing this. It may be helpful to have a nasogastric tube in place or use intraoperative endoscopy if tissue planes are distorted to aid in identification. Irrigation under saline may help identify subtle injuries.

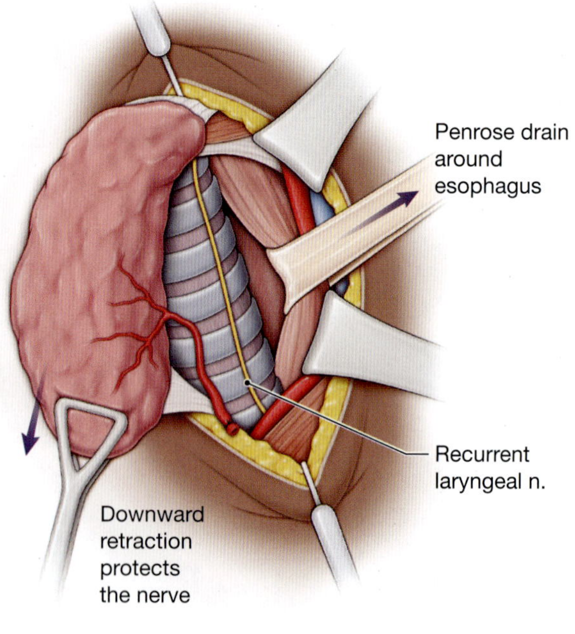

D

Figure 9-2 C, D

Exposure

Repair of Defect

Any nonviable tissue edges should be debrided back to healthy tissue. Importantly, the extent of mucosal defect may not be clear and the myotomy may need to be extended. The defect should then be closed in one to two layers with absorbable monofilament suture. If possible, pedicled muscle flap is rotated to buttress the repair.

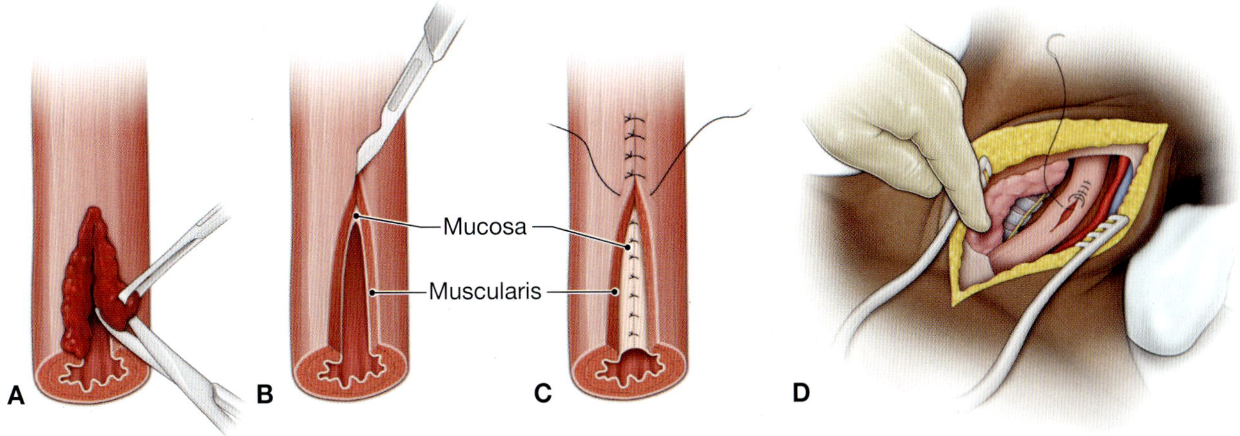

Figure 9-3 A-D

Esophagostomy/Gastrostomy with Jejunostomy

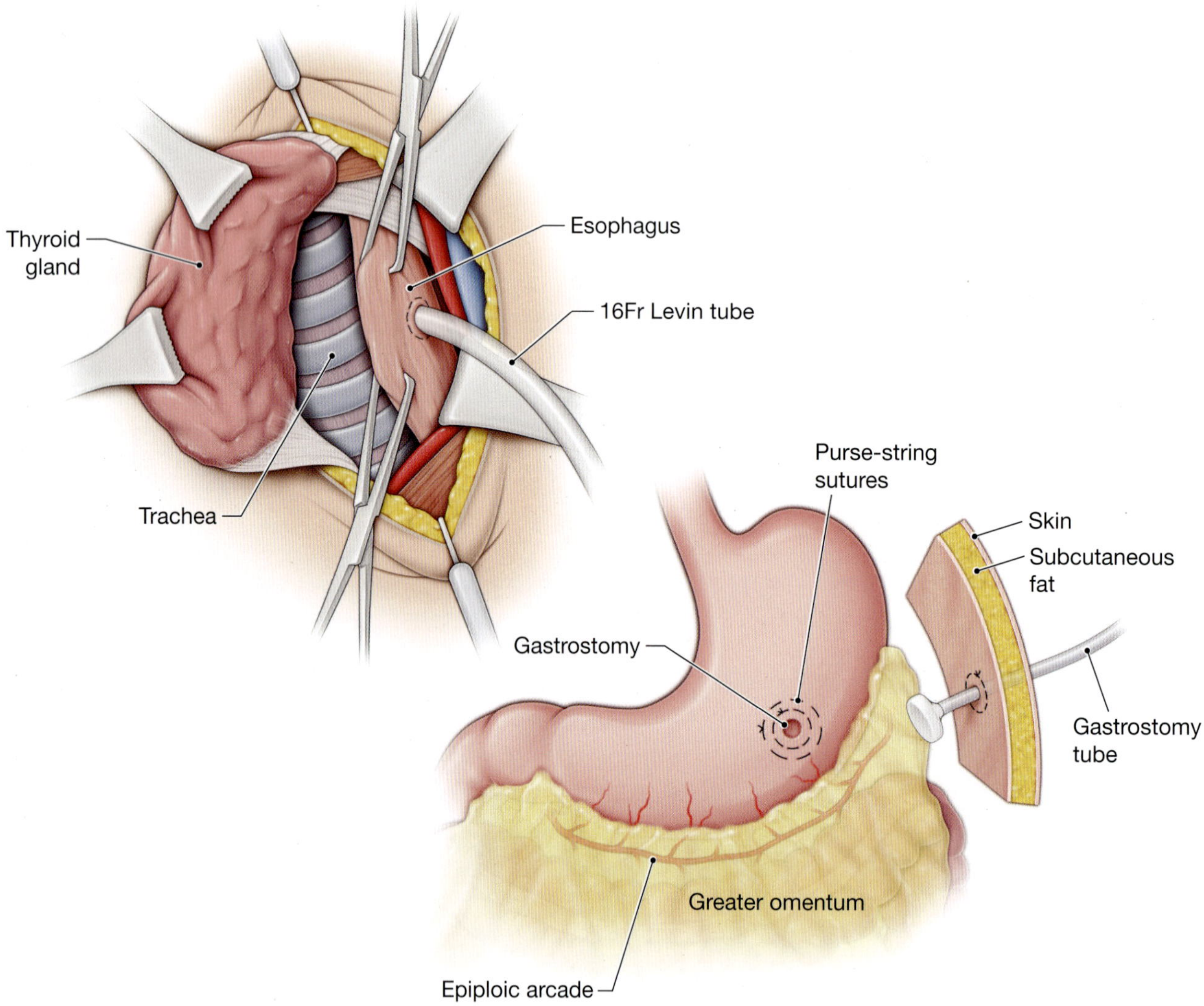

Figure 9-4

If the injury is not amenable to primary repair due to tissue loss and necrosis, drainage or exteriorization of the injury as a lateral esophagostomy is performed for damage control and exclusion.

This can be accomplished by mobilizing the proximal end of the esophagus to the skin or, in cases where there is insufficient length, using a large T-tube secured to the skin for a tube esophagostomy.

An esophagostomy prevents further leakage from above. Enteral access is performed using a gastrojejunostomy (GJ) tube via an open or laparoscopic technique. Double, concentric purse-string sutures using nonabsorbable sutures are placed in the stomach, and a gastrotomy is made in the central portion of the purse strings. The GJ tube is inserted through a left subcostal stab skin incision and into the gastrotomy. The jejunostomy limb is advanced distally until the tip is palpated past the ligament of Treitz. The balloon is inflated with sterile water and the tube pulled snug and then the sutures are secured. A gastropexy is then performed by anchoring the stomach to the anterior abdominal wall using interrupted 2-0 silk suture at four points. The outer purse-string suture strands are left long with the needle attached and can be used as one of the gastropexy sutures.

Complications

The key to minimizing complications is prompt and individualized diagnosis and treatment. The esophagus has no serosal layer, and uncontrolled leak is the most frequent complication. Cervical esophageal leak is better tolerated than in the thorax or abdomen. Placing a pedicled flap as a buttress and meticulous technique during primary repair may help prevent this complication. Esophageal fistula, stenosis, infection, injury to recurrent laryngeal nerve, and mediastinitis may occur as well.

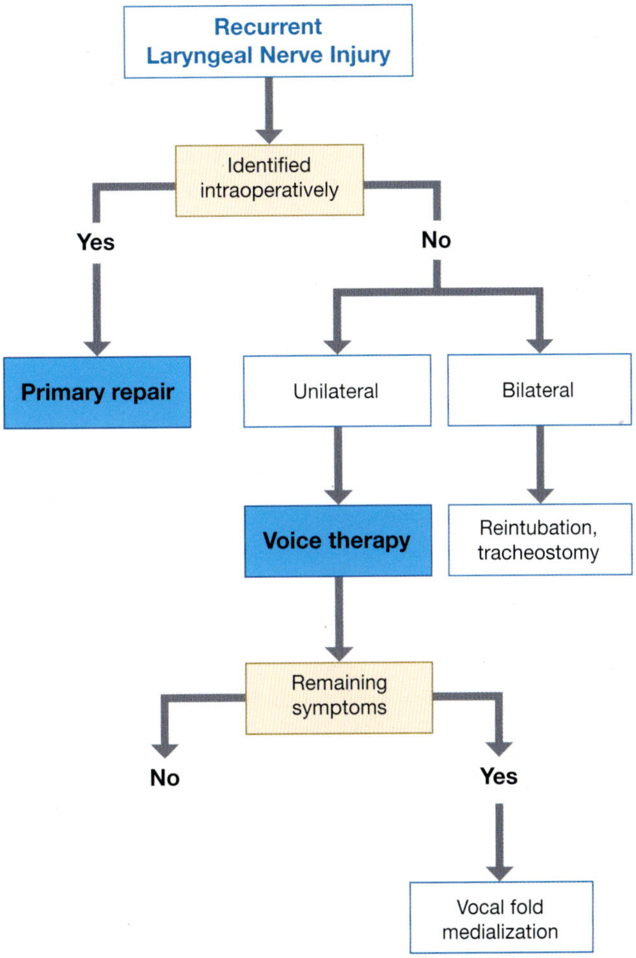

Figure 9-5

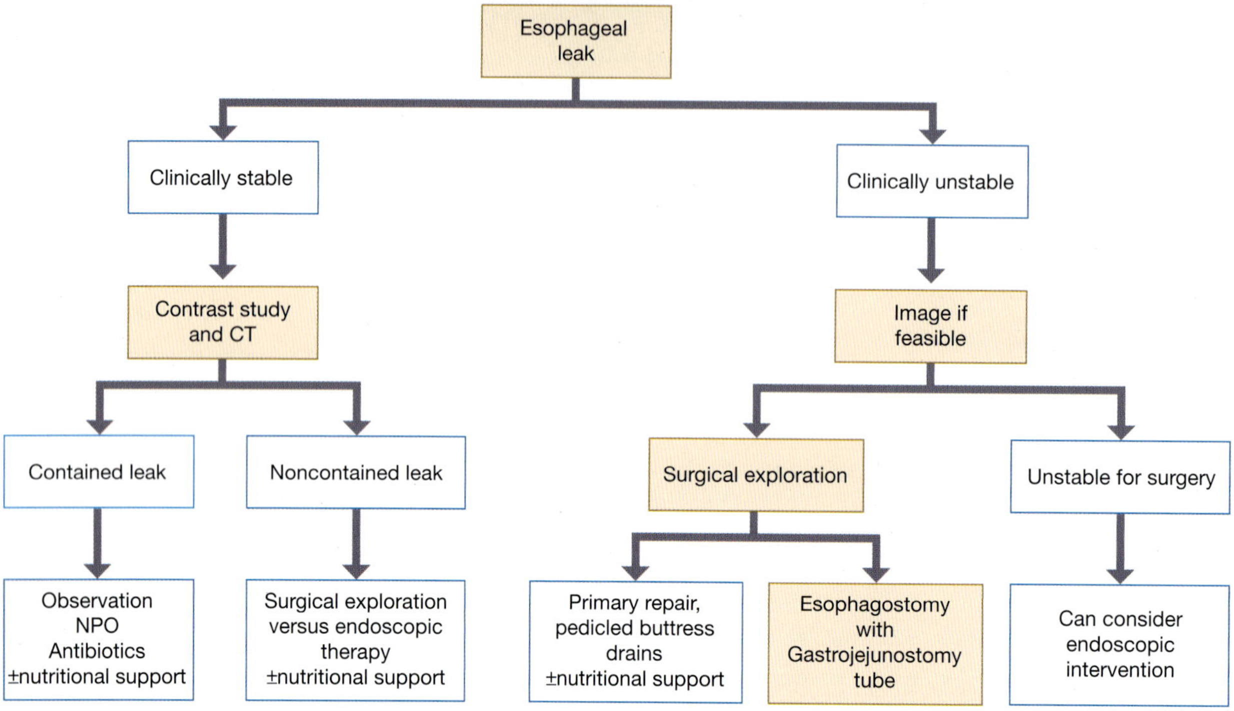
Esophageal leak
Clinically stable
Clinically unstable
Contrast study and CT
Image if feasible
Contained leak
Noncontained leak
Surgical exploration
Unstable for surgery
Observation
NPO
Antibiotics
±nutritional support
Surgical exploration versus endoscopic therapy
±nutritional support
Primary repair, pedicled buttress drains
±nutritional support
Esophagostomy with Gastrojejunostomy tube
Can consider endoscopic intervention

Figure 9-6

10

ESOPHAGUS

Leon Ray White, DO, MS

TIPS

1. Ninety-eight percent of patients with penetrating thoracic esophageal injuries have at least one other associated injury.
2. Esophageal repair is performed in two layers, with absorbable sutures to repair the mucosa and permanent sutures for the muscular layer.
3. An intercostal muscle pedicle should be used to reinforce repairs to the thoracic esophagus.

THORACIC

Introduction

Traumatic injuries, especially blunt injuries, to the thoracic esophagus are rare but usually significant in nature. In particular, traumatic injuries to the thoracic esophagus will often present with concomitant injuries to surrounding vital structures (eg, hemothorax, pneumothorax, rib fractures). If there is high suspicion for esophageal injury, appropriate diagnostic tests and procedures must be performed.

Options for diagnosis include computed tomographic (CT) esophagram, fluoroscopic contrast esophagram, and esophagoscopy. Esophagogastroduodenoscopy (EGD) alone has a greater than 98% negative predictive value for esophageal injury; additionally, the combination of EGD and a contrasted imaging study has a diagnostic accuracy of nearly 100%. The contemporary approach begins with a CT angiogram (CTA) and a subsequent adjunctive endoscopic and/or fluoroscopic esophagram if there is periesophageal air or fluid on CTA.

As opposed to cervical esophageal injury, management with open surgical exploration of the thoracic esophagus is significantly more morbid and thus should not be indiscriminate. Previously, it was suggested that delays to operative repair resulted in excessive morbidity and mortality. Recent studies have concluded that although the rates of primary repair may be lower, delayed diagnosis and treatment of a thoracic esophageal injury did not necessarily lead to adverse outcomes. Thus, an efficient diagnostic evaluation is recommended in the stable patient to rapidly confirm an injury.

Furthermore, the classical tenet of performing primary repair when less than 24 hours from perforation and avoiding primary repair when more than 24 hours has been disproven in clinical studies. If expertise is available, endoscopic endoluminal stents may be considered as is described in Chapter 11.

Anatomy

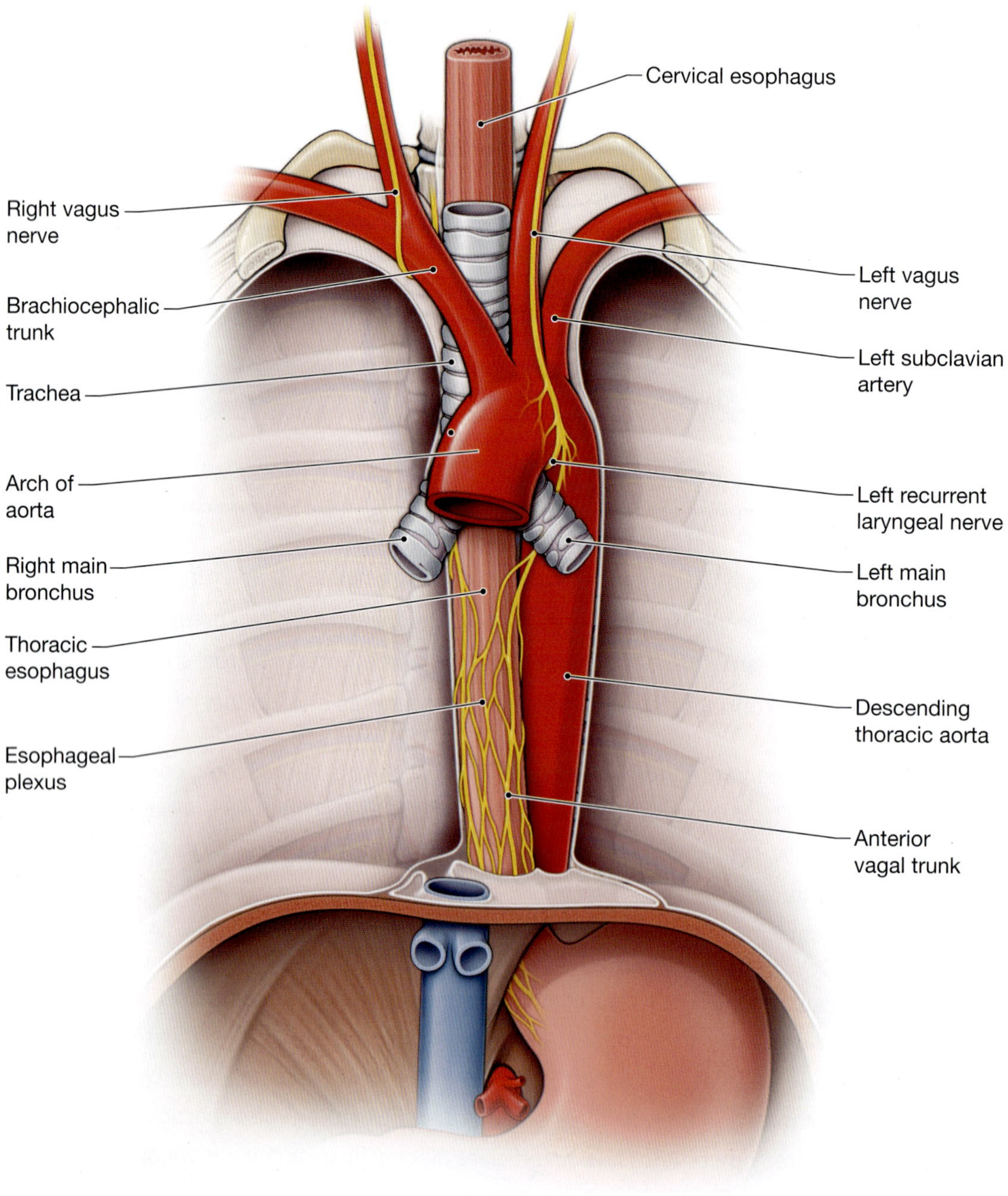

Figure 10-1

TABLE 10-1. American Association for the Surgery of Trauma (AAST) Organ Injury Scale

Grade	AAST Injury Scale - Esophagus
Grade: I Contusion/hematoma or partial-thickness laceration	
Grade: II Laceration <50% circumference	
Grade: III Laceration >50% circumference	
Grade: IV Segmental tissue loss or devascularization <2 cm	
Grade: V Segmental tissue loss or devascularization >2 cm	

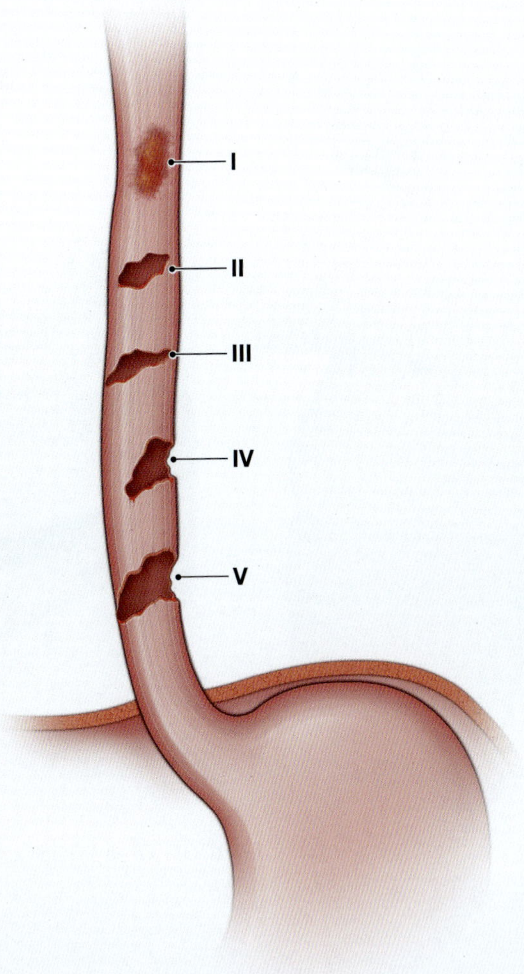

Operative Steps with Illustration

1. Right posterolateral thoracotomy

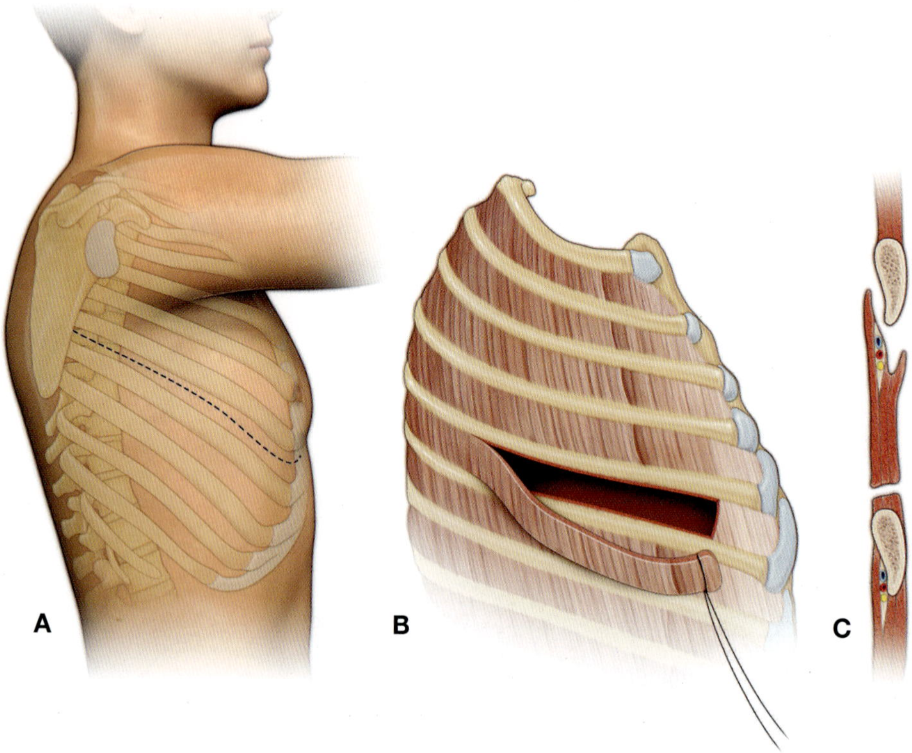

Figure 10-2. Creation of a musculopleural flap.

2. Division of the azygous vein and exposure of the esophagus

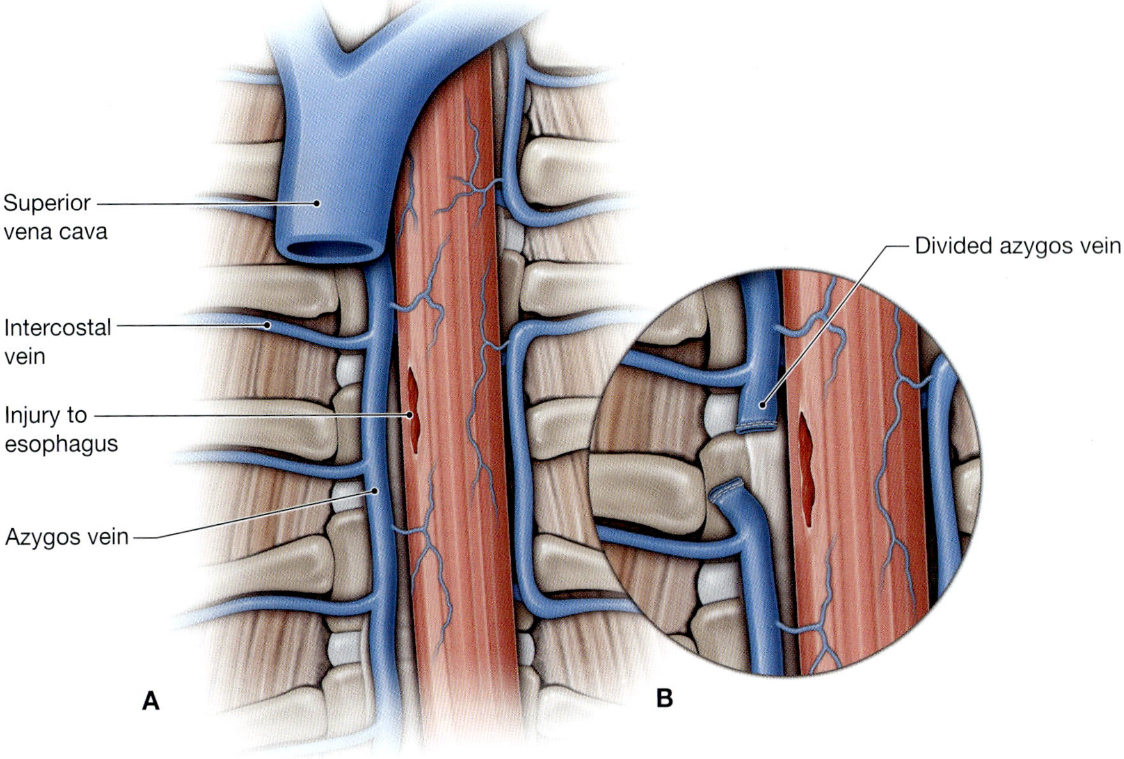

Figure 10-3

3. Fully expose the esophageal injury

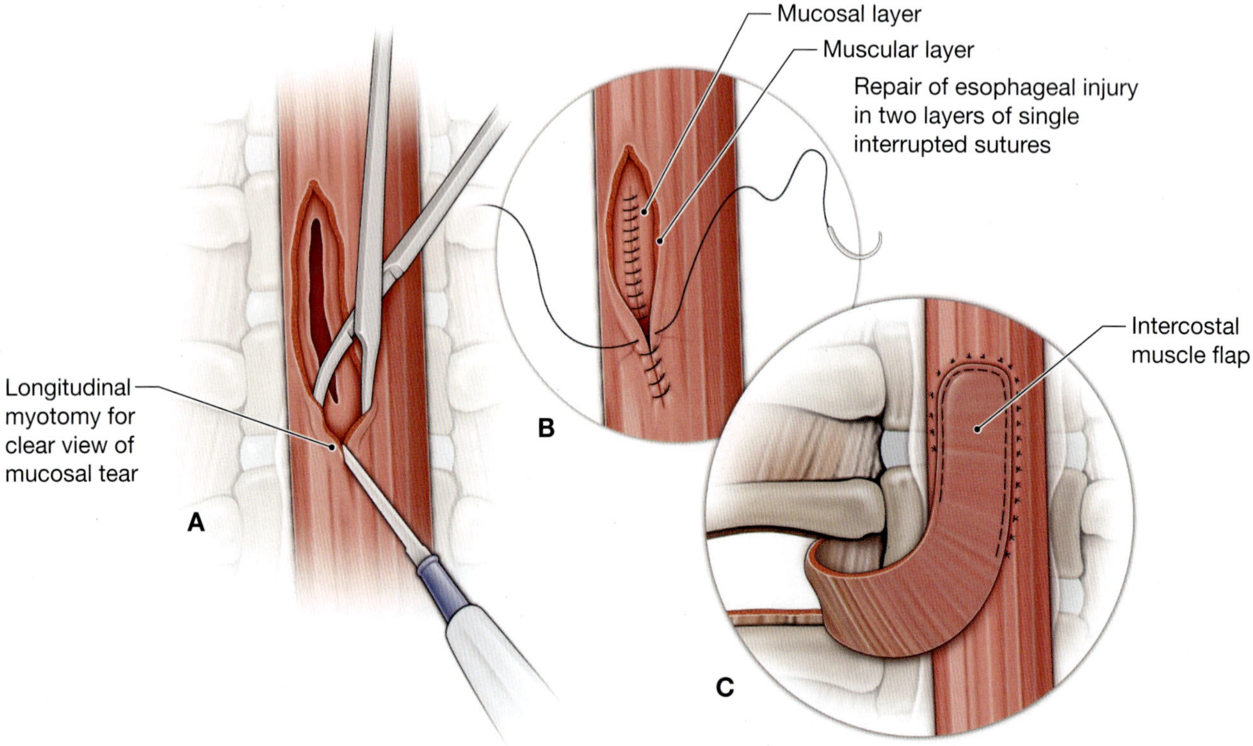

Figure 10-4 A-C

Repair the defect in two layers, buttress repair with intercostal flap, and close the chest.

4. Damage control in the unstable patient

In the unstable trauma patient, or if primary repair with flap coverage is not feasible, a damage control operation must be performed.

One option for damage control is esophageal diversion and exclusion. This involves creation of a cervical esophagostomy, exclusion of the gastroesophageal junction, placement of gastrostomy and jejunostomy tubes, as well as wide mediastinal drainage.

Another option when primary repair is not possible is creation of a controlled fistula with a T-tube. A large T-tube is placed in the perforation and exits the chest wall. If practical, the operating surgeon may elect to reinforce the T-tube with a muscle flap. An nasogastric tube is then inserted through the T-tube for gastric decompression, and the chest/mediastinum is widely drained.

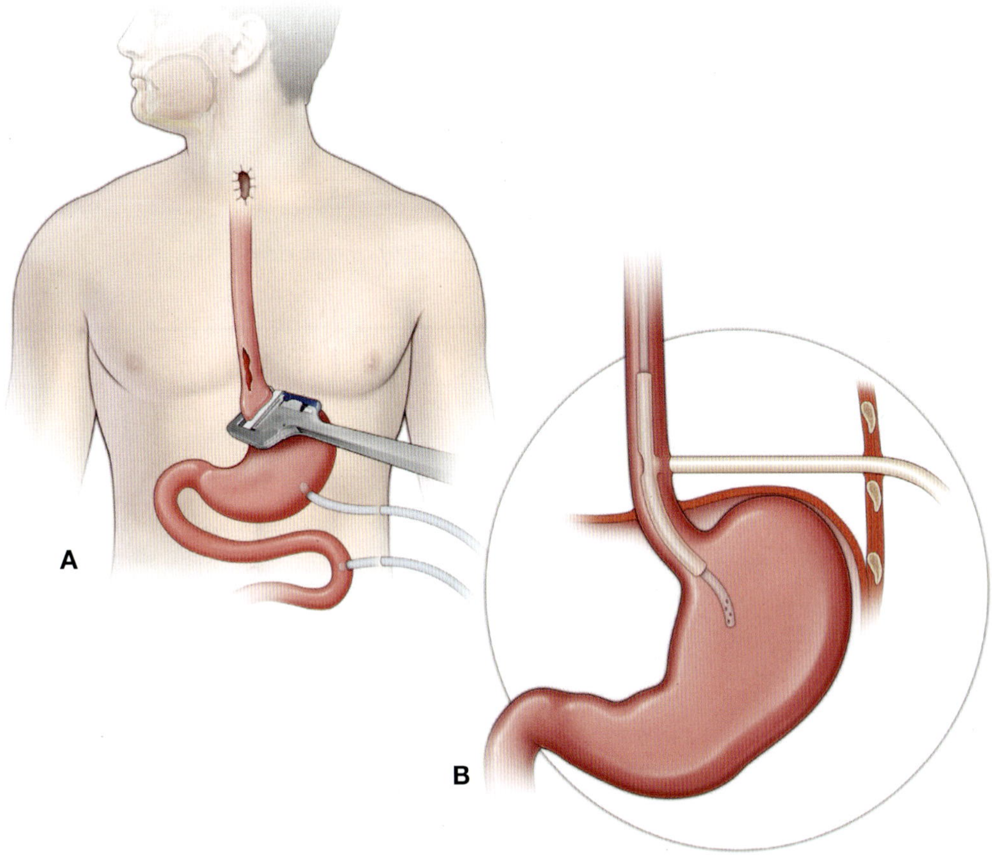

Figure 10-5 A, B

Complications

The complication rate after esophageal trauma ranges from 38% to 66%, and rates are often higher in patients who had delays in diagnosis and higher-grade injuries.

Potential early complications after primary thoracic esophageal repair include postoperative leak, bleeding, and chylothorax. Esophageal stenosis is a potential late complication.

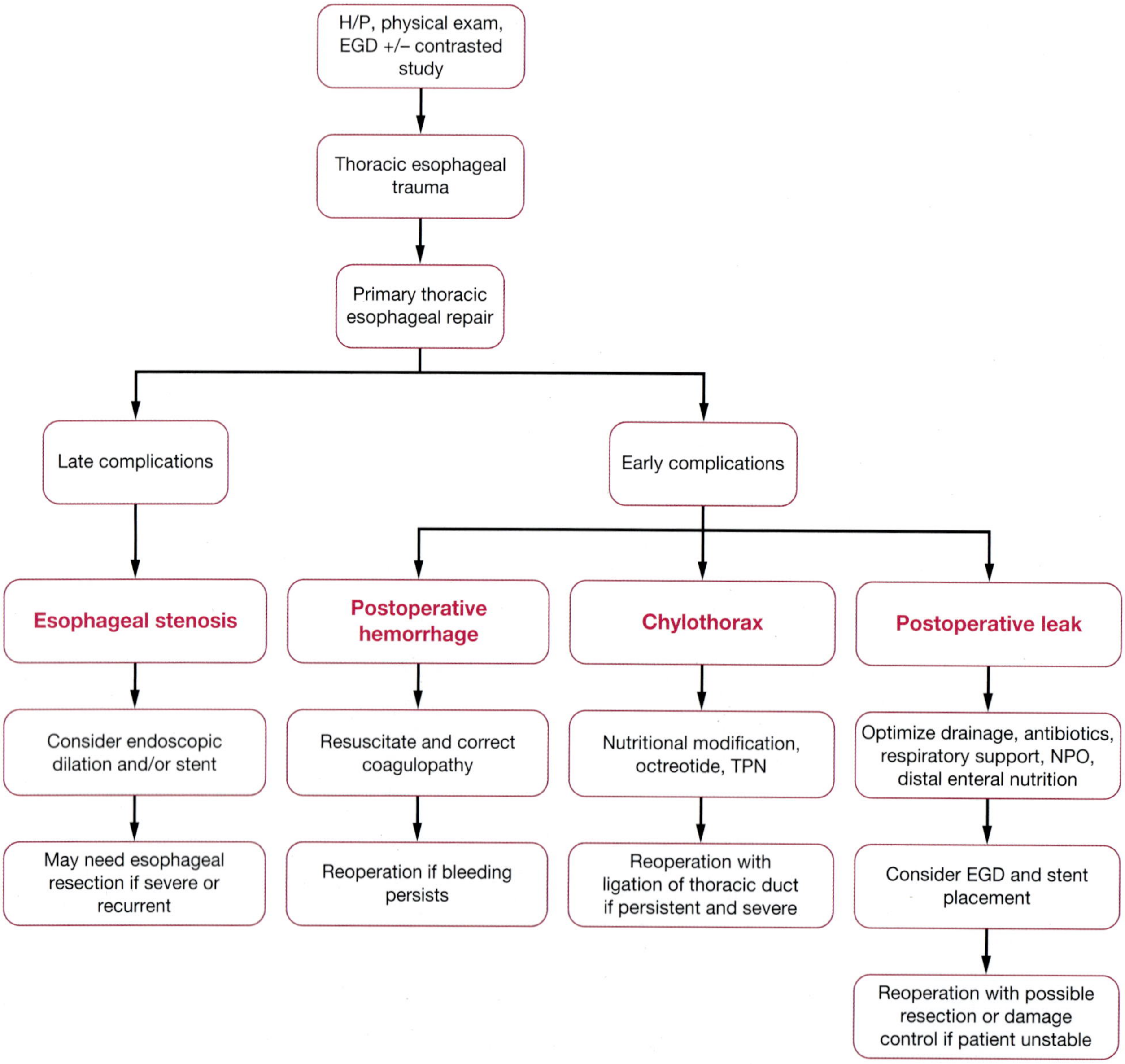

Figure 10-6

ABDOMINAL ESOPHAGUS

While uncommon, injuries to the abdominal esophagus mandate a high degree of suspicion and are often accompanied by extensive associated intra-abdominal or intrathoracic injuries. Management principles are similar to cervical and thoracic esophageal injuries; however, there are key differences. Abdominal esophageal injuries can be associated with left pleural effusions. They are best approached through a midline laparotomy incision (with the left chest prepped in the operative field should a thoracotomy be required). Perforations to the distal esophagus should be closed primarily in one or two layers with nonabsorbable sutures. The layered closure should be buttressed with either a fundoplication over a 50- to 60-French bougie, a gastric serosal ("Thal") patch, or a diaphragm flap. Injuries not amenable to primary closure should be primarily closed with a diaphragm flap. The area of repair should be adequately drained. Surgical decompression with a gastrostomy tube and distal enteral access with a jejunostomy tube should be placed. Alternatively, a gastrojejunostomy tube is placed.

Approach

The left triangular ligament of the liver is taken down, and the left lateral lobe is folded up. The gastrohepatic ligament is divided, and then the posterior peritoneum overlying the esophagus is opened, enabling encircling the esophagus with a finger. Occasionally, if a posterior injury in the distal esophagus cannot be exposed, the anterior wall of the stomach is opened longitudinally near the cardia, and the injury is repaired from within the stomach. Division of the short gastric vessels may provide better exposure.

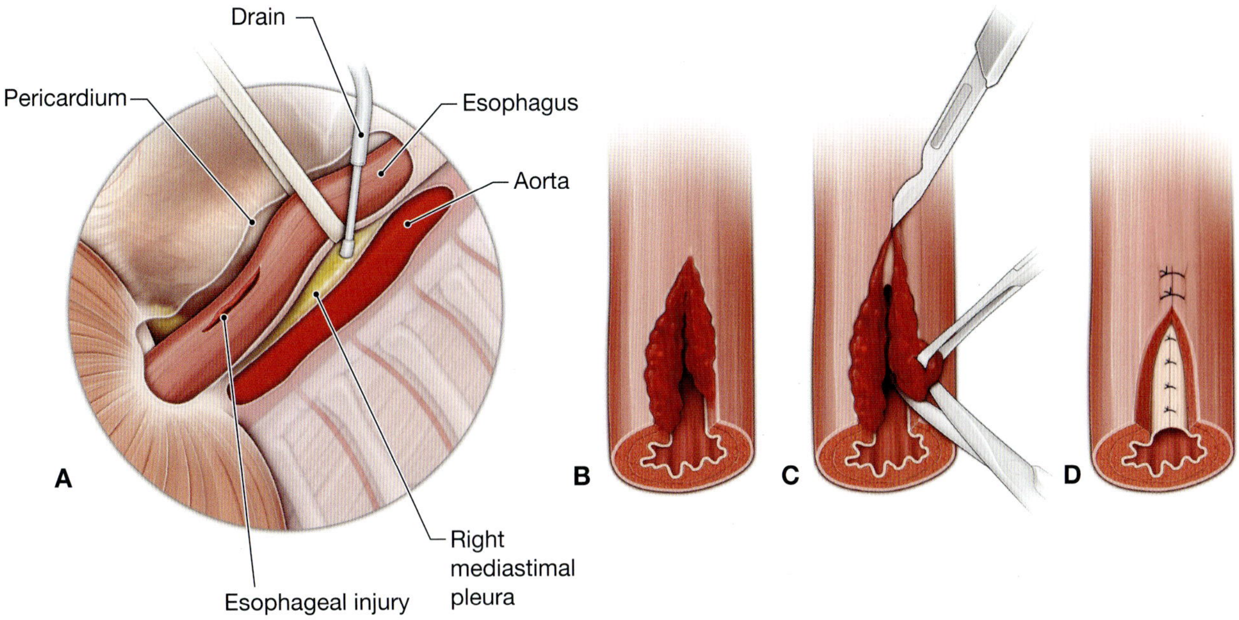

Figure 10-7 A-D. Fundoplication, when performed, requires mobilization of the gastric fundus, which necessitates division of several of the vasa brevia along the greater curvature, as well as branches of the left gastric vessels along the lesser curvature. The mobilized fundus is wrapped circumferentially around the esophageal repair, and the wrap is generally much longer than the usual Nissen fundoplication utilized for gastroesophageal reflux disease. Seromuscular bites of the gastric wall to include the submucosa are used to create the fundoplication using synthetic interrupted nonabsorbable sutures.

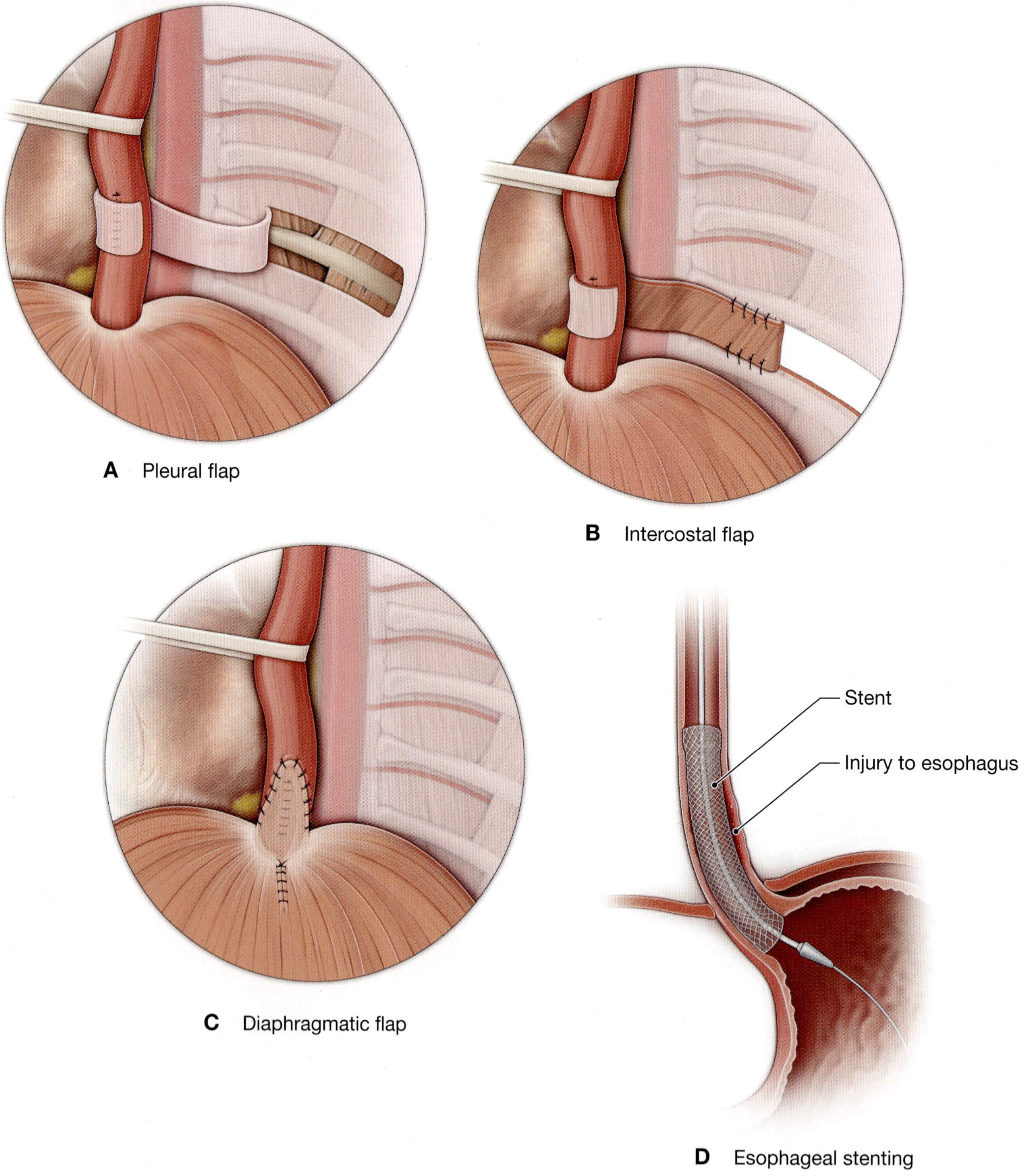

Figure 10-8 A-D

Esophageal Stenting

Smaller perforations may be amenable to closure and sealing by endoluminal stents. The vast majority of patients studied in various series have sustained iatrogenic or spontaneous perforations and not external trauma. Covered plastic stents are placed endoscopically. Fluoroscopic guidance is helpful but not necessary. The stent is placed and extracted after surveillance esophagram after 4 to 6 weeks to document healing. Marking the proximal and distal ends of the tumor with contrast injections or endoscopic clips or use of external fluoroscopic markers, such as coins, paperclips, or other metallic objects is helpful. The use of these proximal and distal markers should be considered optional, and many physicians prefer to use contrast injection alone to delineate the lesion more clearly or fluoroscopic markers, such as the position of the endoscope when it is located at the proximal and distal ends of the defect, when deciding on stent length and to guide stent placement. Proximal stents may be more prone to migration and interference with swallowing, but they have been placed successfully in some cases of high esophageal injury.

Time to healing is uncertain, and complications including exacerbation of tears, esophageal perforation due to the device, bleeding, and stricture and the reported mortality rates (13% overall) remain unclear. If these strategies are used, it is important to debride the perforation site and provide adequate drainage. This may be done thoracoscopically. As always, establishing enteral nutritional access must be achieved using either a nasogastric tube or gastrostomy/jejunostomy tubes.

Occasionally, major devastating injuries of the esophagus occur and require a damage control option if repair is not feasible. These include resection, T-tube placement, and cervical esophagostomy with or without esophageal exclusion.

In rare circumstances, esophageal resection may be indicated such as in severe caustic injuries. Delayed reconstruction using gastric or colonic interposition would be the treatment of choice.

Large defects in the esophagus that cannot be closed are managed with onlay muscle flaps or by creation of a controlled fistula using a T-tube brought out through the abdominal wall. Cervical esophagostomy may complicate reconstruction so if possible, a loop esophagostomy is preferred. If diversion is performed, distal esophageal ligation is unnecessary so as to avoid a distal obstruction. If the injuries are severe enough to require exclusion then resection may be a better option.

Complications

Development of anastomotic leaks and subsequent mediastinitis, sepsis, and pulmonary failure present significant management challenges. Shock, extensive mobilization, inadequate debridement, and excessive tension are all established risk factors for suture line dehiscence and esophageal leakage.

Approximately 50% of esophageal leaks are asymptomatic and are diagnosed subclinically on postoperative esophagrams. Once a leak is identified, the administration of broad-spectrum antibiotics, adequate drainage, and limited oral intake with distal feeding access are crucial. Most leaks do not require further operative intervention with the advent of radiologic and percutaneous techniques. More recently, endoluminal stents have been used to manage leaks as well.

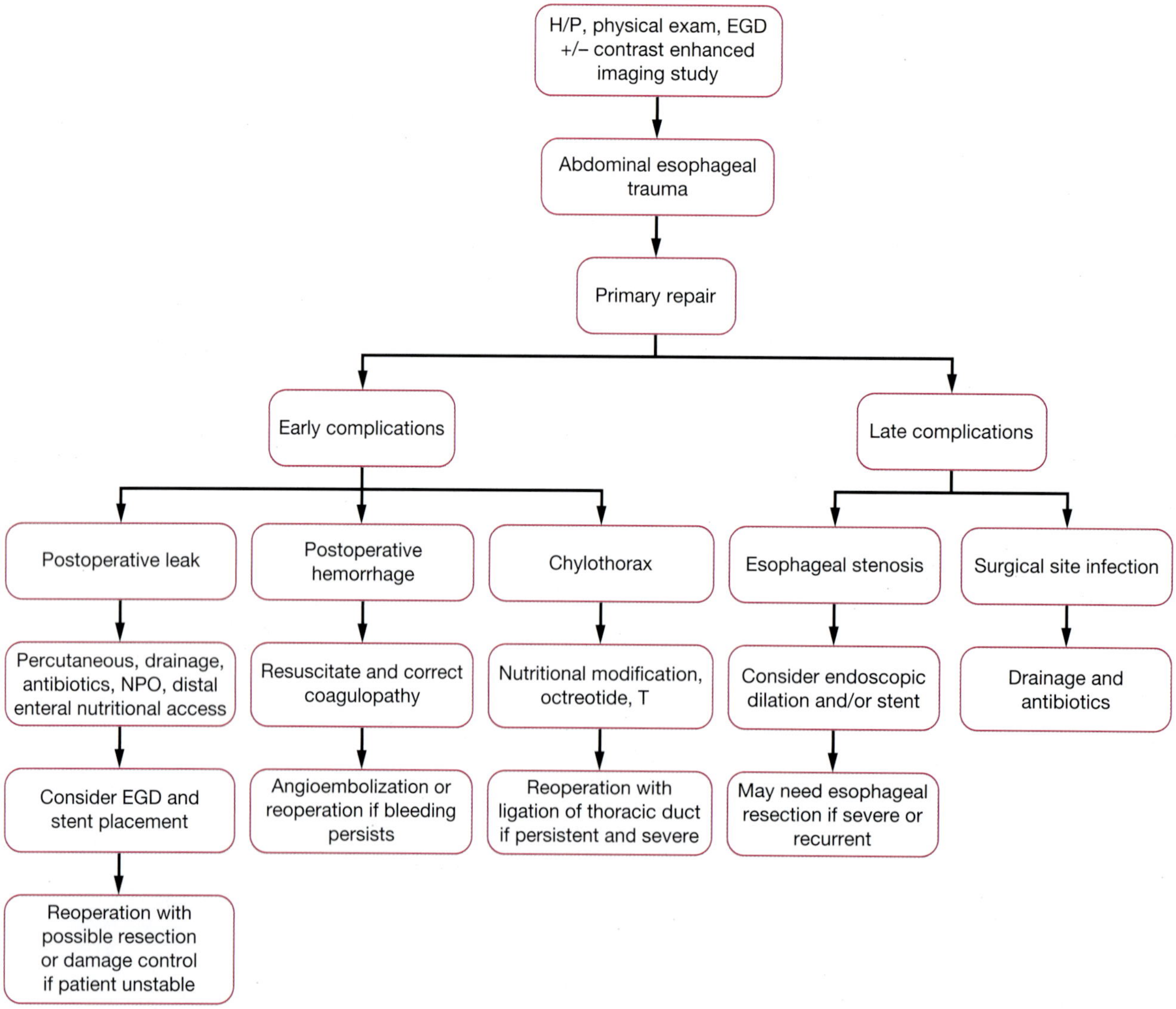

Figure 10-9

11

DIAPHRAGM INJURY

Dale A. Dangleben, MD, FACS
Kathleen Koesarie, MD

TIPS

1. **Utilize Babcock or Kocher forceps to grab the edges of the injury to facilitate pulling them together to make repair easier.**
2. **Toward the end of the case, prior to the last stitch, place a red rubber into the chest and suck out the air, and as the last stitch is thrown, pull out the tube.**
3. **In situations of hostile abdomen from previous surgery, the chest approach is more favorable.**

Introduction

Traumatic diaphragmatic injury incidence is low. Diagnosis can be difficult, and presentation may vary. Blunt traumatic injury tends to be higher compared to penetrating mechanisms. In significantly hemodynamically unstable patients, damage control may be required and diaphragm repaired after full resuscitation. In blunt trauma, a sudden increase in peritoneal pressure results in diaphragmatic disruption. This tends to be on the left side due to an area of congenital weakness during embryologic development (Figure 11-1A). On the right side, it is less affected due to the position of the liver. Also noteworthy, penetrating injuries are smaller in size.

Anatomy

Diaphragmatic injuries occur in about 1% of blunt trauma cases. These injuries are often associated with other significant injuries and result in considerable morbidity and mortality. Initial chest X-rays show abnormalities in 75% of cases, but only 50% of these cases are diagnostic for diaphragmatic injury. Other diagnostic options include computed tomography scan, thoracoscopy, and laparoscopy. Note that many of these injuries are often only discovered during surgery for other associated injuries. The position of the diaphragm varies during the respiratory cycle, extending from the fourth intercostal space in the front to the seventh or eighth space at the sides and the back (Figure 11-1B). This variation places the diaphragm at risk for injuries from penetrating trauma to the lower chest.

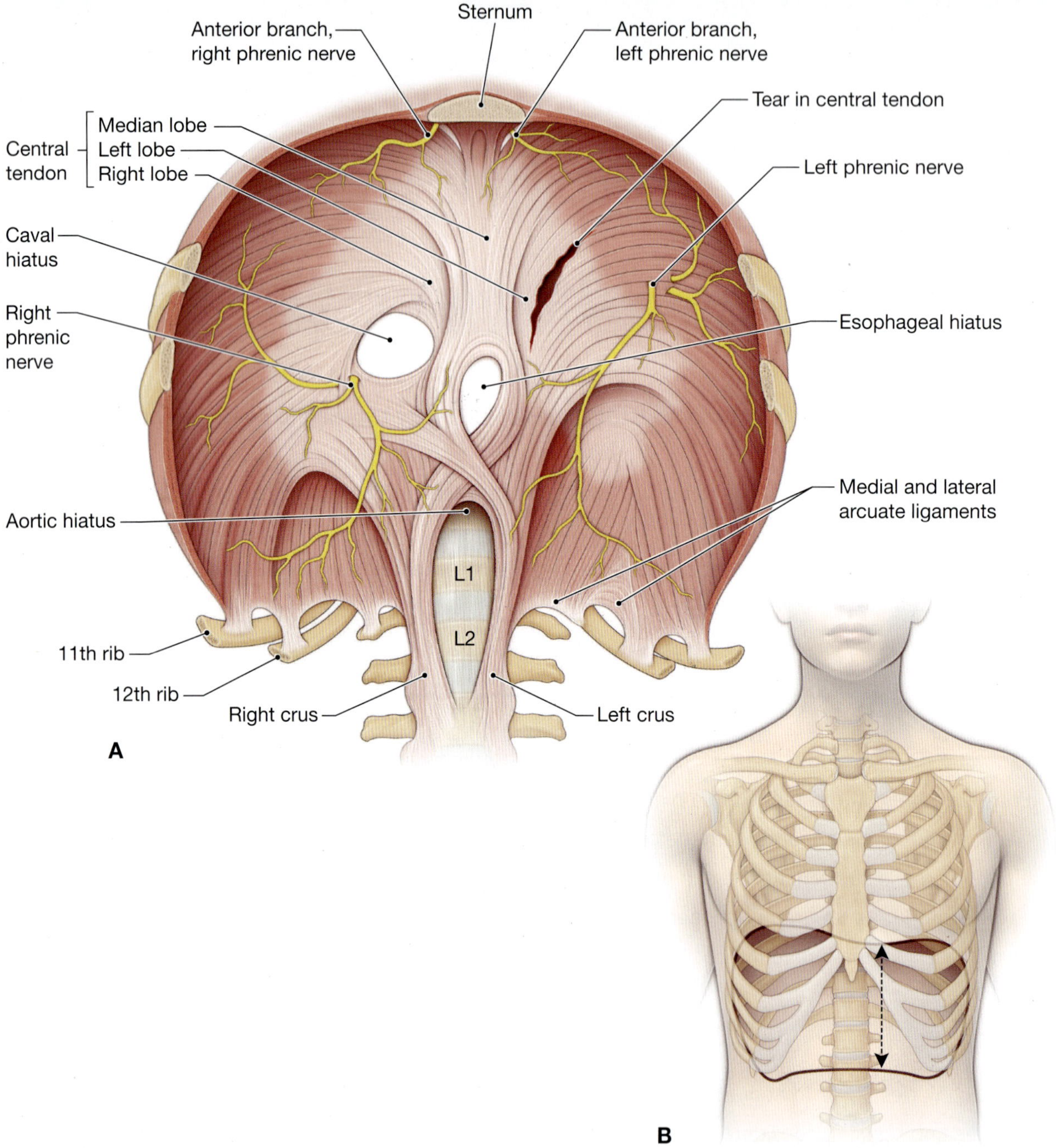

Figure 11-1 A, B

Mechanism of Injury

Blunt diaphragmatic injuries are typically caused by increased abdominal pressure from high-energy impacts and are frequently associated with other injuries such as intra-abdominal trauma and pelvic fractures (Figure 11-2).

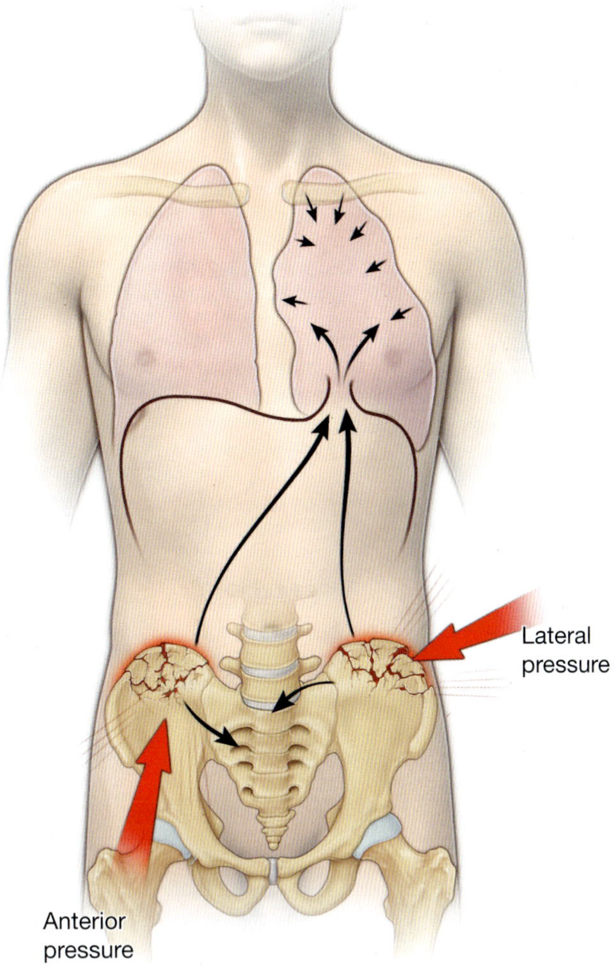

Figure 11-2

Operative Exposure

A midline incision provides optimal exposure to repair either side of the diaphragm. It also allows access to the abdomen for a thorough exploration to check for any additional injuries. The right hemidiaphragm is exposed by releasing the left and right diaphragmatic ligaments (Figure 11-3A, B).

By pulling the stomach and spleen downward, the left side of the diaphragm becomes visible (Fig. 11-3D). The damaged edges of the diaphragm can be grasped using specialized clamps, such as a Babcock or Allis clamp. The defect is closed with a monofilament suture, using either a running or interrupted stitch technique (Figure 11-4A).

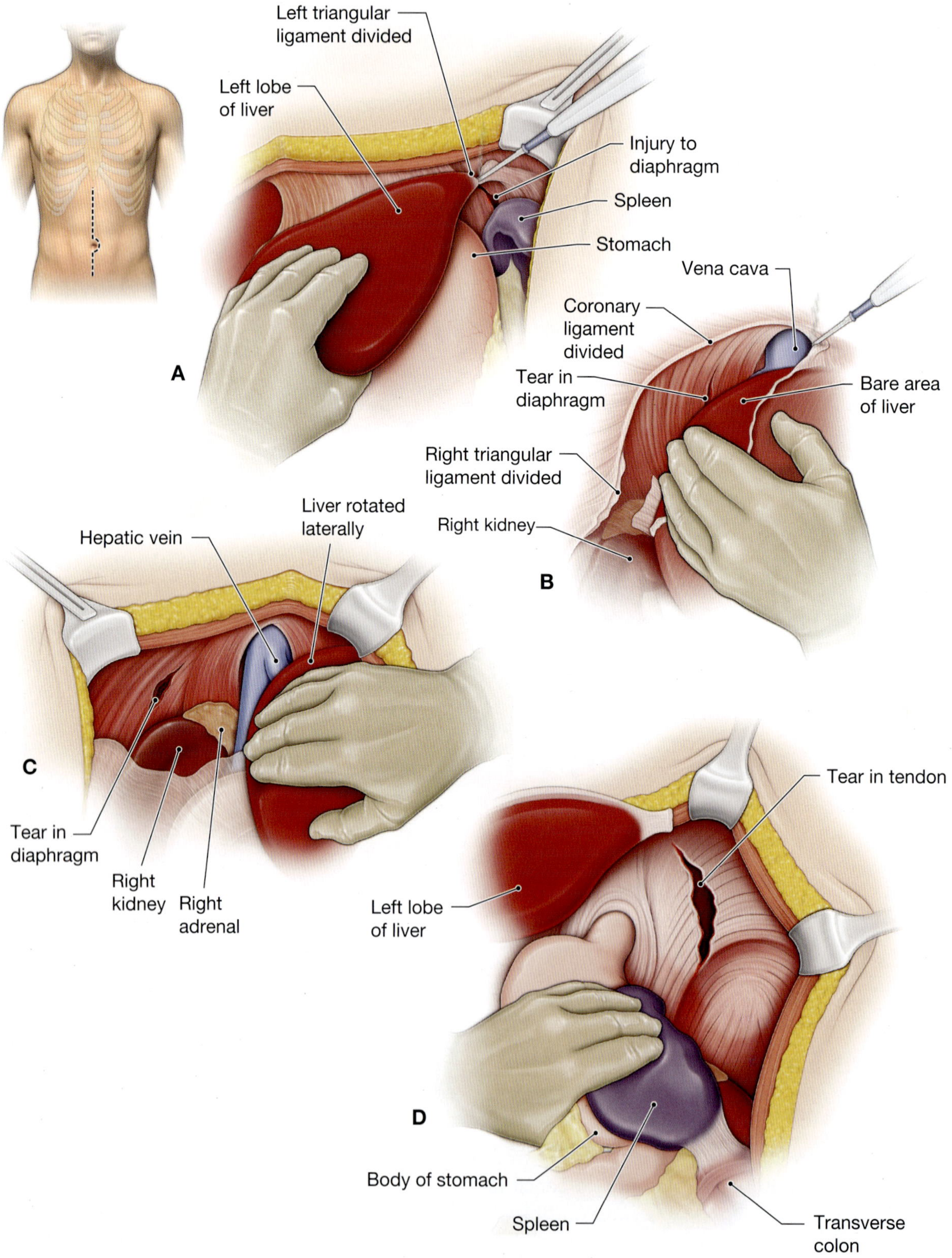

Figure 11-3 A-D

Defects without significant tissue loss can be closed easily without tension, and in most cases, pledgets are unnecessary. For cases involving tissue loss, prosthetic material may be used to achieve a tension-free repair (Figure 11-4D). If there is contamination of the chest from an abdominal injury, thoroughly irrigating the chest is vital to reduce the risk of postoperative infection.

After irrigation, the lung is reinflated while directly observing through the diaphragmatic injury. A chest tube is inserted via the repair (Figure 11-4A) to ensure proper suction and lung expansion. This step involves close coordination between the surgeon and anesthesiologist and may eliminate the need for a postoperative chest tube. During the final stitch closure, the tube is removed while the patient is on continued suction (Figure 11-4B). Alternatively, the chest tube can be placed in the chest before the diaphragm is fully closed.

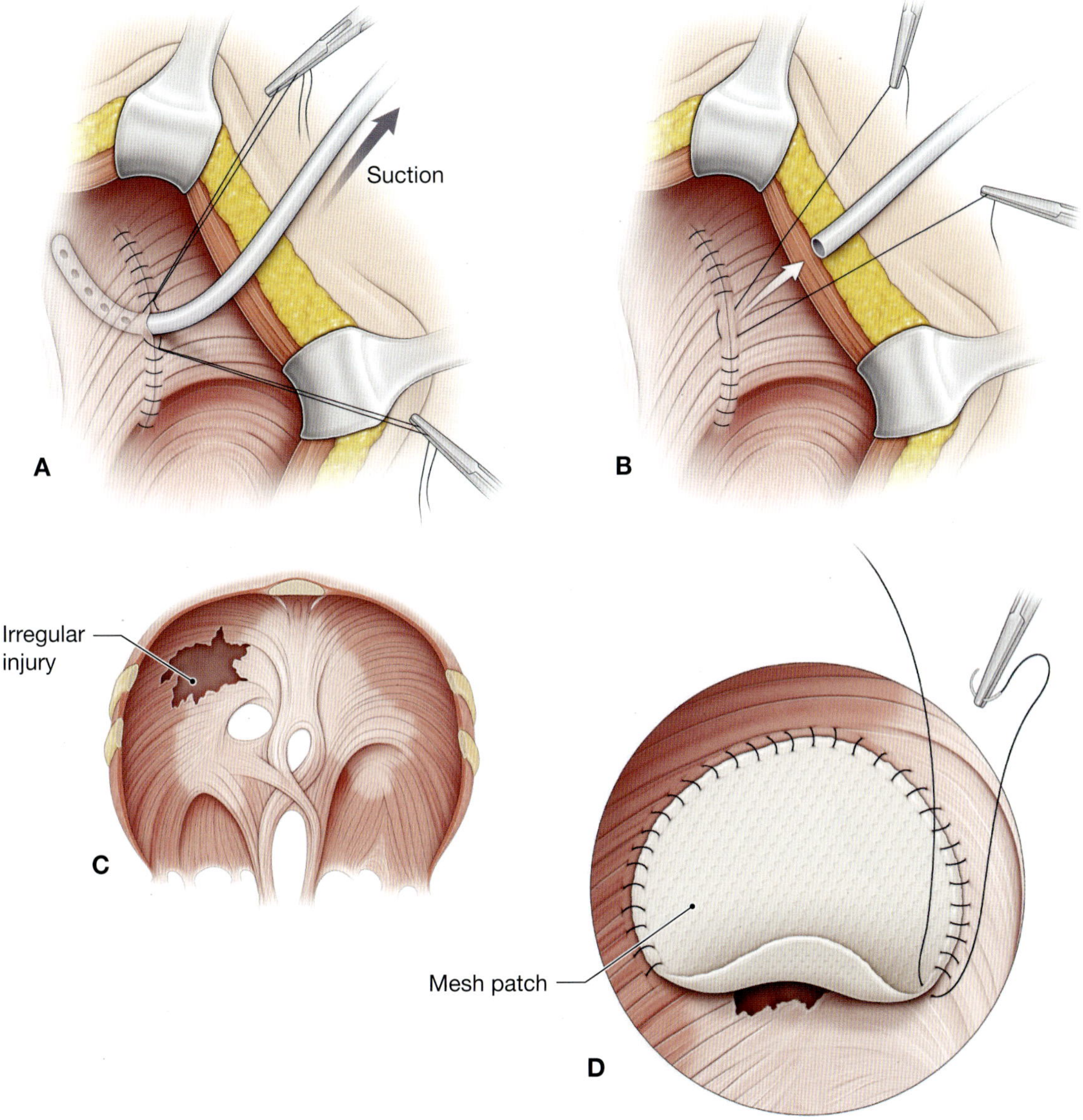

Figure 11-4 A-D

Thoracic Approach (Chronic Hernia)

Chronic diaphragmatic hernias are commonly linked to both blunt and penetrating trauma. The progression of these injuries can vary, ranging from an asymptomatic state to serious complications such as strangulation of the herniated abdominal organs. Since intra-abdominal injury is not a major issue, these chronic diaphragmatic injuries are typically repaired using a posterolateral thoracotomy. The lung may often be stuck to the stomach, necessitating careful dissection of the stomach and other abdominal organs (Figure 11-5A). This allows the intra-abdominal contents to be repositioned (Figure 11-5B), with the diaphragm being closed using prosthetic material (Figure 11-5C).

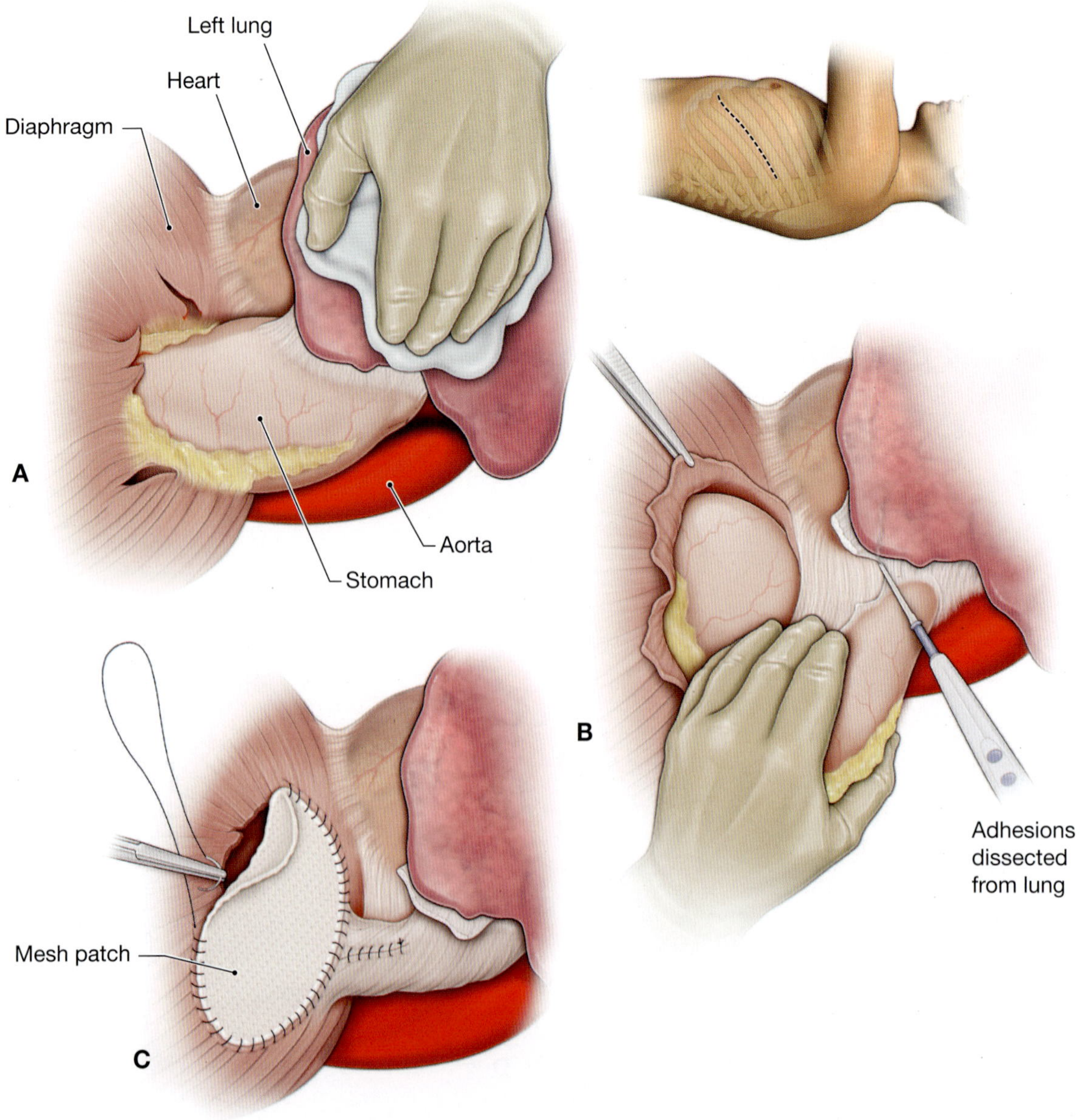

Figure 11-5 A-C

Complications

In scenarios when the diaphragmatic injury is missed, a larger diaphragmatic defect will occur with time. This allows for a larger amount of intraperitoneal content to migrate into the chest, posing a greater challenge. This increases morbidity and mortality because there is greater risk of obstruction, ischemia, and even necrosis. These can be approached laparoscopically or transthoracically.

STOMACH

12

Ginger L. Justice, MD
Dale A. Dangleben, MD, FACS

TIPS

1. **Priority is to control bleeding and spillage of gastric contents.**
2. **Control of gastric spillage can be performed without resection.**
3. **Damage control resection without reconstruction is often imperative.**

Introduction

Gastric trauma is commonly associated with penetrating injuries to the abdomen and lower chest wall. These includes gunshot wounds and stabbings (approximately 20% and 10%, respectively). Gastric rupture due to blunt trauma is much less common and is associated with a higher severity of mechanism such as motor vehicle collisions and pedestrians struck due to increased luminal pressure, crush against the spine, and shear forces. Often, patients with gastric injuries are hypotensive due to the vast blood supply to the stomach and their likelihood of injury to adjacent organs. This may include spleen, liver, small bowel, colon, and diaphragm. This is particularly seen with gunshot wounds.

Many patients with gastric injury will have evidence of peritonitis on exam. Early operative intervention is essential with a damage control mindset for unstable patients. Focused assessment with sonography in trauma (FAST) exams are often negative as there may only be a small amount of fluid, especially if posterior into the lesser sac. Plain film imaging frequently does not reveal free air, even with blunt mechanism. Only hemodynamically stable patients without peritonitis should proceed to computed tomography imaging because this is the more sensitive study for free air and free fluid.

Mortality associated with gastric injury is rarely from the gastric injury itself (approximately 30%) with a reported range of approximately 28% to 66%. It is highly dependent on shock, transfusion requirements, and the associated severe injuries and mechanism. Complications are noted to be anastomotic leakage, abscess, and fistula formation. These complications may lead to multisystem organ failure.

Anatomy

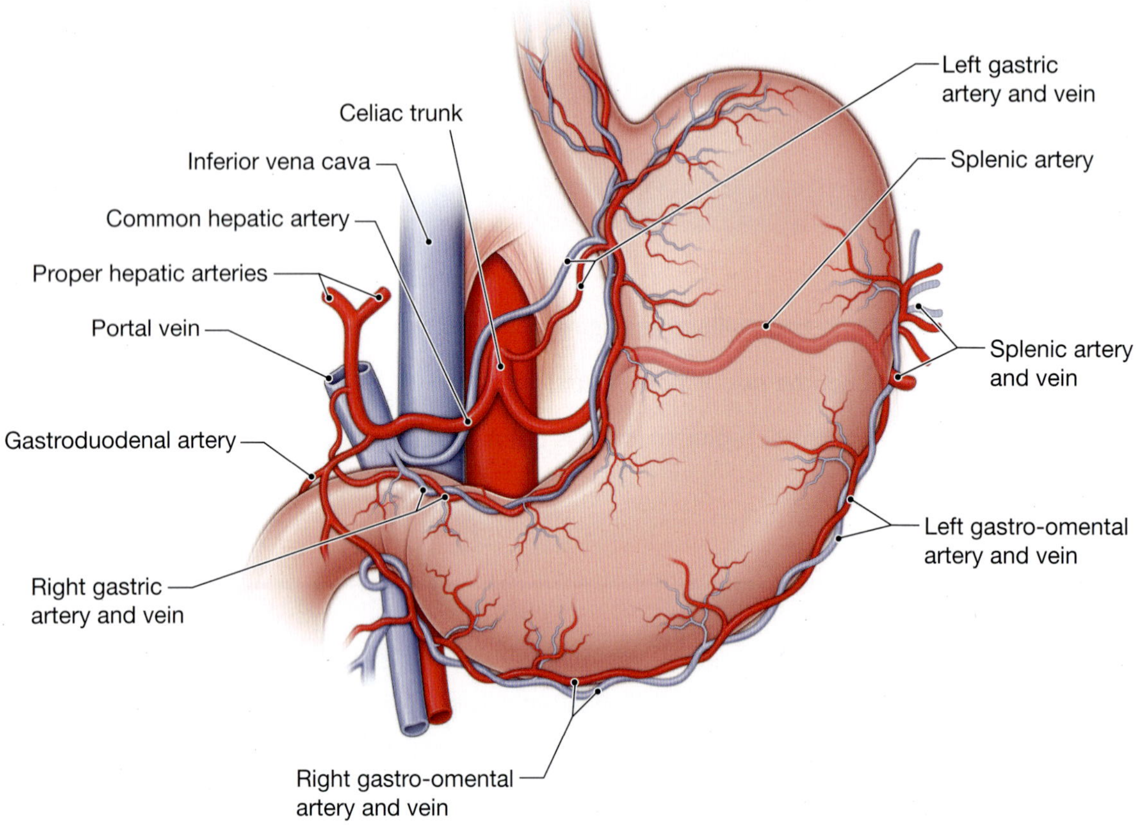

Figure 12-1

TABLE 12-1. American Association for the Surgery of Trauma (AAST) Organ Injury Scale

Grade	AAST Injury Scale - Stomach	
I	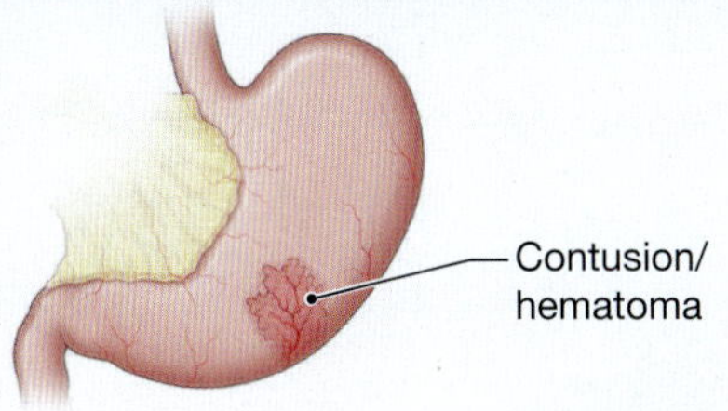	Grade I: Contusion/Hematoma or Partial Thickness Laceration with no gastric spillage
II	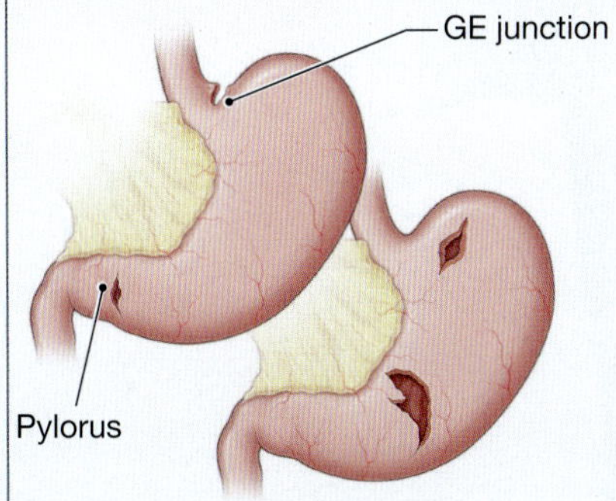	Grade II: Laceration < 2 cm in gastroesophageal junction or pylorus Laceration < 5 cm in proximal 1/3 stomach Laceration < 10 cm in distal 2/3 stomach
III	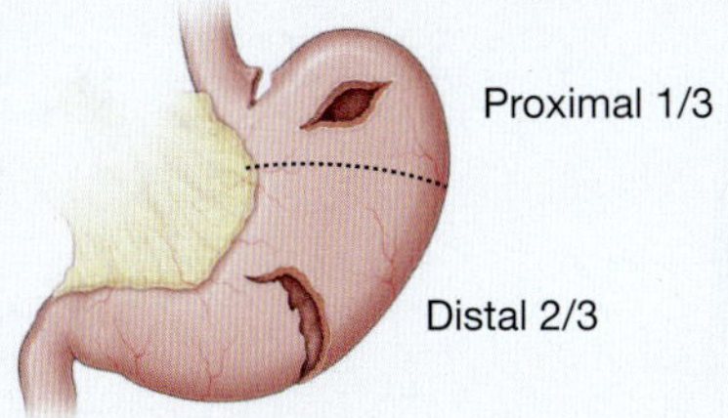	Grade III: Laceration > 2 cm in gastroesophageal junction or pylorus Laceration > 5 cm in proximal 1/3 stomach Laceration > 10 cm in distal 2/3 stomach
IV	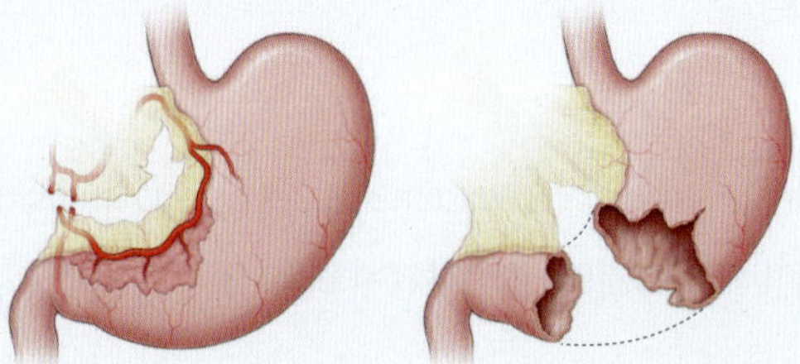	Grade IV: Tissue Loss or Devascularization < 2/3 stomach
V	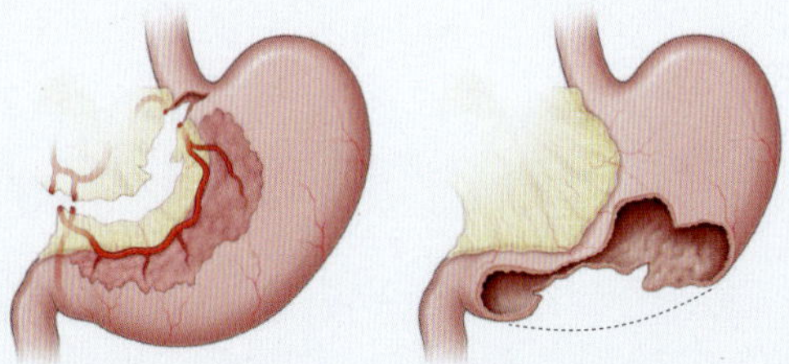	Grade V: Tissue Loss or Devascularization > 2/3 stomach

Source: Data from Organ injury scaling. VI: Extrahepatic biliary, esophagus, stomach, vulva, vagina, uterus (nonpregnant), uterus (pregnant), fallopian tube, and ovary. Moore EE, Jurkovich GJ, Knudson MM, et al. *J Trauma*. 1995;39(6):1069-1070.

Operative Steps

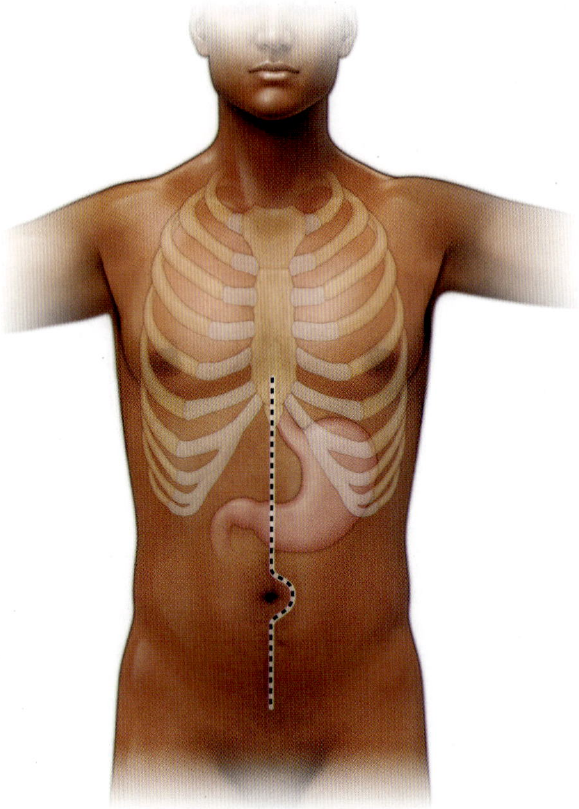

Figure 12-2

Place the patient in the supine position with the arms out 90 degrees. Prep from the chin to knees and proceed with a midline laparotomy incision. Note that you may need to extend toward xiphoid.

Adequate exposure is key, and a retractor system can be very helpful. Always enter the lesser sac to examine the posterior wall of the stomach (Figure 12-3A, B).

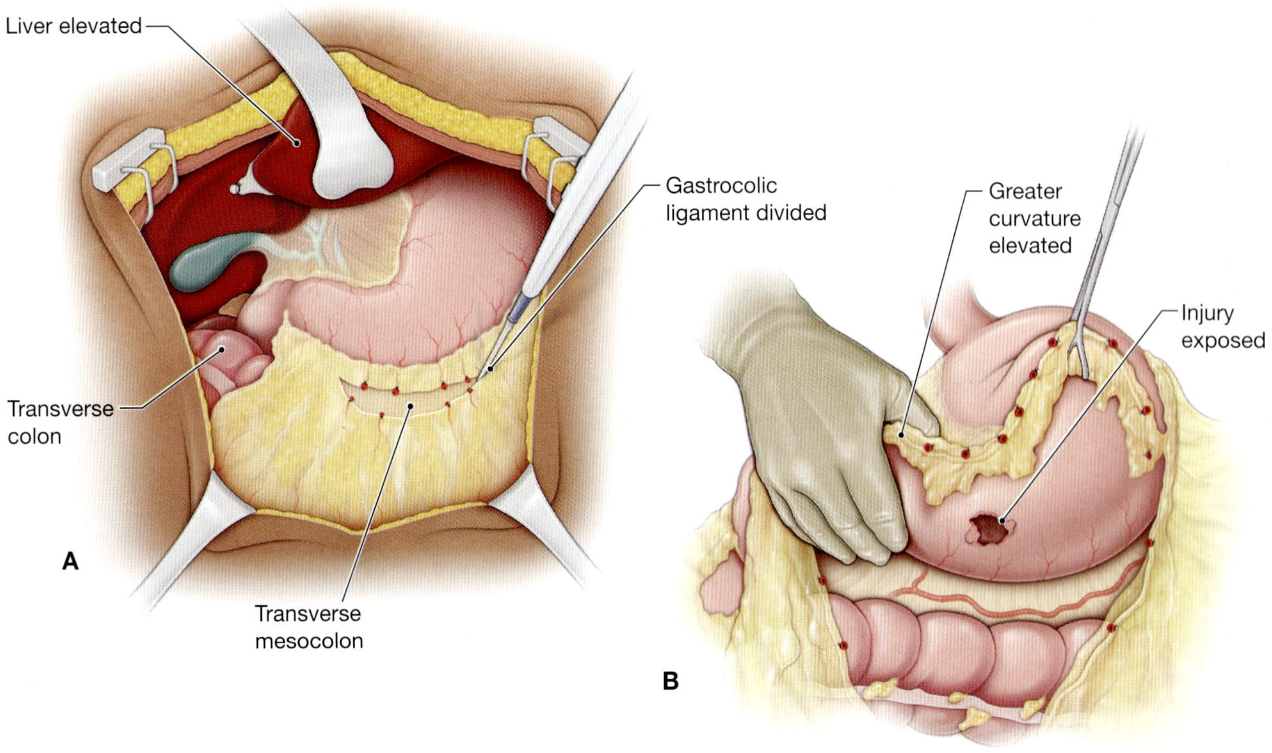

Figure 12-3

Gastrorrhaphy

Gastrorrhaphy is performed primarily with single- or two-layered closure after debridement of devitalized tissue. The first layer is running and must be full-thickness bites with eversion of the mucosa using 3-0 Vicryl. The second layer is composed of interrupted 3-0 silk Lembert sutures (Figure 12-4).

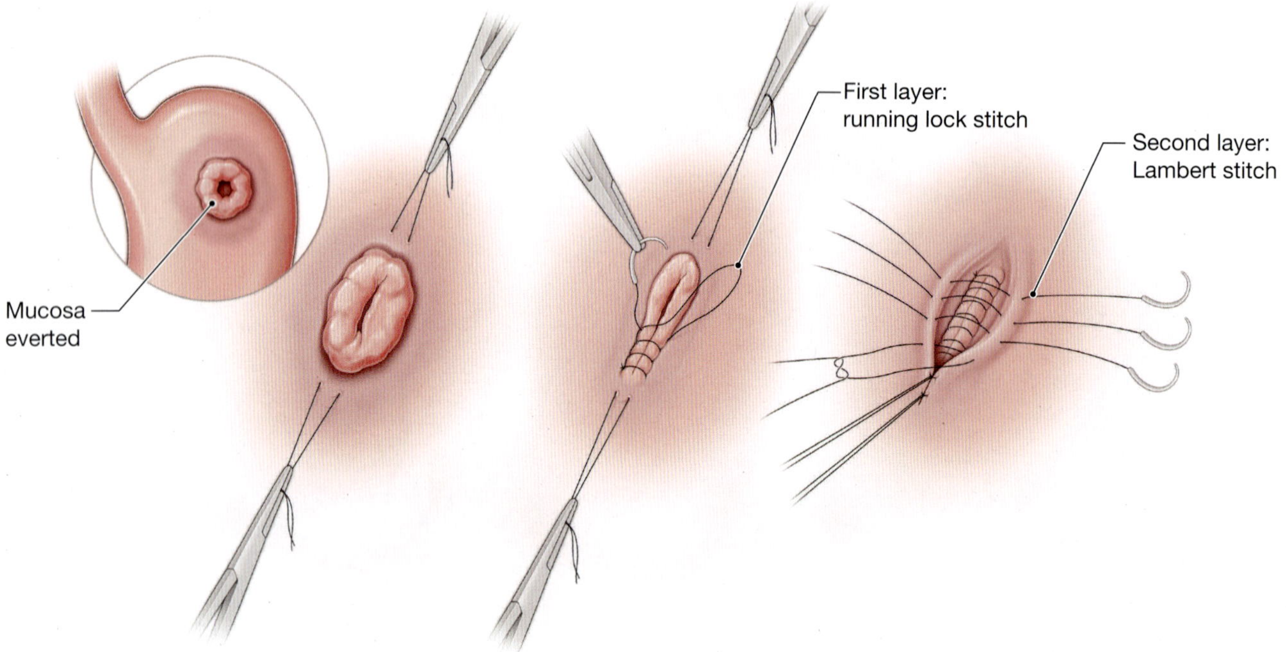

Figure 12-4

Wedge Resection

Wedge resection with a linear cutting stapler can be used for single lacerations or multiple lacerations near each other. This is particularly useful on the body of the stomach and often can be taken with one firing of the stapler (Figure 12-5).

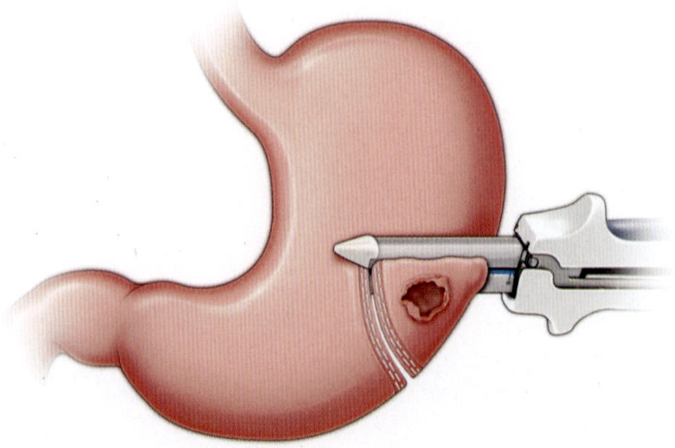

Figure 12-5

Antrectomy

Injuries at or near the pylorus require antrectomy with Billroth I or II reconstruction. This is necessary because primary repair frequently leads to stenosis. The gastrocolic ligament and lesser omentum are incised at the midpoint of the curvature. A Penrose drain can be used for retraction. Gastroepiploic vessels are divided along the greater curve toward the duodenum. A Kocher maneuver is performed to fully mobilize the duodenum. Dissection continues along the lesser curve dividing vessels until the level of the third vein. The duodenum is divided with a linear cutting stapler. The distal stomach is divided just proximal to the injury with a TA90 stapler (Figure 12-6A, B).

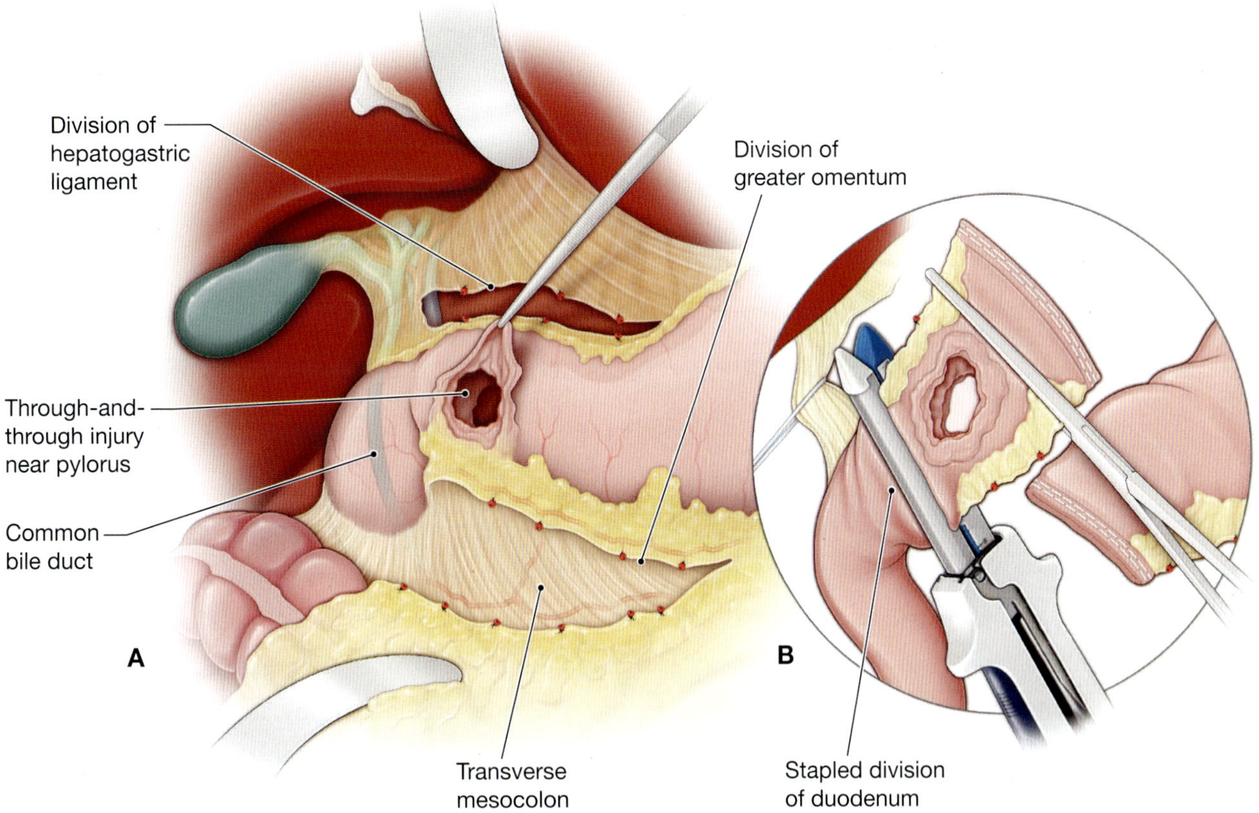

Figure 12-6 A, B

Billroth I

A gastrotomy is performed at the lower portion of the gastric remnant, and enterotomy is performed on the adjacent lying duodenum. A posterior layer of 3-0 silk interrupted Lembert sutures is placed. The inner layer is then closed with a running layer of 3-0 Vicryl. An anterior layer of 3-0 silk interrupted Lembert sutures is placed. The anastomosis is checked for patency.

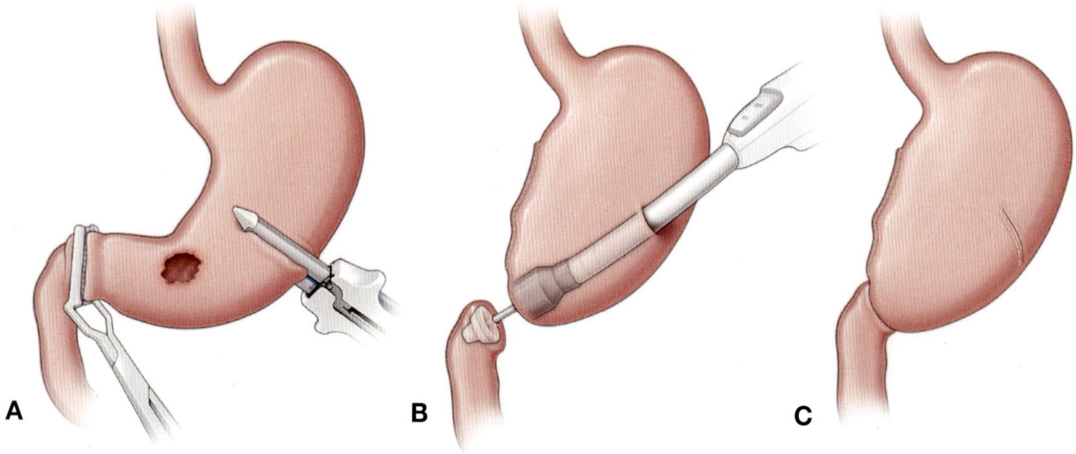

Figure 12-7. Billroth I reconstruction using staplers.

Billroth II

The ligament of Treitz is palpated and a mobile piece of jejunum brought up to lie adjacent to the gastric remnant in an antecolic fashion. Stay sutures are used to maintain this relationship. A gastrotomy is performed along the greater curve of the gastric remnant and enterotomy on the adjacent lying jejunum. A posterior row of 2-0 sutures is placed between the jejunum and the stomach. Then, an inner running absorbable suture is used. This stitch is continued to the anterior wall for complete closure. A set of Lembert sutures completes the anastomosis. Place a stay suture at the anastomosis to the mesocolon to anchor it.

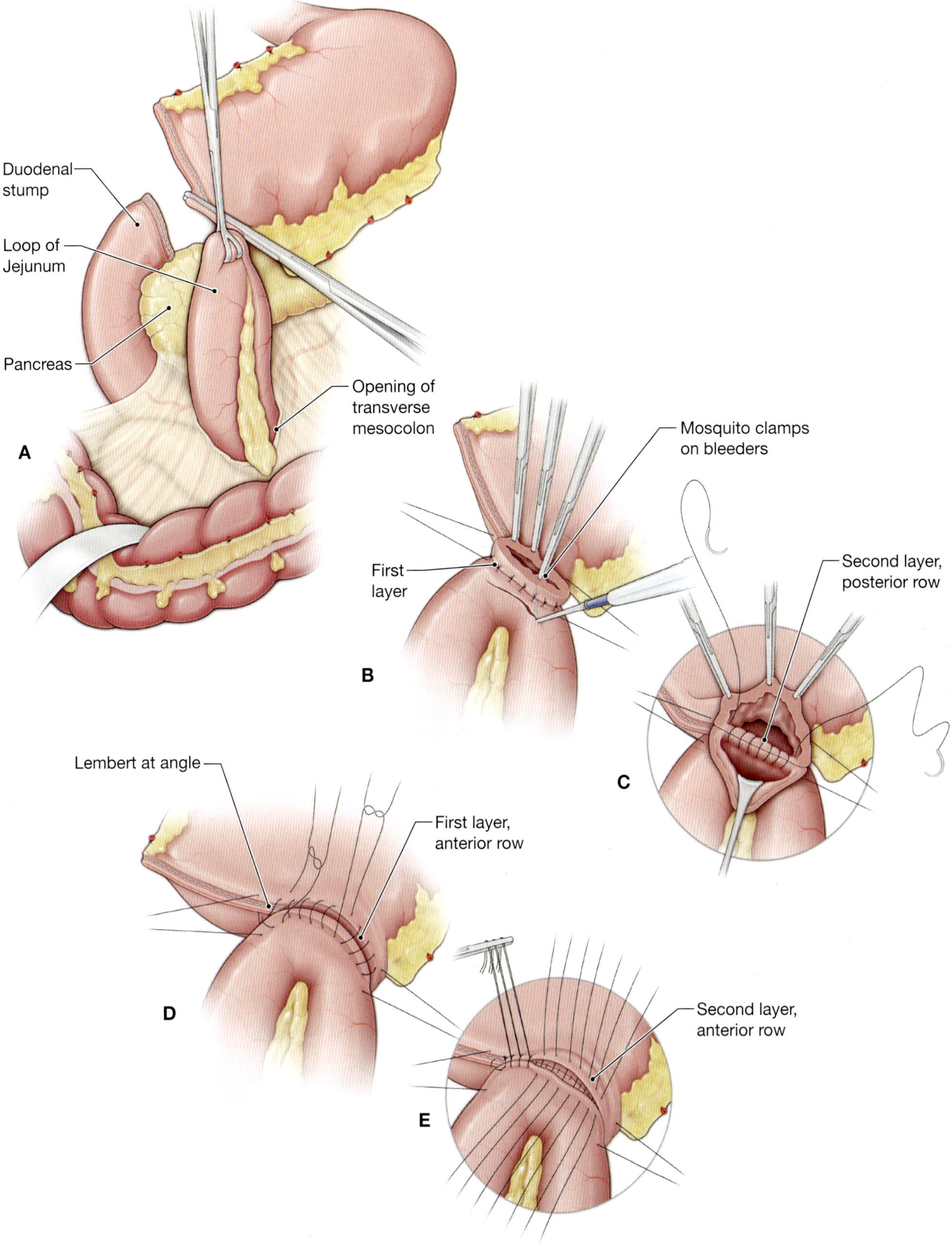

Figure 12-8 A-E

A linear cutting stapler is used to create a common lumen. The common enterotomy is closed with a linear cutting stapler. Of note, two-layered suture closure can be substituted for the two fires of the stapler. Note that the duodenal stump must be oversewn as shown in a Billroth II reconstruction.

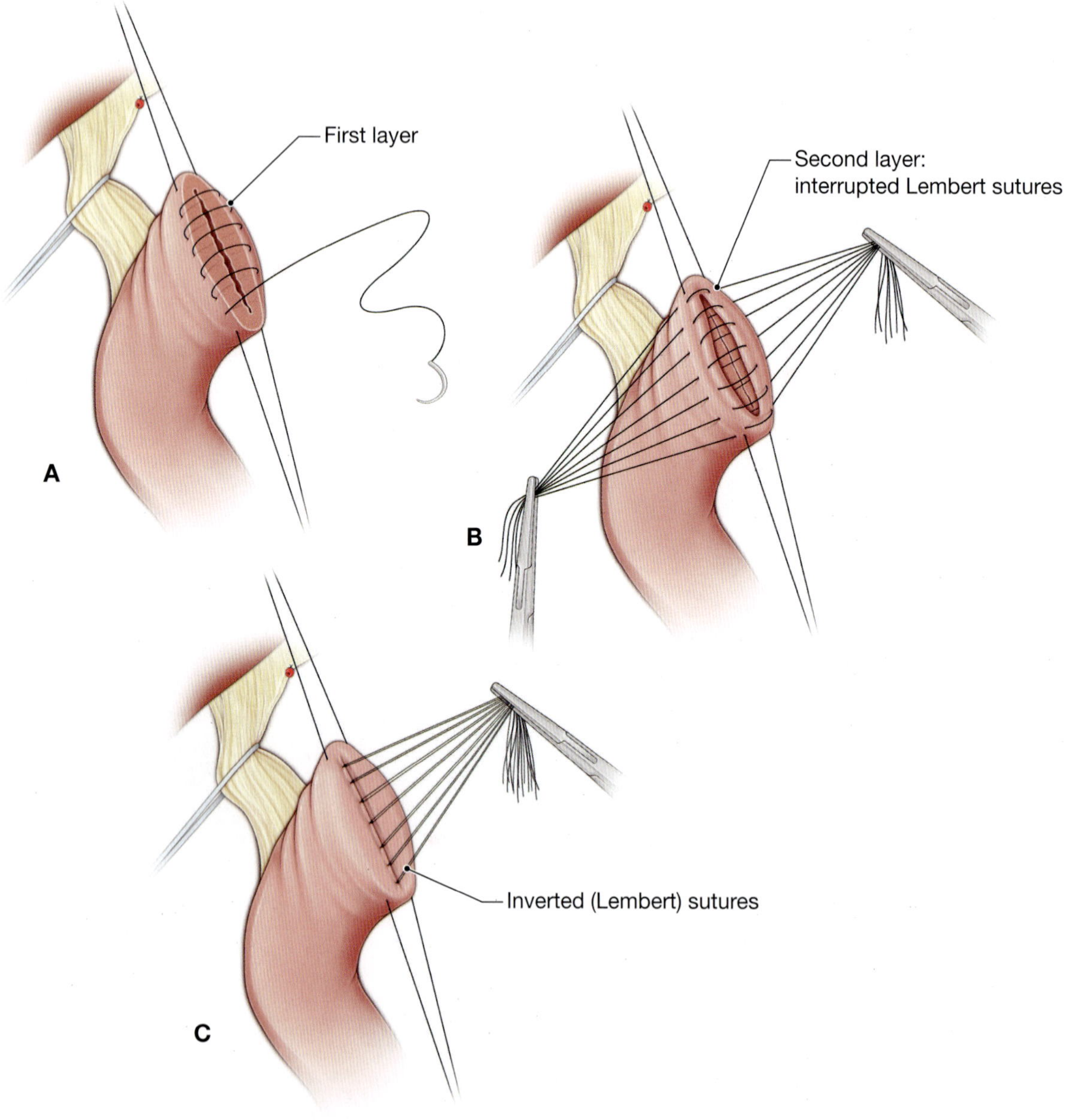

Figure 12-9 A-C. Closure of the duodenal stump.

A GIA staple can be used to close the duodenum, and an EEA staple can be used for the anastomosis.

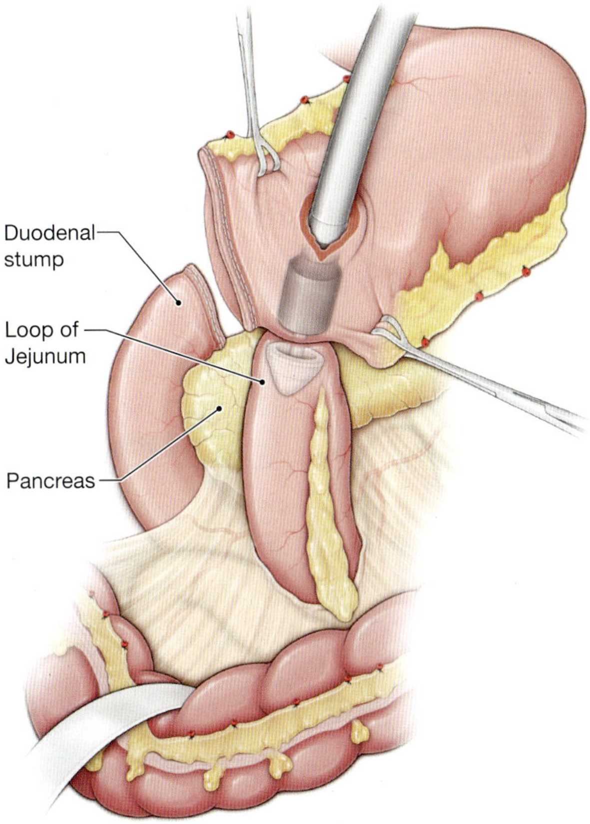

Figure 12-10

Gastrectomy

Proximal or total gastrectomy can be necessary due to position of injury or extent of devitalization (Figure 12-11). Similar dissection and division are continued as above for antrectomy. The triangular ligament is taken down and the left lobe of the liver folded upon itself. Dissect the posterior peritoneal attachments to free the esophagus circumferentially. An EEA stapler can be used to create a common lumen between the esophagus and gastric remnant or esophagus and jejunum. The anvil is placed in the distal esophagus and purse string tied. A gastrotomy or enterotomy is made and the stapler inserted. The pin perforates the wall and is secured to the anvil. After firing the stapler, check for continuity of the two rings (Figure 12-12A-C).

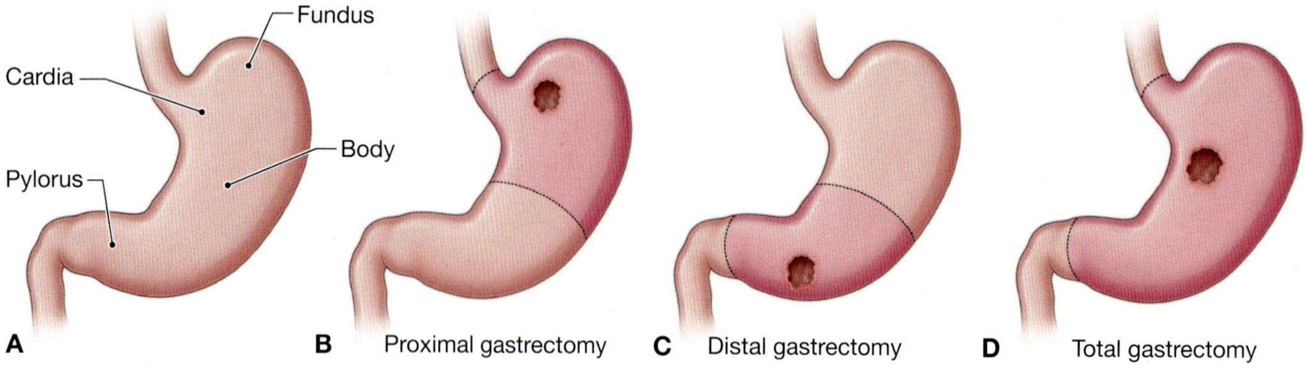

Figure 12-11

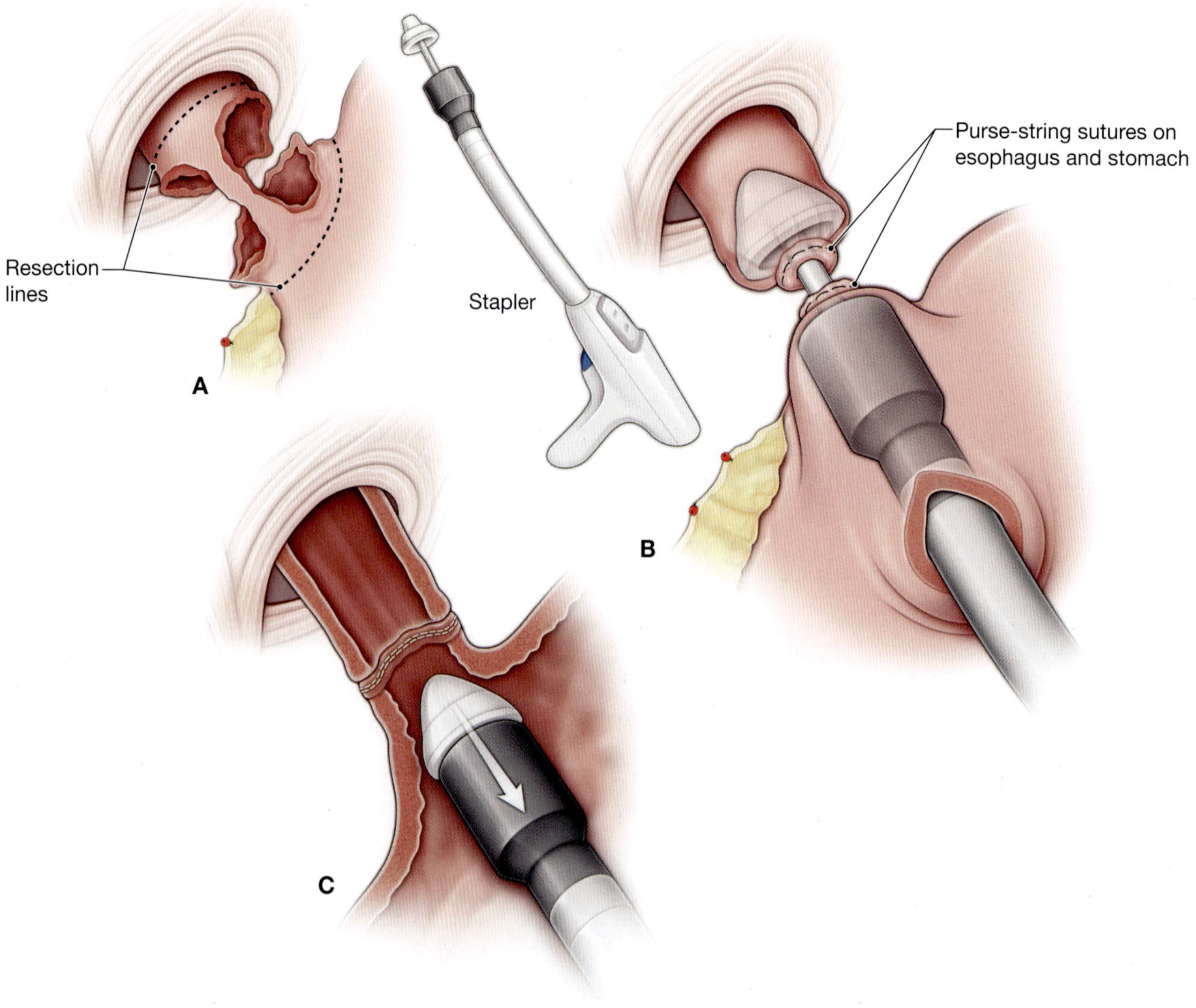

Figure 12-12 A-C

Roux-en-Y

In addition to the Billroth I and II reconstructions, the Roux-en-Y reconstruction can also be utilized. It requires two anastomoses and the duodenal stump, which can confuse the postoperative picture if any of the three staple lines leak (Figure 12-13A, B).

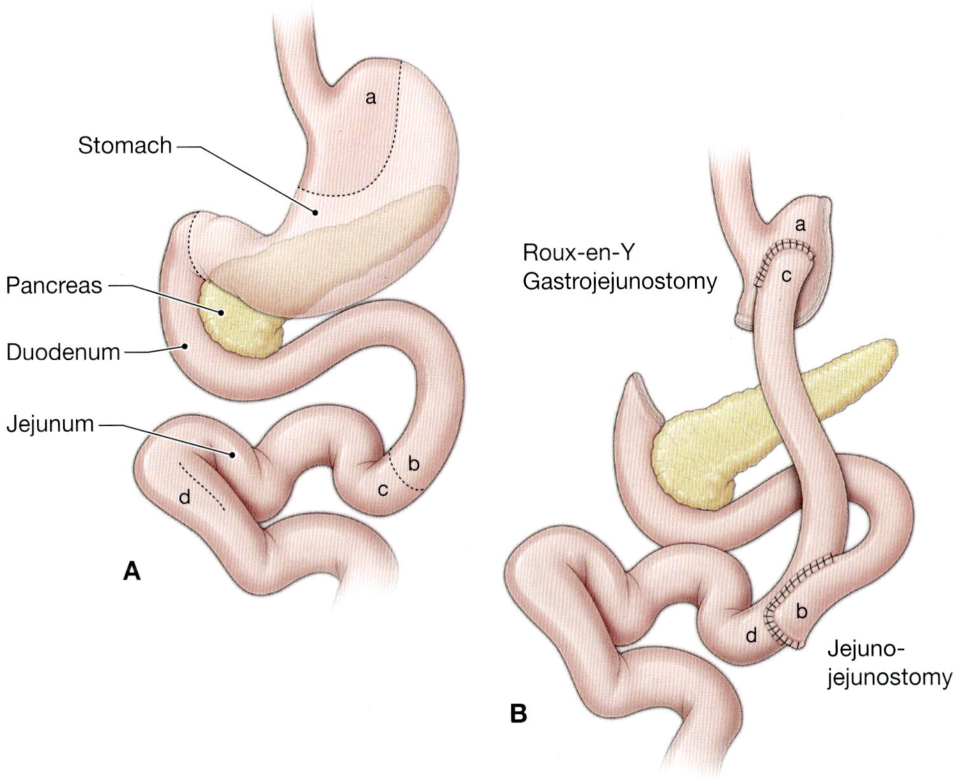

Figure 12-13 A, B

Complications

Due to the high acidity of the stomach, there are not too many bacteria, so acute bacterial growth is low on perforation. However, spillage of gastric content will produce severe peritonitis due to the acidity. Many of these patients will quickly develop an acute abdomen and signs of peritonitis on exam. Even after exploration and repair, a copious amount of irrigation must be undertaken. The spillage content will cause an inflammatory reaction with possibility of abscess formation. If missed or left untreated, the patient will develop sepsis that can quickly lead to multiorgan failure.

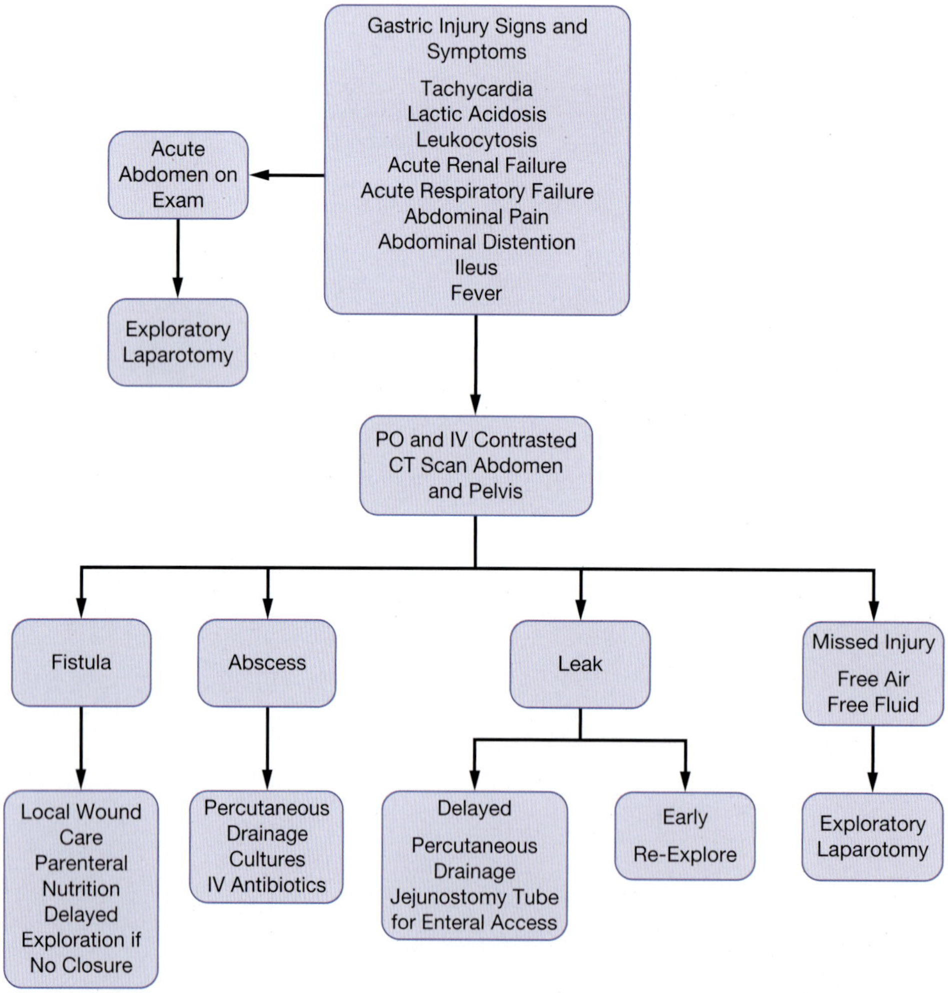

Figure 12-14

13 DUODENAL TRAUMA

Dale A. Dangleben, MD, FACS
Anthony Lam, DO

TIPS

1. **Up to 90% of patients with duodenal injury have at least one other associated intra-abdominal organ injury (most frequently involving the liver and pancreas).**
2. **The treatment of duodenal hematomas can be conservative (with nasogastric suction and intravenous fluids) until the hematoma resolves.**

Introduction

Duodenal trauma accounts for 0.5% of blunt abdominal trauma and 0.1% all blunt trauma mechanisms. Despite being an uncommon injury, it can be extremely devastating if missed. It is imperative that the diagnosis is made promptly. Imaging with computed tomography scan is the main modality for diagnosis in hemodynamically stable blunt trauma patients. The mainstay for penetrating injuries is thorough surgical exploration. During exploration, duodenal injury is identified in up to 5% of patients. A deep understanding of duodenal anatomy is important, along with knowing that the majority of these injuries are at the second portion.

During laparotomy, there are key findings that raise suspicion for an associated duodenal injury. These are bile staining, edema or fluid in the lesser sac, retroperitoneal hematoma, saponification, and peripancreatic edema, especially in the head of the pancreas.

Mortality in duodenal injuries (2%-5%) is due to delay in diagnosis leading to sepsis and multiorgan failure and other associated injuries. It has been shown that associated pancreatic, splenic, thoracic, or abdominal vascular injury, hypothermia <35°C, Injury Severity Score >25, and >5 units of blood transfusion portend high risk of mortality.

It is imperative to identify all critical injuries in a timely manner and follow the principles of damage control where indicated.

Anatomy

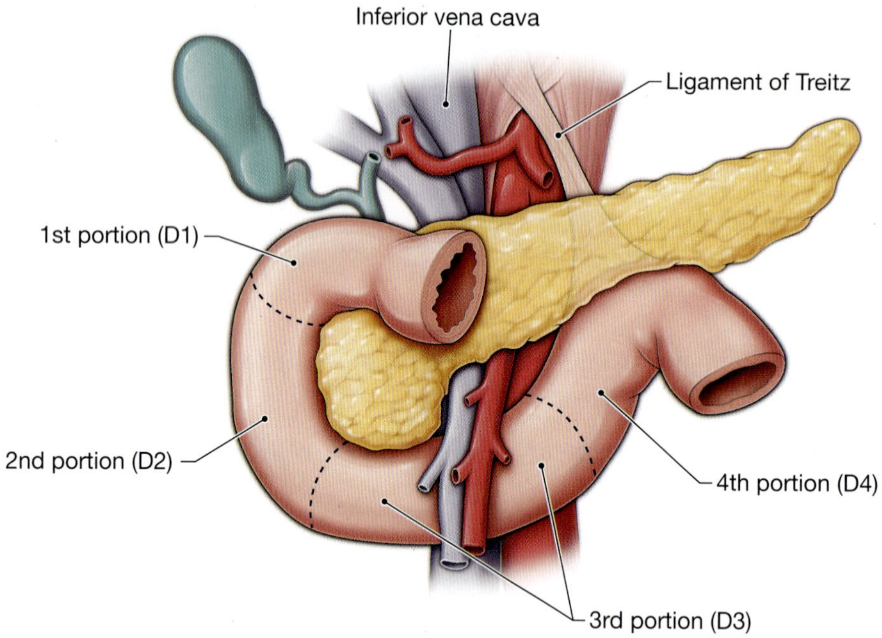

Figure 13-1

TABLE 13-1. American Association for the Surgery of Trauma (AAST) Injury Grades

Grade	AAST Injury Scale - Duodenum
Grade I	• Intramural hematoma < 50% length • Partial-thickness leak 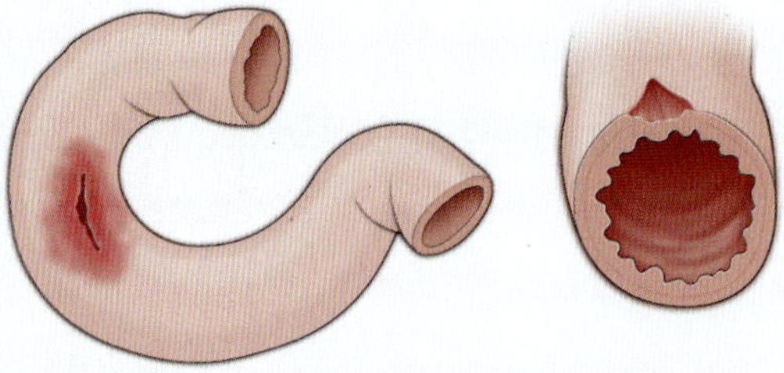
Grade II	• Intramural hematoma > 50% length • Laceration < 50% circumference 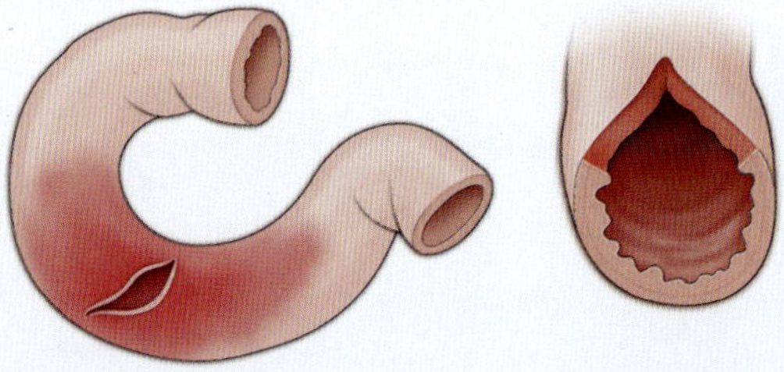
Grade III	• Laceration > 50% circumference, any segment • Transection of D1, D3, D4 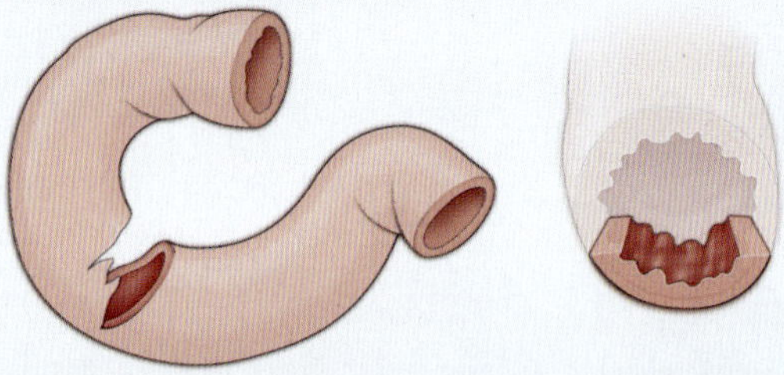
Grade IV	• Laceration > 75% circumference of D2 • Partial-thickness leak 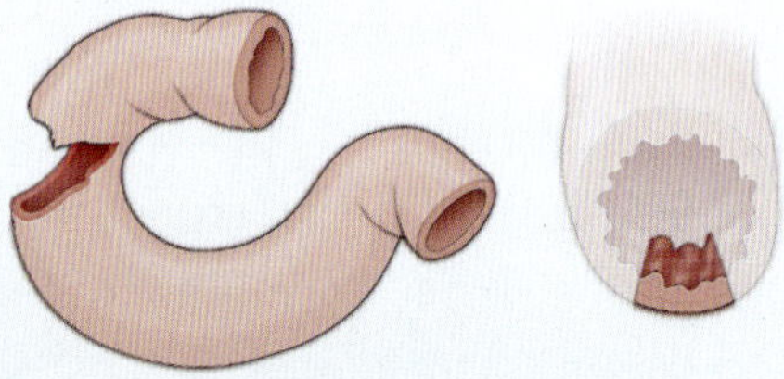 • Transection of ampulla 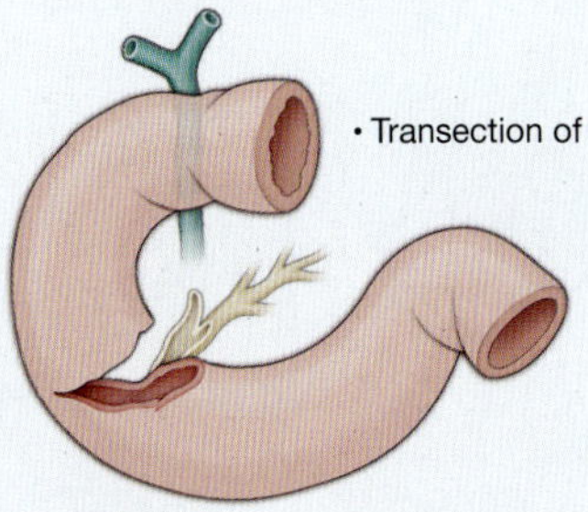 • Transection of intrapancreatic common bile duct 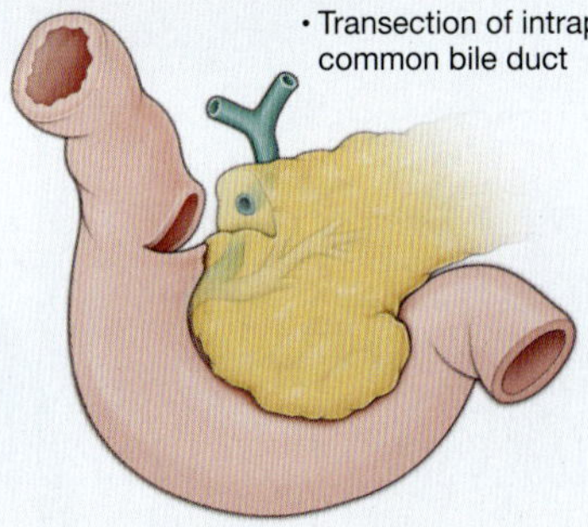
Grade V	• Duodenal devascularization • Combined duodeno-pancreatic injury 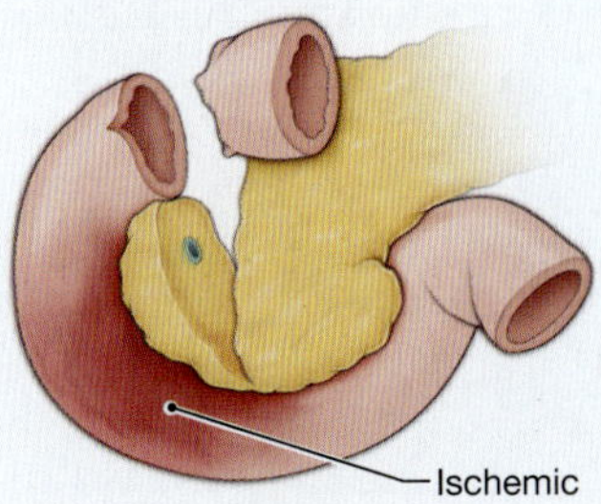

Source: Reproduced with permission from Moore EE, Cogbill TH, Malangoni MA, et al. Organ injury scaling, II: Pancreas, duodenum, small bowel, colon, and rectum. *J Trauma*. 1990;30(11):1427-9..

Duodenal Mobilization

The first step in the operative management of the injured duodenum is to perform the Kocher maneuver (Figure 13-2A). This mobilization allows the duodenum to be medialized. The duodenum is dissected from the common bile duct to the superior mesenteric vein (SMV). This allows exposure of the pancreatic head and the second and some of the third portions of the duodenum. This will allow access to the underlying vena cava in that area (Figure 13-2B). Further exposure of adjacent structures and an improved workspace can be developed by extending the incision in the posterior peritoneum caudad along the white line of Toldt and mobilizing the right colon (Figure 13-2A, B).

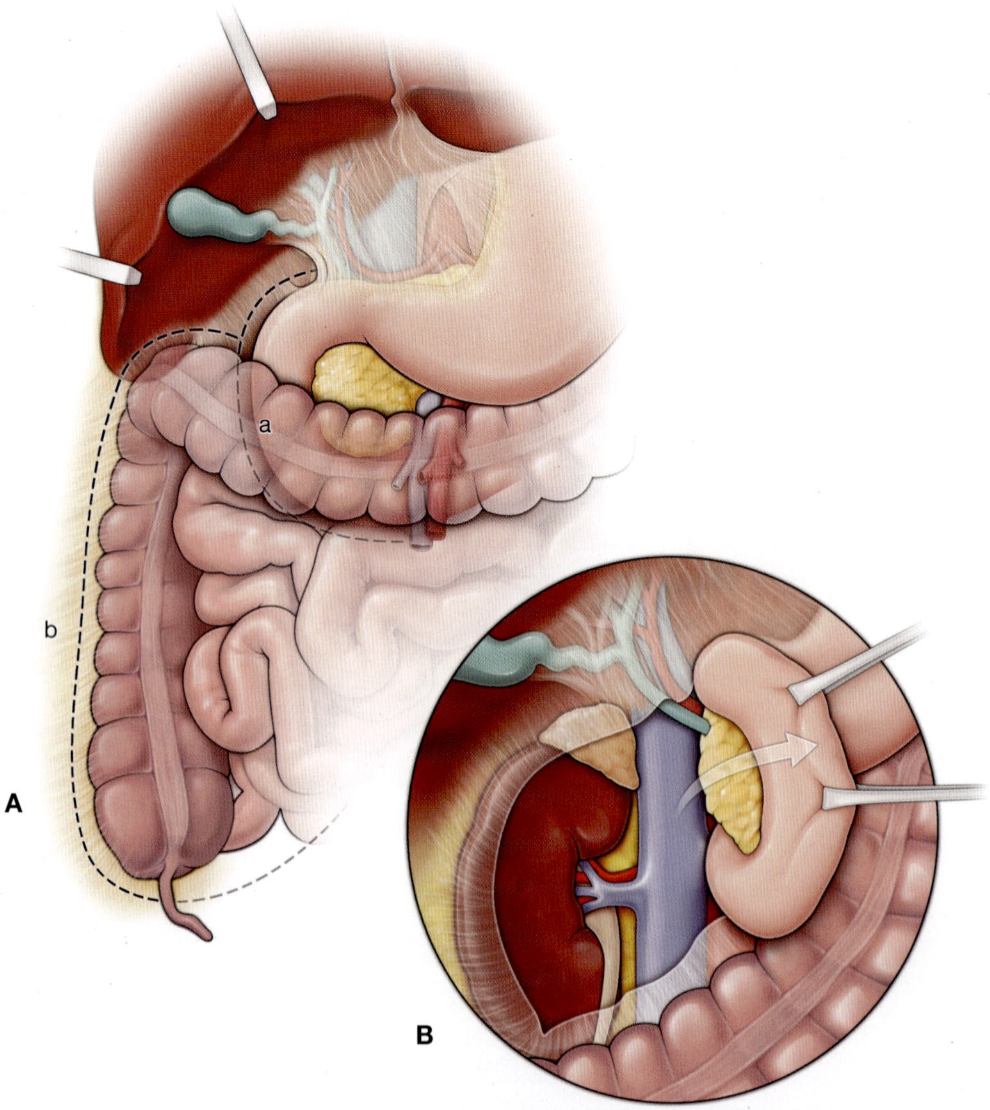

Figure 13-2 A, B

Cattell-Braasch Maneuver (Right Medial Visceral Rotation)

This exposes the entire inframesocolic retroperitoneal organs, including the inferior vena cava (IVC), the right renal pedicle, the right iliac vessels, the duodenum, and the head of the pancreas. The maneuver begins with dissecting the hepatic flexure and then dividing along the white line of Toldt (Figure 13-3A). This allows for the incision of the avascular plane between the small bowel mesentery and the posterior peritoneum. At this stage, gentle traction in the cephalad direction permits the extensive medial mobilization of the entire right colon and small bowel (Figure 13-3B).

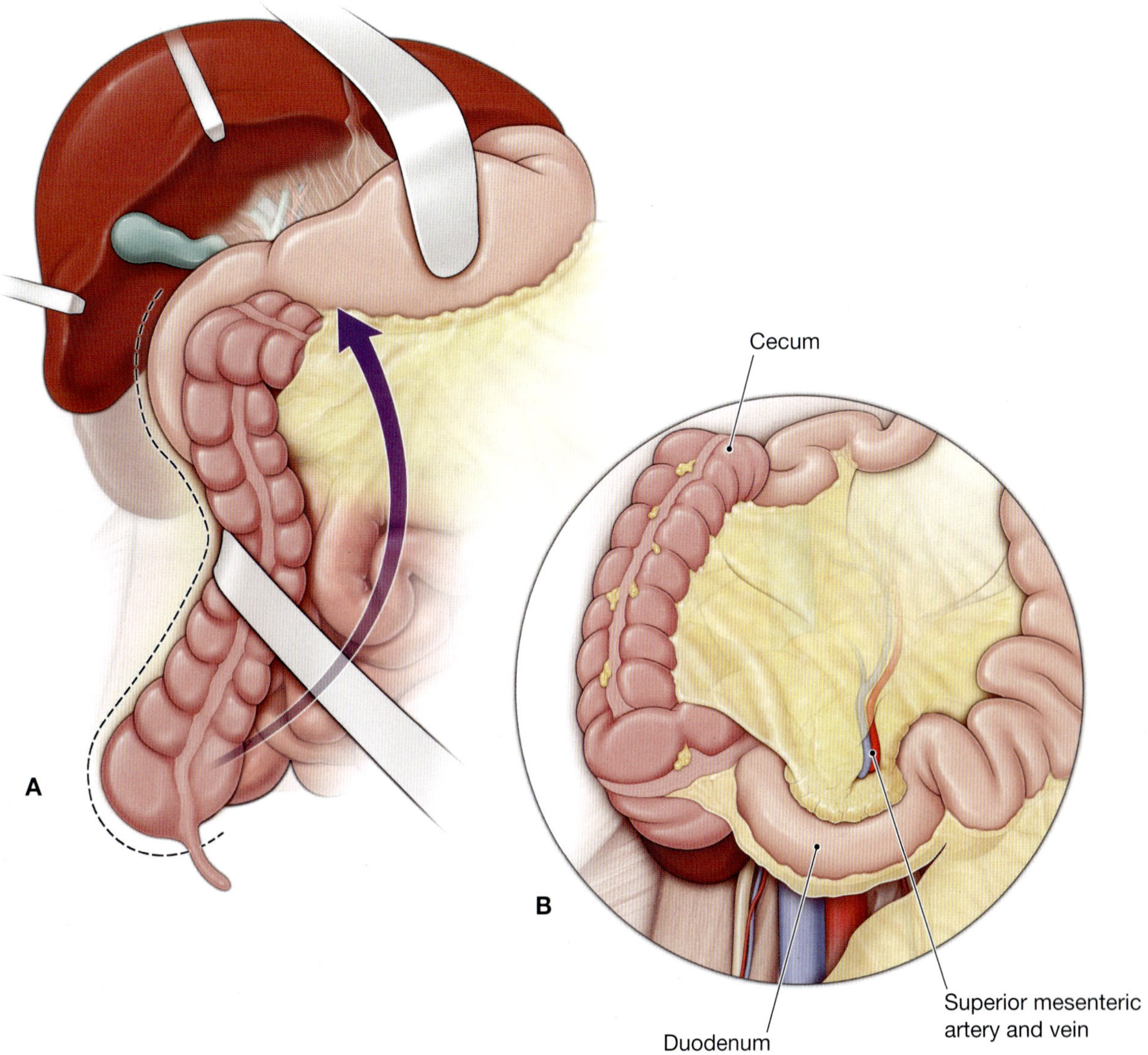

Figure 13-3 A, B

Duodenal Hematoma

In the case of intraoperative identification of a duodenal hematoma, a Kocher maneuver or Cattel-Braasch maneuver should be performed, and the duodenum should be extensively evaluated for any evidence of perforation. If no evidence for perforation is identified, the duodenal hematoma can be managed conservatively. If a high suspicion of a full-thickness injury or narrowing of the small bowel lumen >50% is suspected, then evacuation of the hematoma is indicated via a seromuscular incision overlying the hematoma (Figure 13-4A, B).

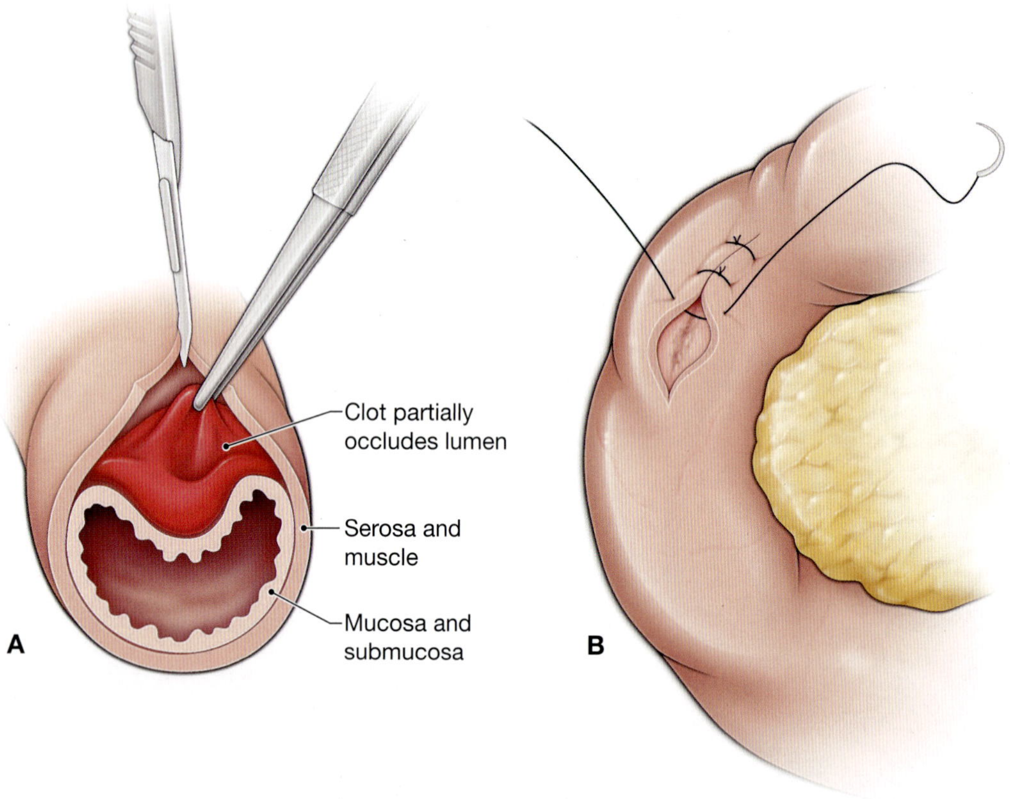

Figure 13-4 A, B

Duodenorrhaphy

For grade II duodenal injuries, primary closure can usually be achieved. A double-layer closure is performed. The inner layer incorporates the mucosa, and that can be achieved with a 3-0 absorbable suture. The seromuscular layer can be done with a 4-0 nonabsorbable such as silk. Of note, close the injury in the direction of the injury itself whether longitudinal or oblique (Figure 13-5).

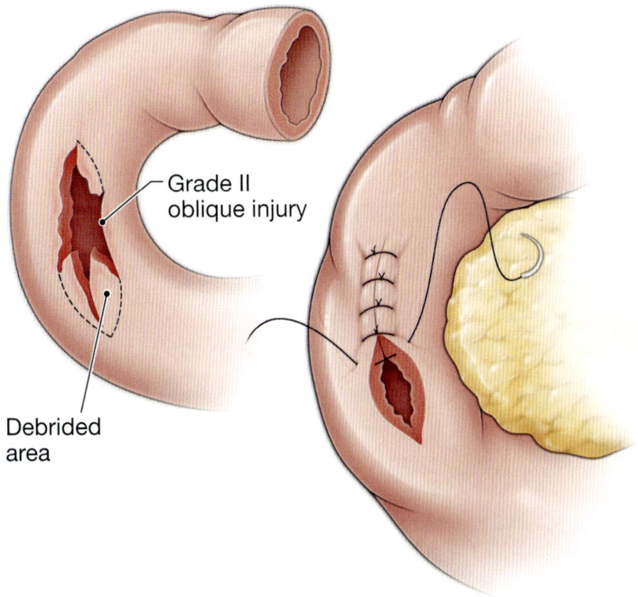

Figure 13-5

Duodenoduodenostomy

If there is a >50% circumference laceration or a transection of D1, 3, or 4, then consider an end-to-end anastomosis (duodenoduodenostomy) (Figure 13-6A). This is achieved with a two-layer closure starting with the posterior wall seromuscular layer in interrupted fashion with 3-0 or 4-0 silk (Figure 13-6B). Once this is done, then the inner layer can be done with a running absorbable suture (Figure 13-6C). The final step of the anastomosis will be the anterior layer using Lembert suture technique (Figure 13-6D).

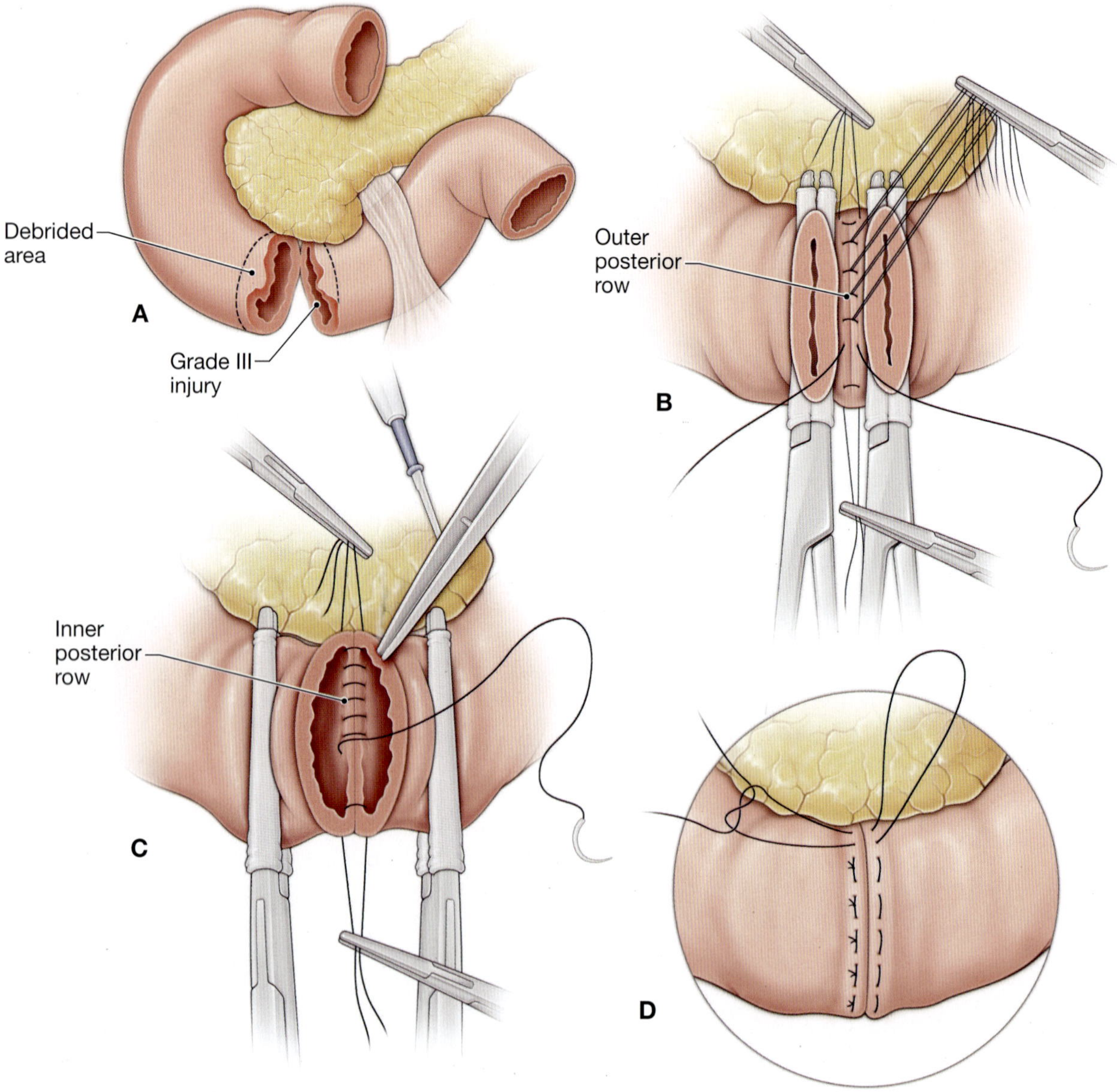

Figure 13-6 A-D

Duodenoenterostomy

There will be circumstances where primary repair or simple anastomosis will not be achieved. Always determine if the ampulla of Vater is intact. If there is disruption, there has to be consideration for pancreaticoduodenectomy. If the ampulla is intact, a jejunal loop can be used as a patch (Figure 13-7A, B), or a Roux-en-Y duodenojejunostomy (Figure 13-8A-C) can be done.

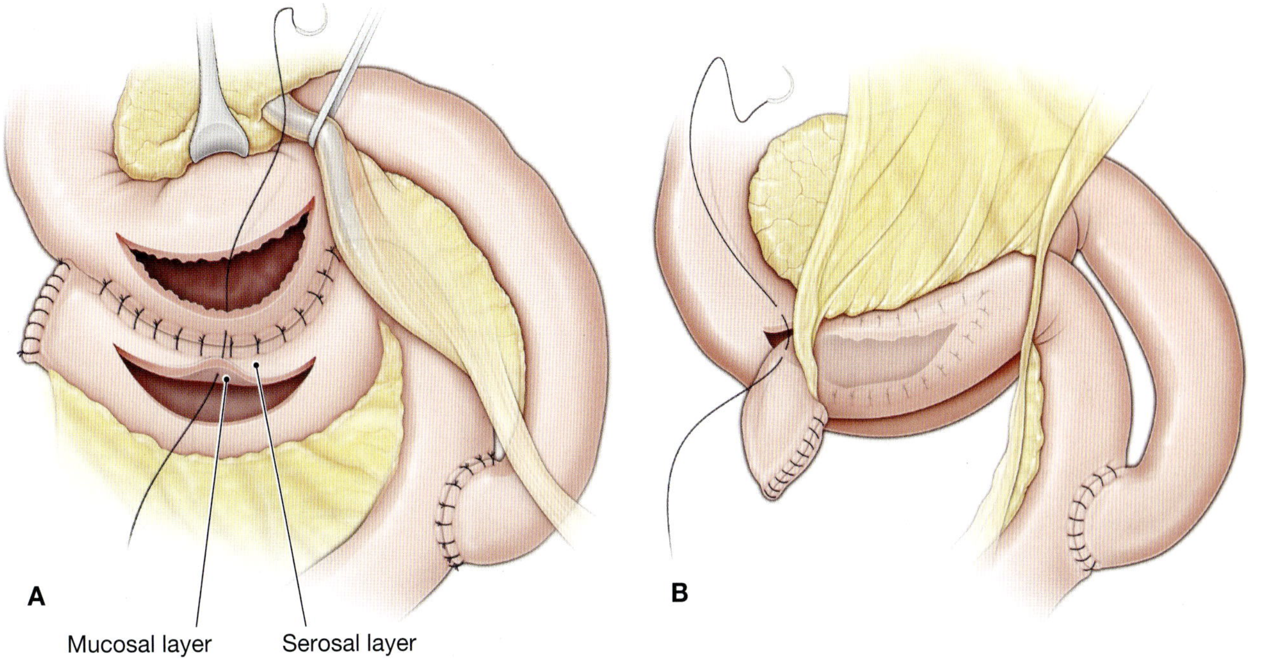

Figure 13-7 A, B

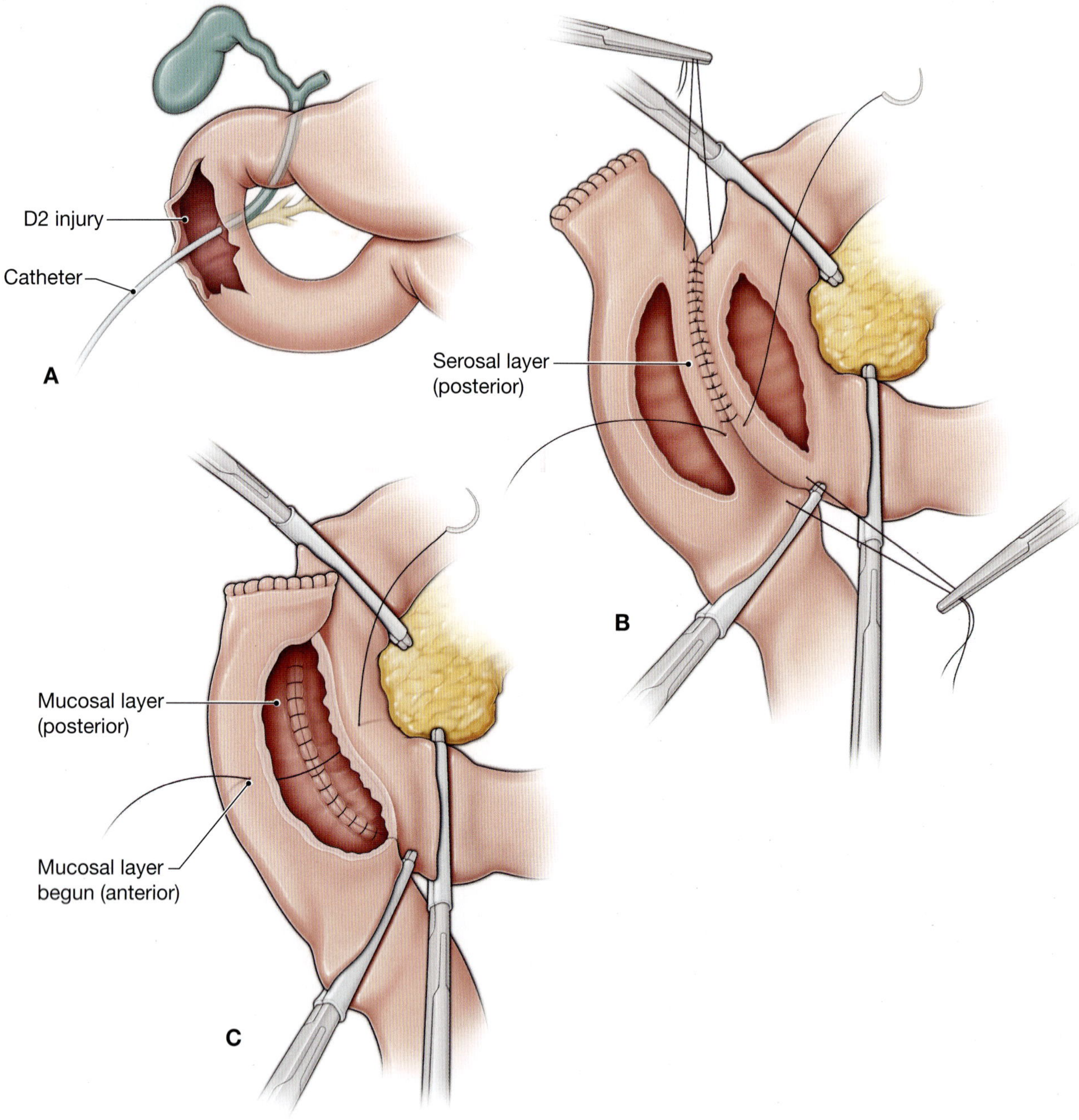

Figure 13-8 **A-C**

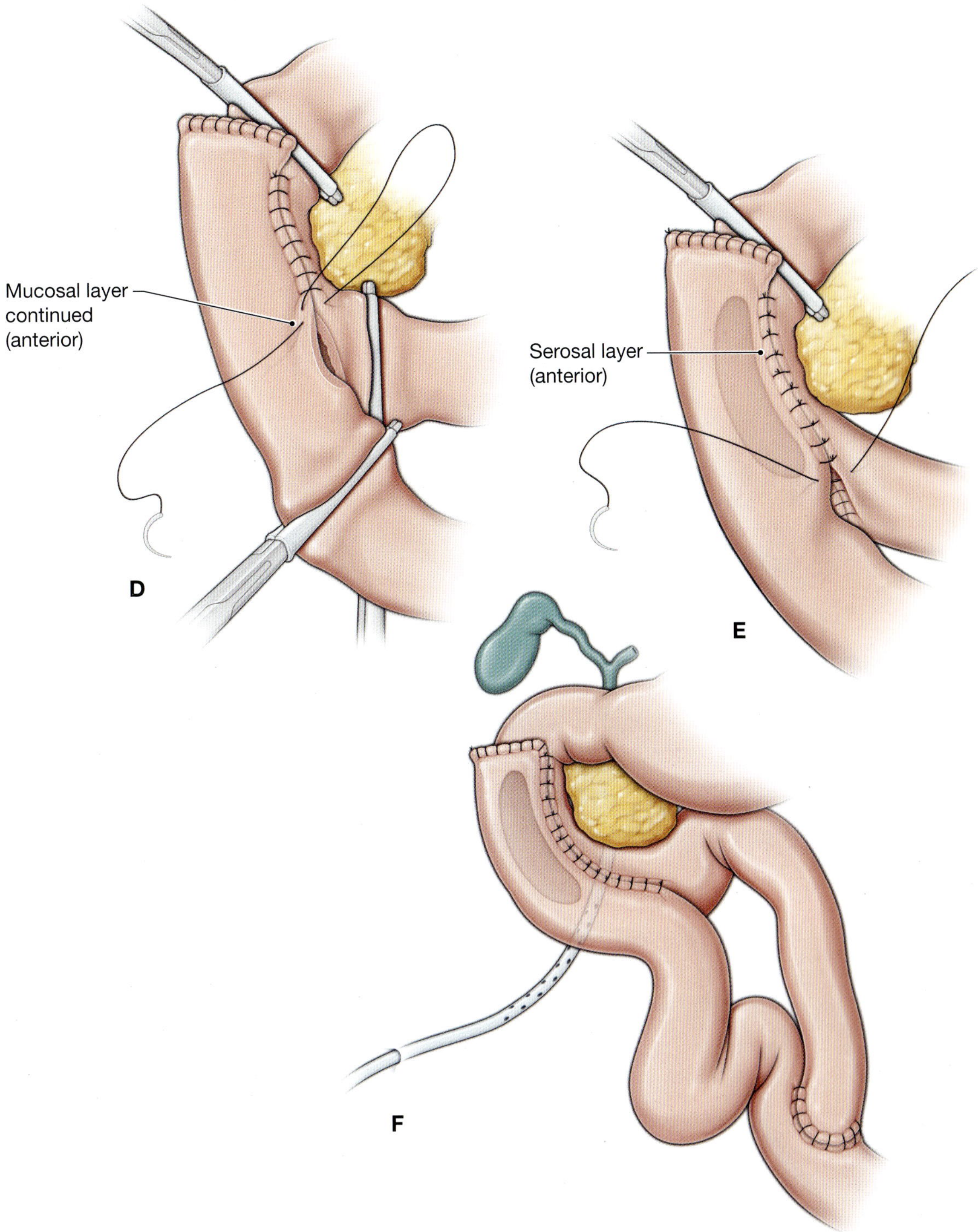

Figure 13-8 D-F

Pyloric Exclusion

There must be a high suspicion of associated hepato-pancreatic injury, especially in grade VI and V injuries. There is a very high complication rate with these injuries. Performing an antrectomy and a gastrojejunostomy is an option here (Figure 13-9A, B). Another option is pyloric exclusion technique. This requires a gastrotomy, grabbing the pylorus with a Babcock, and oversewing the pylorus with an absorbable suture (Figure 13-10A-C). The duodenal injury can be oversewn and drained. A gastro-jejunostomy is then performed.

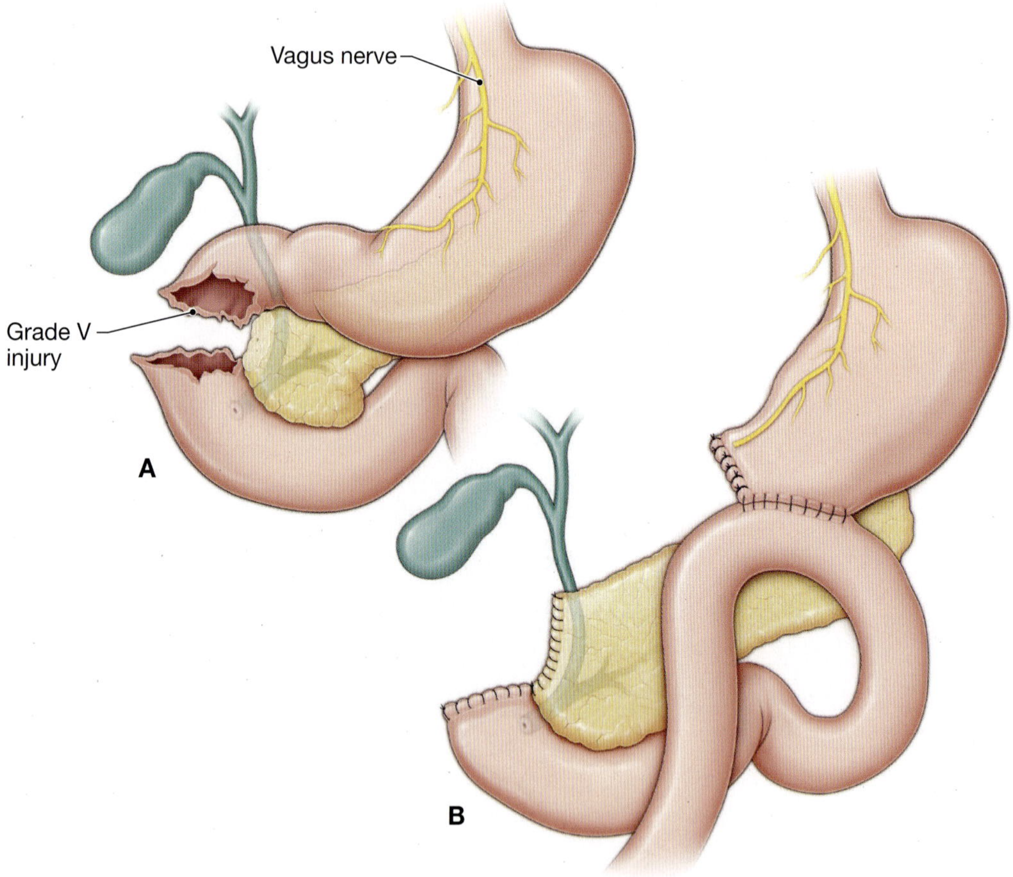

Figure 13-9 A, B

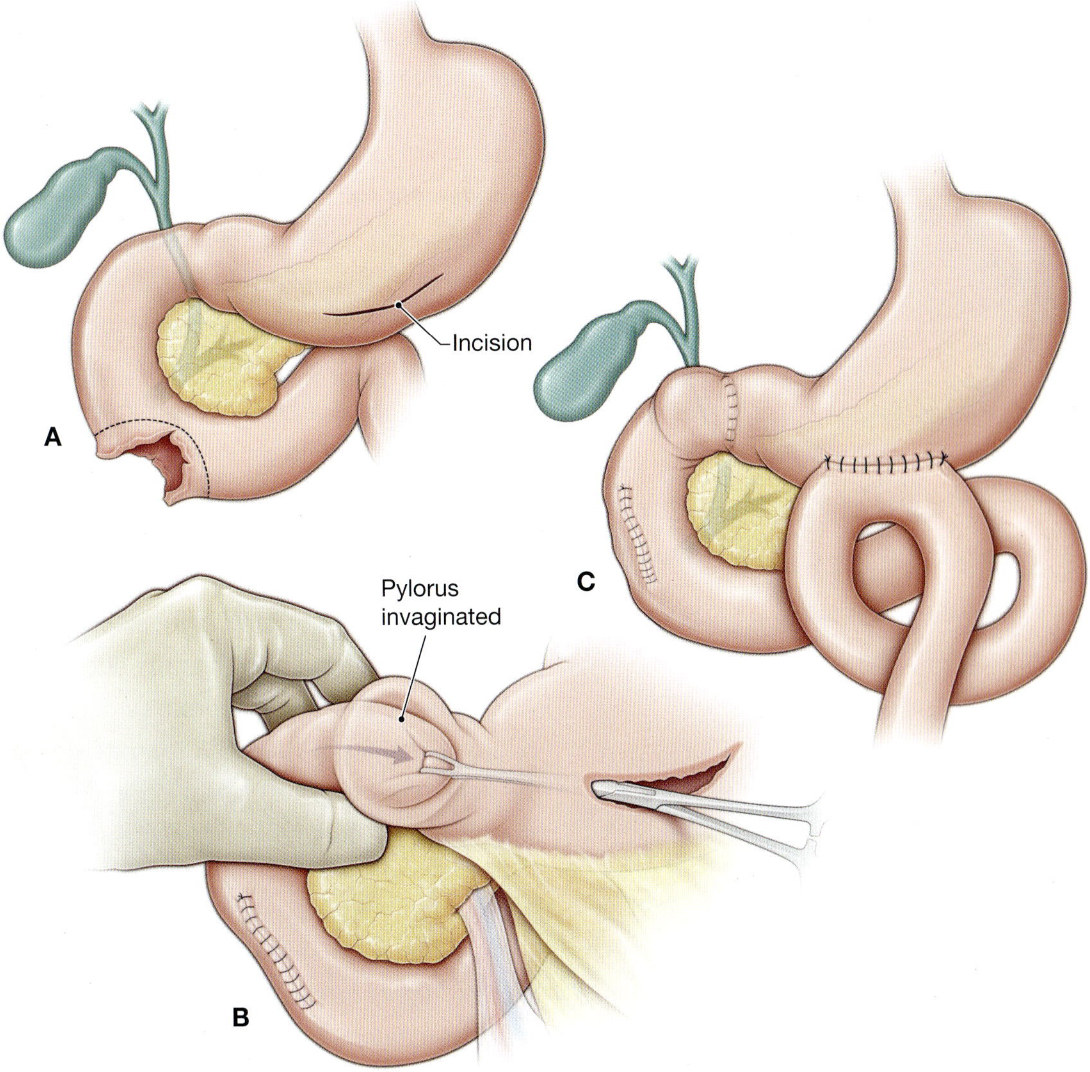

Figure 13-10 A-C

An alternate approach for pyloric exclusion is to utilize a TA stapler and fire at the pylorus without dividing the stomach staple line (Figure 13-11).

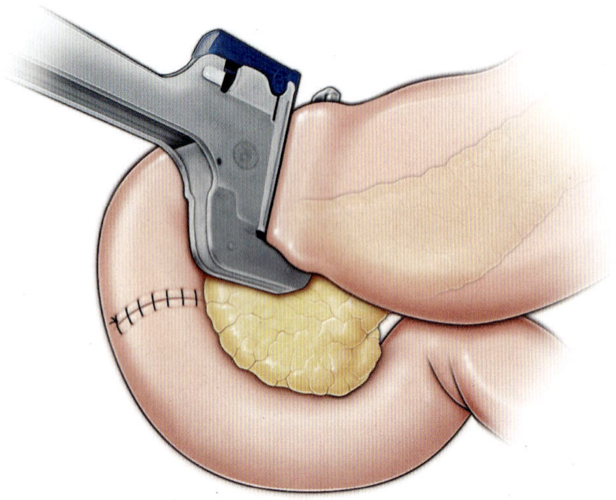

Figure 13-11

Complications

Duodenal trauma can lead to several complications, including bleeding, infection, obstruction, and fistulas (abnormal connections between the duodenum and other organs). In addition, the long-term consequences of duodenal injury can include malnutrition, weight loss, and chronic diarrhea.

Simple duodenal hematomas (American Association for the Surgery of Trauma Organ Injury Scale grade I or grade II) identified on imaging can lead to narrowing of the bowel lumen and thus subsequent duodenal obstruction. In the absence of other injuries requiring operative exploration in hemodynamically stable patients, these injuries can be managed nonoperatively. Initial conservative management consists of placing a nasogastric tube for proximal decompression along with total parenteral nutrition until the small bowel edema and swelling resolve. A marked drop in nasogastric tube output preludes resolution of the hematoma and resolving obstruction, which is typically seen within 2 weeks. To evaluate the progression and/or resolution of obstruction, consider performing an interval upper gastrointestinal contrast study. If the obstruction fails to resolve within 3 weeks, surgical interventions may be warranted.

Most duodenal lacerations can be managed with debridement and primary repair in a transverse fashion. If a transverse repair is not feasible, consider repairing the defect in a longitudinal fashion if able to be conducted without significant narrowing of the lumen. If luminal stenosis is of concern, then a gastrojejunostomy should be created along with the primary repair to assist in diverting flow. With injuries that are concerning for >50% circumferential tissue loss or if excessive tension is anticipated, the injury may require segmental resection and advanced reconstruction with a duodenoduodenostomy, duodenojejunostomy, or Roux-en-Y duodenojejunostomy. The second portion of the duodenum is highly susceptible to vascular compromise due to the proximity of the ampulla of Vater and shared blood supply with the pancreas, which may require complex biliary reconstruction of the duodenopancreatic complex.

Development of duodenal fistulas typically results from a failure of surgical repair due to suture line dehiscence. Multiple factors can include inadequate closure of injury, devascularization, inflammation of surrounding tissue, or increased luminal pressure due to distal obstruction. Duodenal fistulas typically heal in 6 to 8 weeks with conservative management of adequate drainage, intra-abdominal sepsis control, and nutritional support. Electrolyte imbalances can often occur and should be carefully monitored. Overall, duodenal fistulas can be one of the more serious and challenging complications associated with intra-abdominal foregut operations. They are coupled with prolonged hospitalization in the postoperative period due to possible related complications of pancreatitis, intra-abdominal abscess formation, surgical site infections, bleeding, severe malnutrition, and dehydration. If conservative management fails, operative reintervention may be required but carries a high perioperative morbidity and mortality rate.

14 SPLEEN

Graham G. Laurence, MD, PhD
Nathan Wong, MD
Dale A. Dangleben, MD, FACS

TIPS

1. **The most expedient maneuver to access the splenic hilum during splenectomy from a midline incision is to medialize the spleen through rapid blunt manual dissection of peritoneal attachments and lateral packing.**

2. **Failure of nonoperative management can best be predicted in those with high-grade injuries with large amounts of hemoperitoneum, concomitant solid organ injury, and splenic vascular abnormalities.**

3. **Missed ligation of transected short gastric arteries is a likely reason for return to the operating room for postsplenectomy bleeding.**

Introduction

Splenic trauma is the most common reason for operative intervention in blunt traumatic injury. This is no surprise given that the spleen is the most commonly injured solid organ. Typically, blunt injury is the most common injury mechanism and results in splenectomy, but penetrating injury to the spleen requires operative intervention. Historic data and randomized trials have shown that nonoperative management of blunt splenic injury is appropriate, and even up to 55% of patients can be managed nonoperatively.

Decisions regarding nonoperative or operative management of blunt splenic injury have been outlined by prior studies, and the American Association for the Surgery of Trauma (AAST) grading scale facilitates this decision to manage nonoperatively (Figure 14-1).

Evaluation of a patient should follow Advanced Trauma Life Support (ATLS) guidelines and resuscitation of the patient based on the expected cause of hemodynamic instability. Hemodynamically unstable patients should be managed in the operating room because of presumed hemorrhagic shock from bleeding, which can be readily confirmed by a focused assessment with sonography for trauma (FAST) exam. Hemodynamically normal patients should be evaluated with a contrast-enhanced computed tomography (CT) scan to identify any injuries. Grading

14 SPLEEN

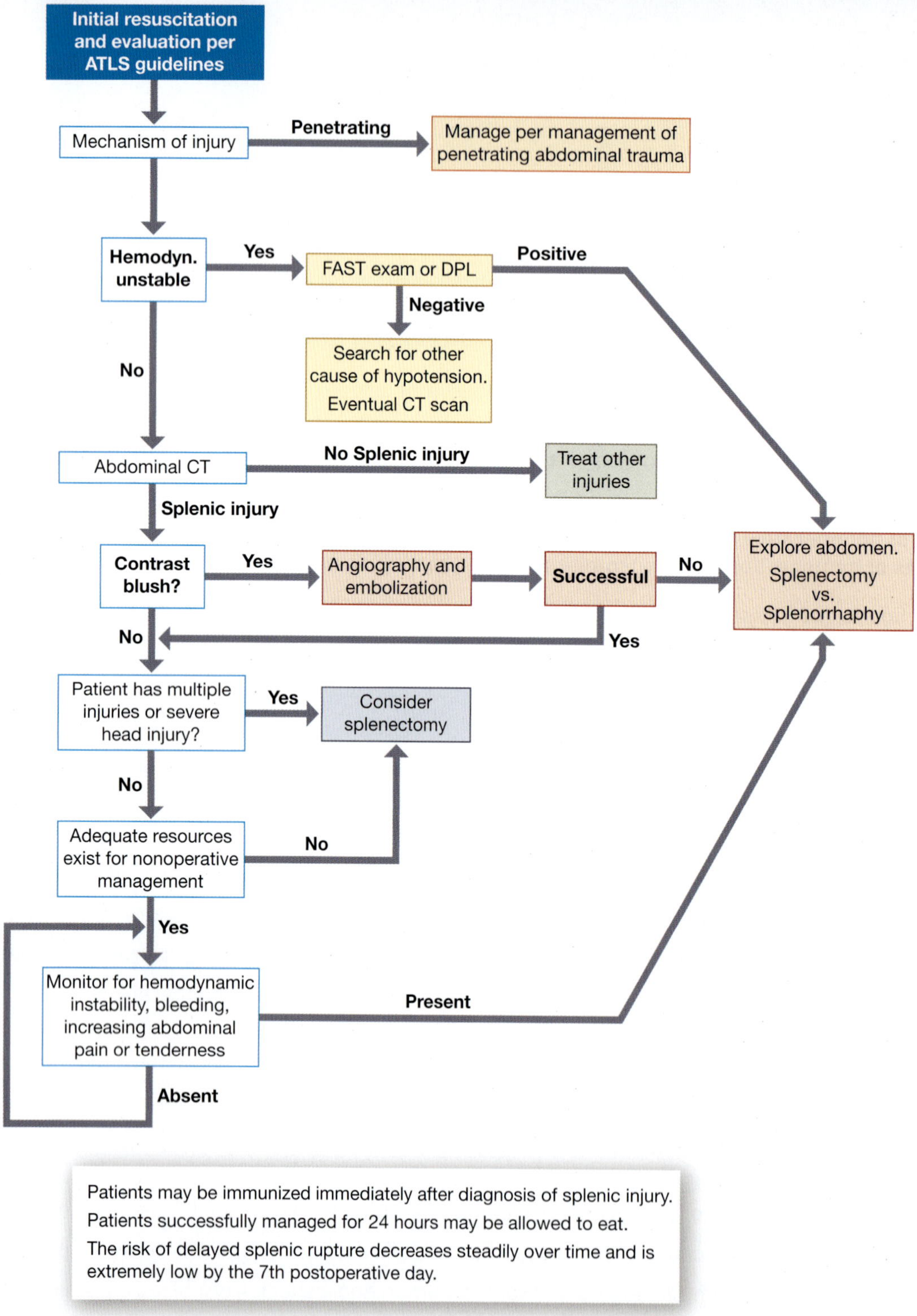

Figure 14-1. (Reproduced with permission from Feliciano DV, Mattox KL, Moore EE, eds. *Trauma*. 9th ed. McGraw Hill; 2021, Figure 34-5.)

of splenic injuries by AAST allows the trauma surgeon to evaluate the extent of injury to the spleen based on radiographic findings. The decision on which patients can be managed nonoperatively is based on clinical factors and the radiographic findings from the abdominal CT scan. Grade I and II splenic injuries usually are managed nonoperatively and are considered low-grade injuries. Grade III, IV, and V injuries are considered high-grade injuries; although many grade III injuries are managed nonoperatively, the higher-grade injuries are expected to need operative intervention. Higher-grade injuries are more likely to have features on CT scan that are suggestive of an ongoing bleed, such as active blush or pseudoaneurysm seen on CT scan. These findings should prompt an urgent call to interventional radiology for angiogram and embolization of the bleeding. Despite embolization, some patients still require operative intervention because of continued bleeding or sudden hemodynamic instability.

Many factors appear to affect the success of nonoperative management of splenic injuries, including age, grade of injury and quantity of hemoperitoneum, concomitant solid organ injury, and vascular abnormalities.

A recent update to the nonoperative management of the spleen in adults by reviewed risk factors for the failure of nonoperative management in splenic trauma. Not surprising, the mortality for patients who fail nonoperative management is 16.5%, which is significantly higher than the mortality rate of patients who were successfully managed nonoperatively (4%).

Studies have specifically looked at the effect of age on failure of nonoperative management and the mortality of splenic injury. It has been demonstrated that age greater than 55 is a risk factor for failure of nonoperative management, with 19% of those older than 55 failing nonoperative management, whereas only 10% of those less than 55 years old failed nonoperative management. Similarly, when the mortality of patients older than 55 years was compared to those younger than 55 years, there was a significant increase in mortality with older age (43% vs 23%, respectively). Thus, the level of suspicion that one has for failure in the older patient must be higher given the higher risk for failure and the attendant increase in the mortality rate that come with increased failure of nonoperative management.

The grade of splenic injury and quantity of hemoperitoneum are also factors that are associated with increased rates of nonoperative failure. Although this is no surprise and, intuitively, most trauma surgeons know this, multiple studies have verified this fact. Specifically, it has been shown that a moderate amount of hemoperitoneum is associated with increased failure of nonoperative management, confirming the suspicion that more bleeding usually leads more often to surgery.

Patients who present with intra-abdominal injuries in addition to splenic laceration usually have a higher Injury Severity Score and multiple areas of bleeding or causes for hypotension. Again, the patient with multiple sites of possible intra-abdominal bleeding is at higher risk for failure of nonoperative management of this bleeding and has a higher chance of requiring surgical interventional to ensure hemostasis.

Finally, abnormalities of the vasculature of the splenic hilum seen on CT imaging confer risk to nonoperative management. Findings such as contrast blushes, pseudoaneurysms, and arteriovenous fistulae are all evidence of vascular injury and have been shown to increase risk of failure of nonoperative management.

Anatomy

Pediatric and adult spleens differ in a few areas. Pediatric spleens tend to have a thicker capsule and tougher parenchymal consistency and thus are more likely to be able to tolerate blunt injury. However, as the spleen matures into that of the adult spleen, it grows in size and its capsule becomes thinner. The spleen also has segmental vessels that fan out from the hilum, and injury in a pattern that traverses these segmental vessels tends to result in more bleeding than if the parenchymal injury was in a pattern that only lacerated the trabeculae (ie, a transverse tear). Additionally, as one ages, there are a number of disease states that can enlarge the spleen and make it more fragile (eg, malaria, leukemia, portal venous hypertension, mononucleosis, lymphoma).

The spleen's location in the posterior left upper quadrant "shielded" by the lower left-sided ribs makes any blunt injury to the area concerning for injury to the spleen and adjacent structures, namely the ribs, splenic flexure of the colon, kidney, and diaphragm. There are variable attachments of the spleen to these adjacent structures by peritoneal reflections, resulting in the splenorenal ligament, splenocolic ligament, and splenophrenic ligament. These attachments keep the spleen in its anatomic position, limit mobilization during a splenectomy, and may require division.

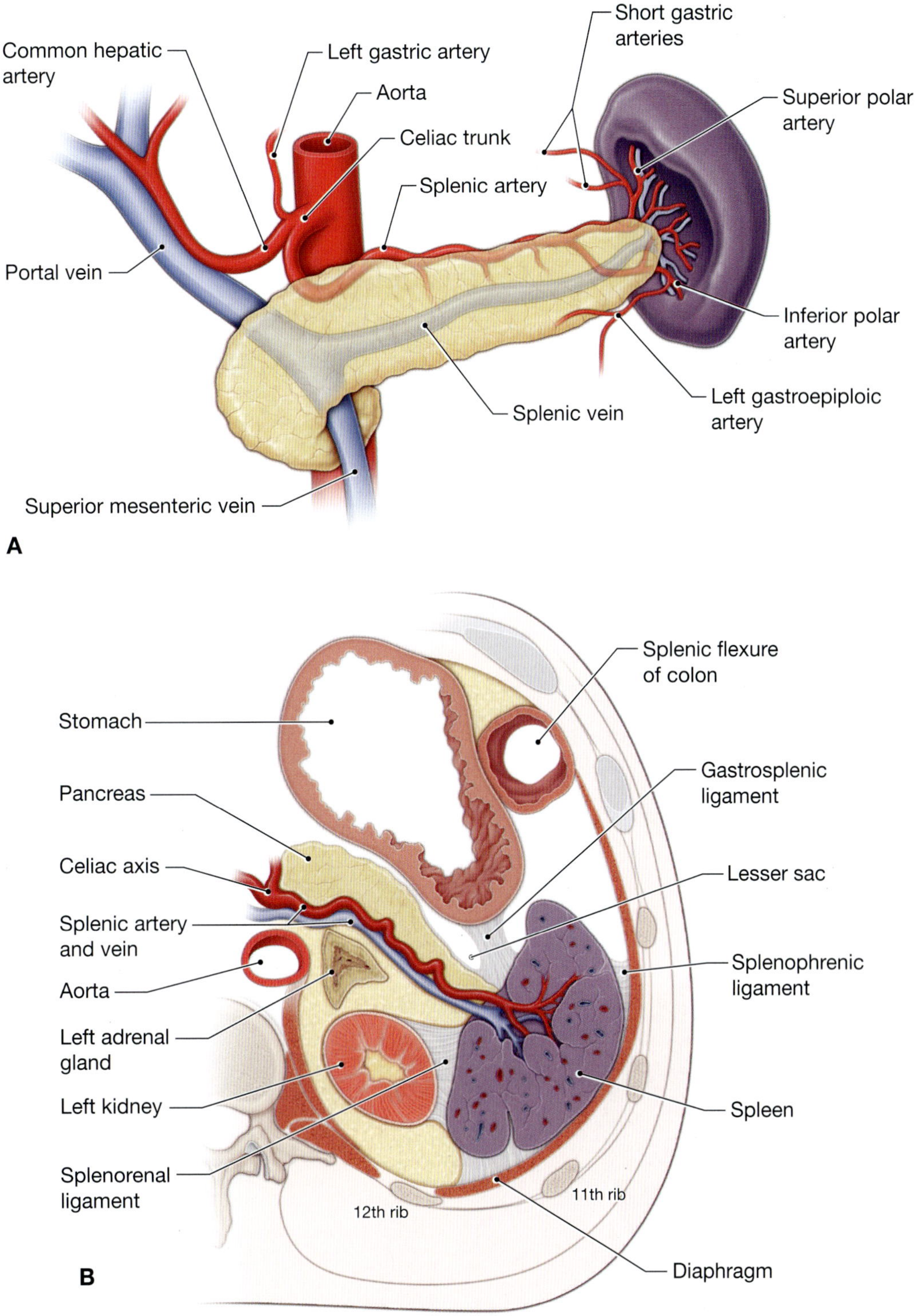

Figure 14-2 A, B

TABLE 14-1. American Association for the Surgery of Trauma (AAST) Organ Injury Grade

Grade	AAST Injury Scale - Spleen	Grade	AAST Injury Scale - Spleen
I	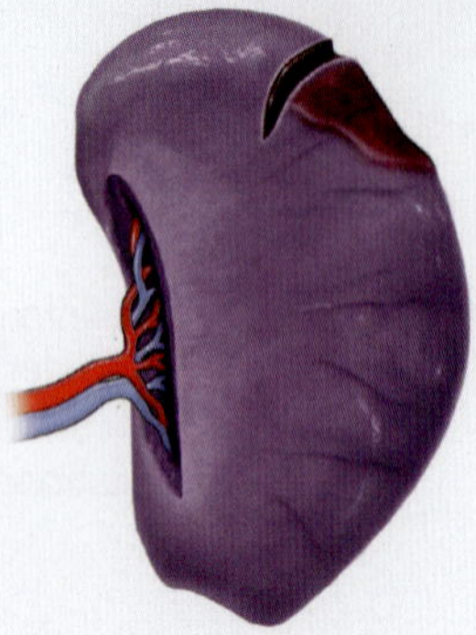	II	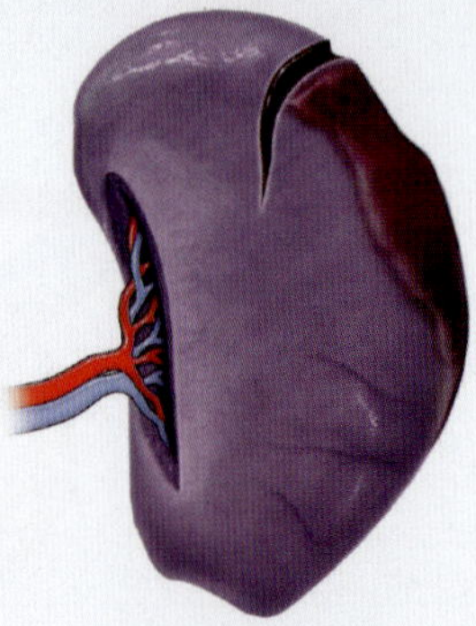
III	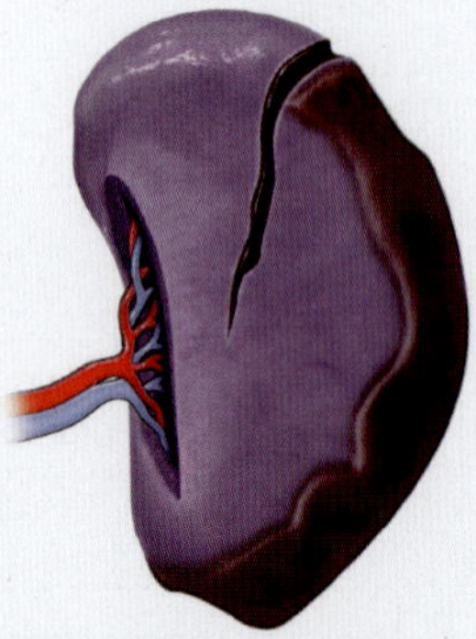	IV	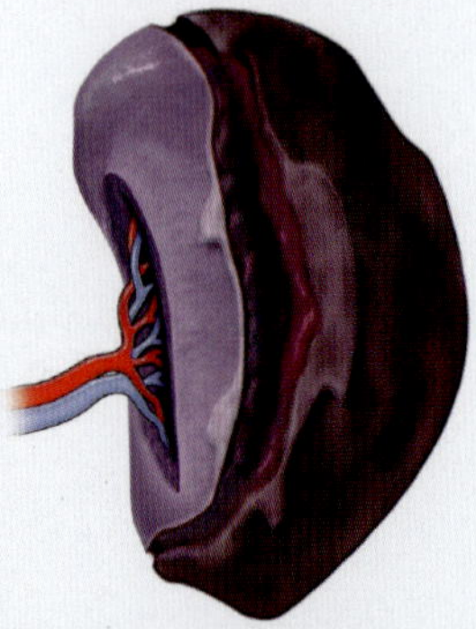
V	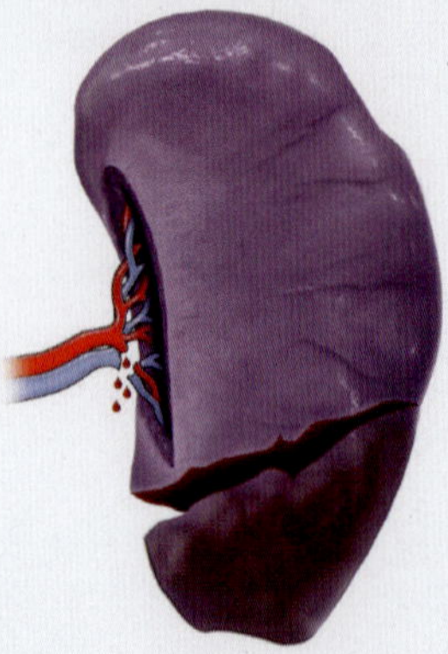		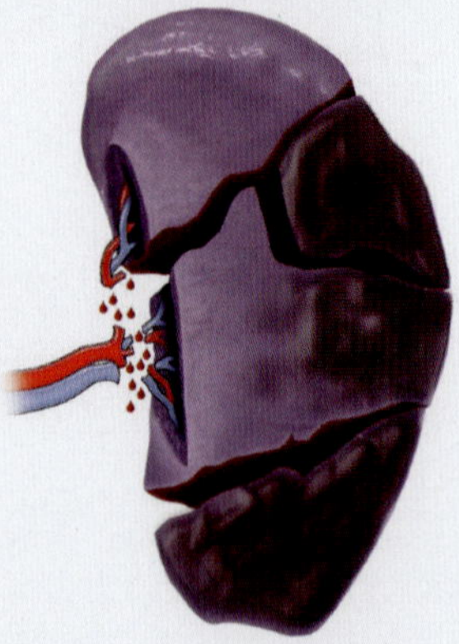

(*Continued*)

TABLE 14-1. Spleen Injury Scale (2018 Revision)

Grade*	AIS Severity	Imaging Criteria (CT Findings)	Operative Criteria	Pathologic Criteria
I	2	Subcapsular hematoma <10% surface area	Subcapsular hematoma <10% surface area	Subcapsular hematoma <10% surface area
		Parenchymal laceration <1 cm depth	Parenchymal laceration <1 cm depth	Parenchymal laceration <1 cm depth
		Capsular tear	Capsular tear	Capsular tear
II	2	Subcapsular hematoma 10%-50% surface area; intraparenchymal hematoma <5 cm	Subcapsular hematoma 10%-50% surface area; intraparenchymal hematoma <5 cm	Subcapsular hematoma 10%-50% surface area; intraparenchymal hematoma <5 cm
		Parenchymal laceration 1-3 cm	Parenchymal laceration 1-3 cm	Parenchymal laceration 1-3 cm
III	3	Subcapsular hematoma >50% surface area; ruptured subcapsular or intraparenchymal hematoma ≥5 cm	Subcapsular hematoma >50% surface area or expanding; ruptured subcapsular or intraparenchymal hematoma ≥5 cm	Subcapsular hematoma >50% surface area; ruptured subcapsular or intraparenchymal hematoma ≥5 cm
		Parenchymal laceration >3 cm depth	Parenchymal laceration >3 cm depth	Parenchymal laceration >3 cm depth
IV	4	Any injury in the presence of a splenic vascular injury or active bleeding confined within splenic capsule	Parenchymal laceration involving segmental or hilar vessels producing >25% devascularization	Parenchymal laceration involving segmental or hilar vessels producing >25% devascularization
		Parenchymal laceration involving segmental or hilar vessels producing >25% devascularization		
V	5	Any injury in the presence of a splenic vascular injury with active bleeding extended beyond the spleen into the peritoneum	Hilar vascular injury with devascularizes the spleen	Hilar vascular injury with devascularizes the spleen
		Shattered spleen	Shattered spleen	Shattered spleen

Vascular injury is defined as a pseudoaneurysm or arteriovenous fistula and appears as a focal collection of vascular contrast that decreases in attenuation with delayed imaging. Active bleeding from a vascular injury presents as vascular contrast, focal or diffuse, that increases in size or attenuation in delayed phase. Vascular thrombosis can lead to organ infarction.

*Grade based on highest grade assessment made on imaging, at operation or on pathologic specimen. More than one grade of splenic injury may be present and should be classified by the higher grade of injury. Advance one grade for multiple injuries up to grade III.

Source: Reproduced with permission from Kozar RA, Crandall M, Shanmuganathan K, et al. Organ injury scaling 2018 update: spleen, liver, and kidney. *J Trauma Acute Care Surg.* 2018;85(6):1119-1122; and Moore EE, Shackford SR, Pachter HL, et al. Organ injury scaling: spleen, liver, and kidney. *J Trauma.* 1989;29(12):1664-1666.

Operative Steps

Many patients who suffer blunt splenic injury may also coincidentally have been anticoagulated because of a chronic medical problem. These patients present to the trauma bay and are more likely to be in hemorrhagic shock because of their drug-induced coagulopathy. Depending on the inciting agent, there may be a need for immediate administration of a reversal agent or an agent to mitigate bleeding like vitamin K, prothrombin complex concentrate, idarucizumab, andexanet alfa, and tranexamic acid.

Positioning and Incisions: Left Subcostal or Midline Abdominal

The best positioning for a trauma patient seems to be supine positioning with arms outstretched; this allows rapid access to most areas of significant bleeding in rapid fashion. This would require that the patient be prepped from chin to knees and would allow placement of rapid tube thoracostomy or vascular control. Most commonly, a midline abdominal incision is made for rapid access to the abdominal cavity, but in the event there is a hostile abdomen from multiple prior laparotomies, a left subcostal incision may be faster (Figure 14-3). Gastric decompression with an orogastric tube is useful to help visualize and mobilize the spleen with a collapsed stomach.

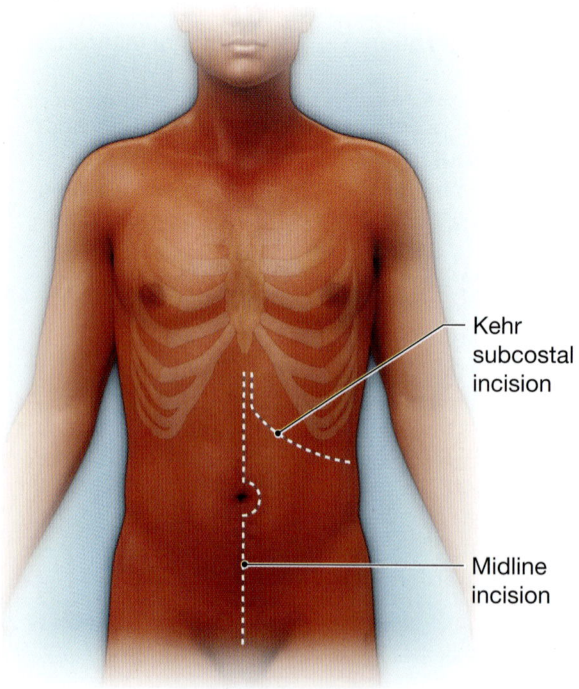

Figure 14-3

Exposure: Divide Ligaments, Medialize the Spleen, and Pack Behind the Spleen

Most commonly, rapid access to the abdomen is achieved by a midline abdominal incision (Figure 14-4A). When the abdomen is initially accessed, the initial phase of a trauma laparotomy would require placement of multiple absorbent lap pads in all four quadrants. Once it has been determined that the only source of bleeding is the spleen, the next step would be to gain rapid control of the hilum to arrest bleeding. Visualize the ligamentous attachments of the spleen to the diaphragm, kidney, and colon; these attachments must first be divided to allow mobilization of the spleen medially to the incision. Given the anatomic relationship, traction is applied to the stomach and spleen medially with the nondominant hand. The dominant hand is used to bluntly divide any attachments to the spleen; however, these attachments are usually divided as part of the traumatic injury. Should these attachments prove stubborn, a long Metzenbaum scissors is usually the fastest means

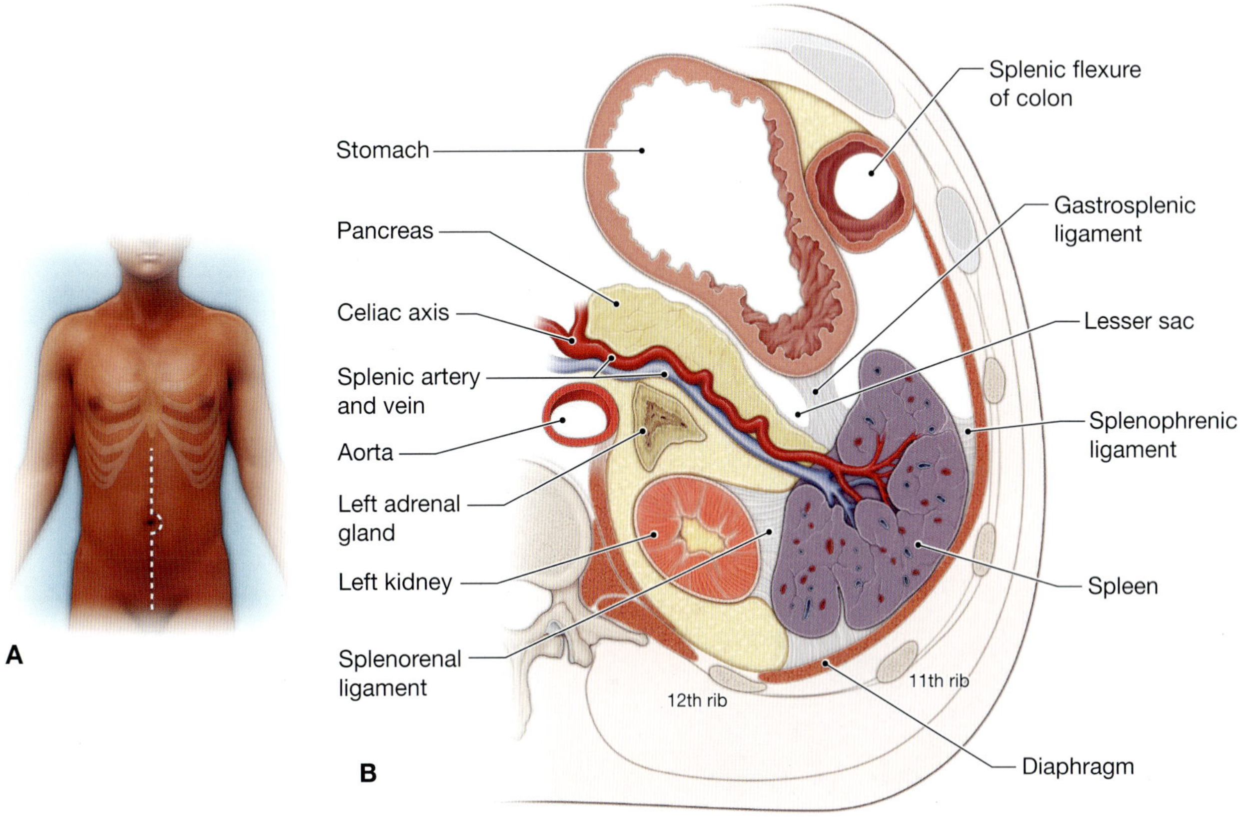

Figure 14-4 A, B

to divide these attachments and mobilize the spleen (Figure 14-5A-C). Continued traction at this point allows the spleen to assume a position in the middle of the incision, while continued packing posterior to the spleen with lap pads helps to render it more anterior.

Control of Bleeding: Ligation of Hilum and Division of Short Gastric Vessels

With enough mobilization and posterior packing, the hilar vessels would be able to be identified posteriorly or via a window in the gastrosplenic ligament. Using a small straight vascular clamp, the splenic hilum is clamped proximal to any branching hilar vessels and hemodynamic stability confirmed with a conversation with anesthesia colleagues. If there is persistent hypotension, continued transfusion of blood products and search for any other causes of hemorrhage are pursued. In a hemodynamically normal patient, the next step would be to separate the artery and vein and to individually ligate these vessels.

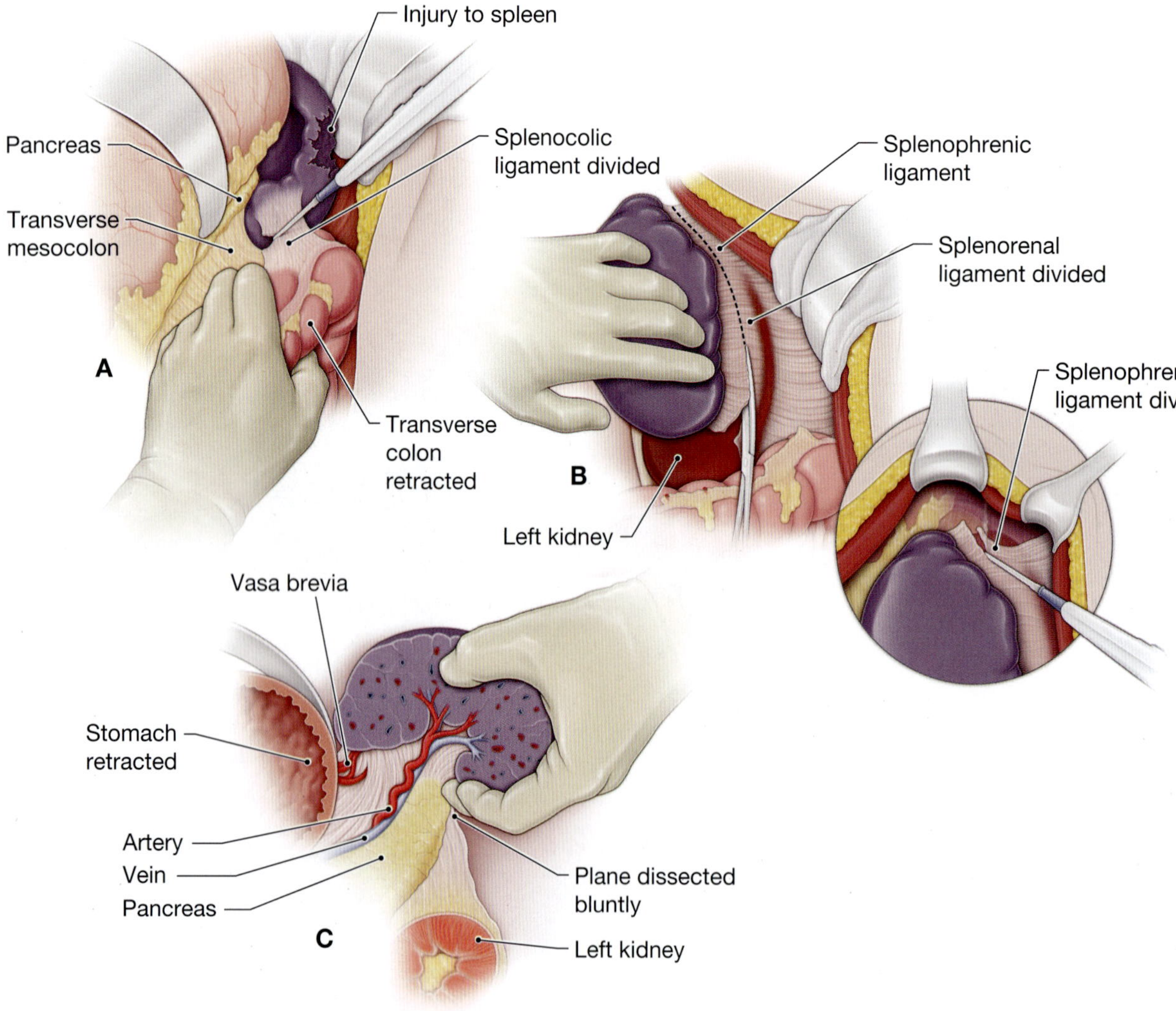

Figure 14-5 A-C

The usual choice would be to initially ligate with 0 silk ties proximally and then suture ligate distal to the ties with 2-0 Prolene.

The short gastric vessels within the gastrosplenic ligament are then usually divided by creating windows in the ligament and clamping and dividing short segments of the ligament containing short gastric arteries (Figure 14-6A-C). These arteries are then ligated with 2-0 silk ties and the clamps removed, being certain to capture all of the short gastric vessels from the left

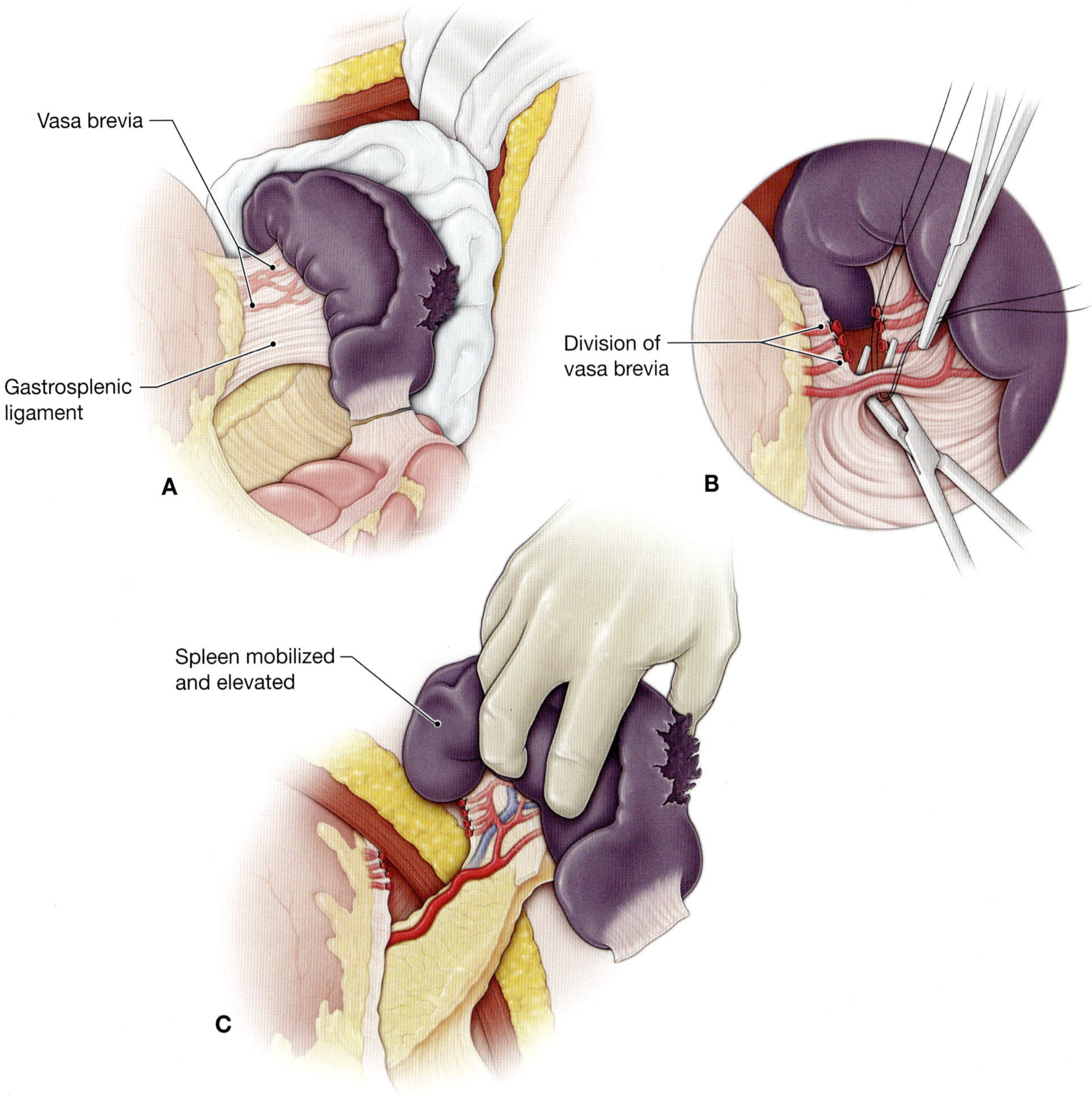

Figure 14-6 A-C

gastroepiploic artery all the way to the fundus of the stomach.

Completion of Procedure: Inspect for Hemostasis and Need for Drain

At this point in the procedure, the spleen has been divided at its hilum and the patient is hemodynamically normal, and care is taken to ensure that there is good hemostasis of the hilum, short gastric vessels, and retroperitoneal attachments of the spleen. Additionally, the splenic hilum is at times intimately attached to the tail of the pancreas, and in the haste to control splenic bleeding, there have been inadvertent injuries to the splenic tail. The tail of the pancreas is ensured to be uninjured; however, should there be a significant injury, placement of a bulb suction drain in the left upper quadrant is usually prudent. Finally, all the packs are removed and the abdomen irrigated to ensure that there is no evidence of bleeding. The abdomen is then closed with a running 0 PDS suture. Regarding postoperative care, given the ligation of short gastric arteries on the greater curve of the stomach, usually maintenance of nasogastric decompression for the first 2 days postoperatively is reasonable. Splenic vaccines are usual postoperative care, and aspirin for a thrombocytosis of greater than 1,000,000 and vaccines are given the day of discharge or on postoperative day 14.

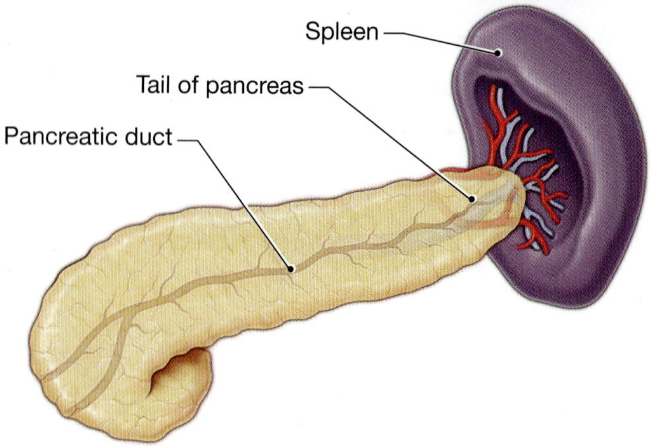

Figure 14-7

Splenorrhaphy/Splenic Conservation

The decision to preserve the spleen suggest that the surgeon thinks that the injury to the spleen and the risk for postoperative bleeding are low enough that it is worth the risk of splenorrhaphy. Note, splenorrhaphy and splenic conservation are rarely done these days. The initial steps of the operation remain the same, and the spleen must be brought up into the field to allow attempts at splenorrhaphy. The laceration to the splenic poles without extension to the hilum may be worthwhile in young patients. The process starts with control of the splenic artery and its inflow with a bulldog clamp or vessel loop. Multiple ways to control bleeding from the site of injury usually start with a topical hemostatic agent and direct compression of the bleeding area with gauze. The use of horizontal mattress sutures and pledgets through the area of bleeding after debridement of the damaged tissue usually can stop bleeding in combination with the application of a topical agent and direct pressure. Splenic mesh wrap and omental wrapping are now more historic in nature.

15

HEPATOBILIARY TRAUMA

Stanley J. Kurek, DO, FACS
Ashley Ludwig, DO, FACS

TIPS

1. **Liver injury is common in both blunt and penetrating trauma, with the majority of these injuries treated nonoperatively. Extrahepatic biliary injuries are less common and often require more complex operative management.**

2. **Liver injuries are graded based on the American Association for the Surgery of Trauma (AAST) Hepatic Injury Scale, and treatment is based on both hemodynamics and grade of injury.**

3. **Postoperative complication rates for AAST grade III or higher liver injuries are high and can manifest in both nonoperative and operative management strategies.**

Introduction

Due to its large size relative to the other abdominal organs, the liver is the most commonly injured solid organ in blunt trauma and the second most commonly injured abdominal organ in penetrating trauma. Because of its fixed location under the diaphragm, it is highly susceptible to shear forces secondary to deceleration injury. The anterior position and large size of the organ also make it prone to penetrating injury. The right lobe is the most frequently injured portion of the liver in both penetrating and blunt mechanisms.

Hepatic injuries result in approximately 5% of total trauma admissions. The degree of injury is graded using the American Association for the Surgery of Trauma (AAST) Hepatic Injury Scale. The majority of liver injuries are treated nonoperatively using interventional radiology techniques such as angioembolization as an adjunct in the setting of active extravasation on contrast-enhanced computed tomography scan. When operative intervention is required due to hemodynamic instability, 80% to 85% of hepatic injuries can be managed by simple techniques to control hemorrhage including packing, application of hemostatic agents, electrocautery, superficial suturing, or drainage. The remaining injuries require more complex surgical techniques, and damage control procedures are frequently utilized.

Treatment of pediatric patients with liver injury mirrors treatment of the adult trauma patient. However, in hemodynamically stable pediatric patients, active extravasation is not an absolute indication for angioembolization and has been associated with higher rates of nonoperative management failure. When angioembolization is not utilized, close follow-up is required to monitor for pseudoaneurysm formation.

15 HEPATOBILIARY TRAUMA

Extrahepatic biliary injuries can involve both the gallbladder and bile ducts. Injuries to the gallbladder are often treated with cholecystectomy. However, injuries to the bile ducts can be difficult to repair due to the small duct caliber in young, healthy patients.

Complication rates after liver injury can be as high as 50% and are especially prevalent in patients with AAST grade III or higher injuries. Liver injury is also the primary cause of death in 10% to 15% of patients. Complications can include hemorrhage, necrosis, abscess, biloma, biliary fistula, pseudoaneurysm, arteriovenous fistula, hemobilia, and intrahepatic biliary strictures. All of the above listed complications can manifest in both nonoperative and operative management strategies.

Anatomy

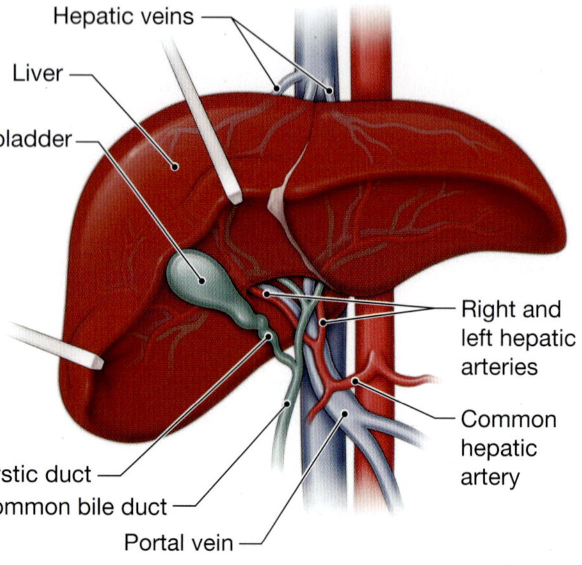

Figure 15-1

TABLE 15-1. American Association for the Surgery of Trauma (AAST) Hepatic Injury Scale

Grade	Injury
Grade I	Hematoma – Subcapsular, <10% surface area Laceration – Capsular tear <1 cm parenchymal depth
Grade II	Hematoma – Subcapsular, 10%-50% surface area Intraparenchymal, <10 cm diameter Laceration – 1-3 cm parenchymal depth, <10 cm in length
Grade III	Hematoma – Subcapsular, >50% surface area or expanding Ruptured subcapsular or parenchymal hematoma Intraparenchymal hematoma >10 cm Laceration – >3 cm parenchymal depth
Grade IV	Laceration – Parenchymal disruption 25%-75% of hepatic lobe 1-3 Couinaud's segments within the single lobe
Grade V	Laceration – Parenchymal disruption >75% of hepatic lobe >3 Couinaud segments within the single lobe Vascular – Juxtavenous hepatic injury (eg, retrohepatic inferior vena cava, central major hepatic veins)
Grade VI	Vascular – Hepatic avulsion

(*Continued*)

TABLE 15-1. American Association for the Surgery of Trauma (AAST) Hepatic Injury Scale (Continued)

Grade	AAST Injury Scale - Liver	Grade	AAST Injury Scale - Liver
I	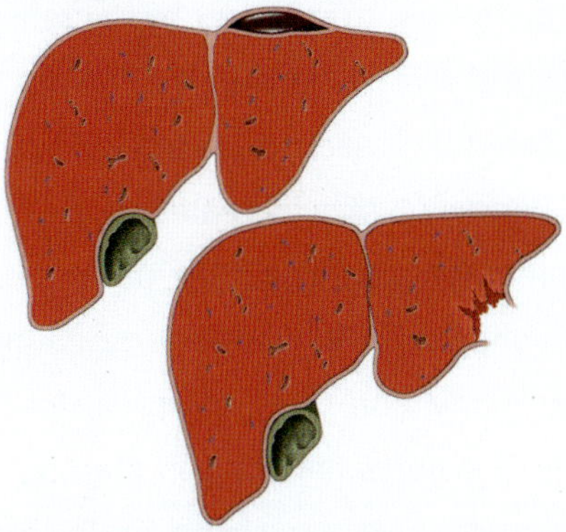	II	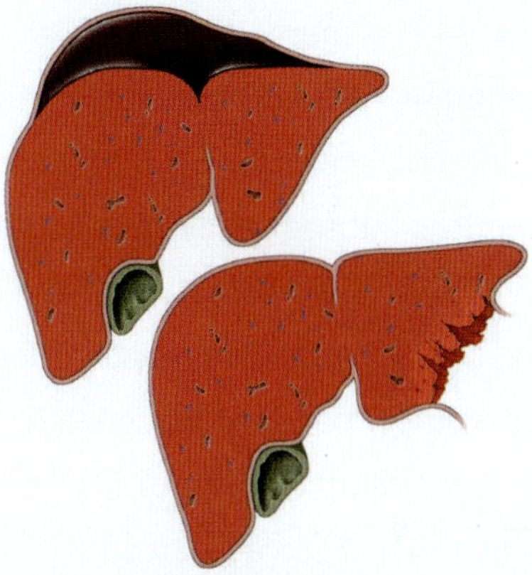
III	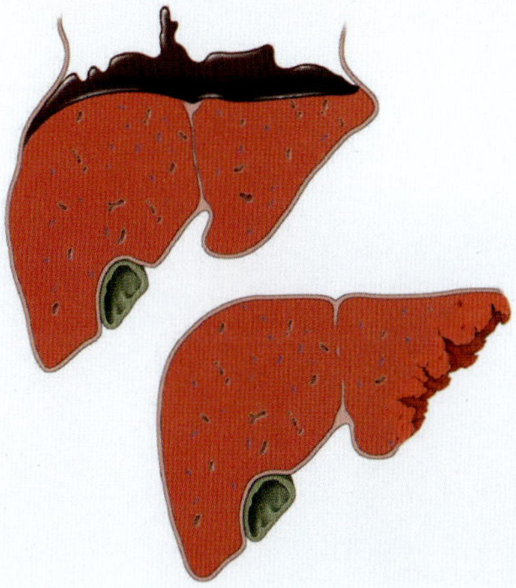	IV	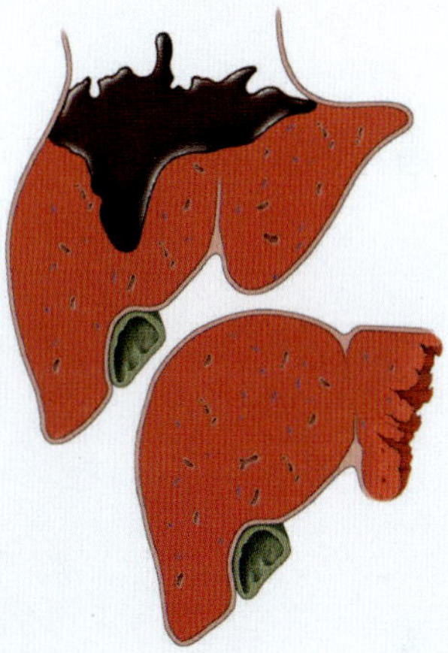
V	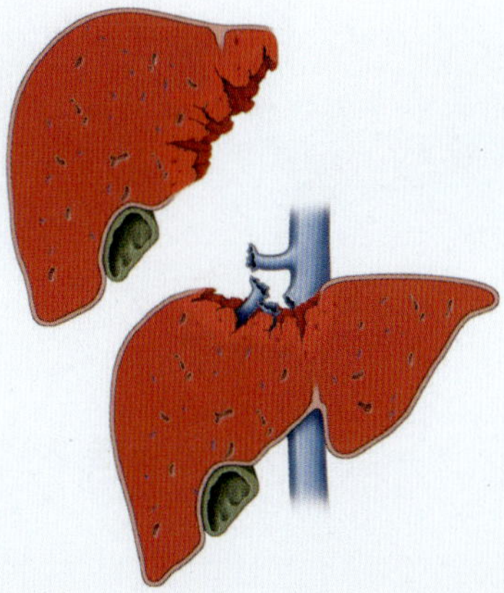		

Source: Reproduced with permission from Kozar RA et al. Organ injury scaling 2018 update: Spleen, liver, and kidney. *J Trauma Acute Care Surg.* 2018;85(6):1119-1122 and Reproduced with permission from Moore EE et al. *J Trauma.* 1989;29(12):1664-1666.

Operative Steps

Liver Mobilization and Packing

The peritoneal cavity is entered through a generous midline incision (Figure 15-2). The falciform ligament is then clamped, divided, and suture ligated near the anterior abdominal wall fascia. The avascular portion of the ligament is subsequently divided with electrocautery. Gentle downward pressure on the liver allows for avoidance of the hepatic veins posteriorly. Next, three to four laparotomy pads are placed behind the liver and under the diaphragm to allow for liver retraction anteriorly and inferiorly (Figure 15-3A-D).

Pringle Maneuver

If temporary compression of the liver wound does not result in hemostasis, the porta hepatis can be cross-clamped (Pringle maneuver) to decrease the vascular inflow to the liver (Figure 15-4). The Pringle maneuver is completed by inserting an index finger into the foramen of Winslow, a space created by the free edge of the lesser omentum containing the porta hepatis anteriorly, inferior vena cava (IVC) posteriorly, caudate lobe of the liver superiorly, and the first portion of the duodenum inferiorly. The porta hepatis can then be controlled with an atraumatic vascular clamp or Rummel tourniquet.

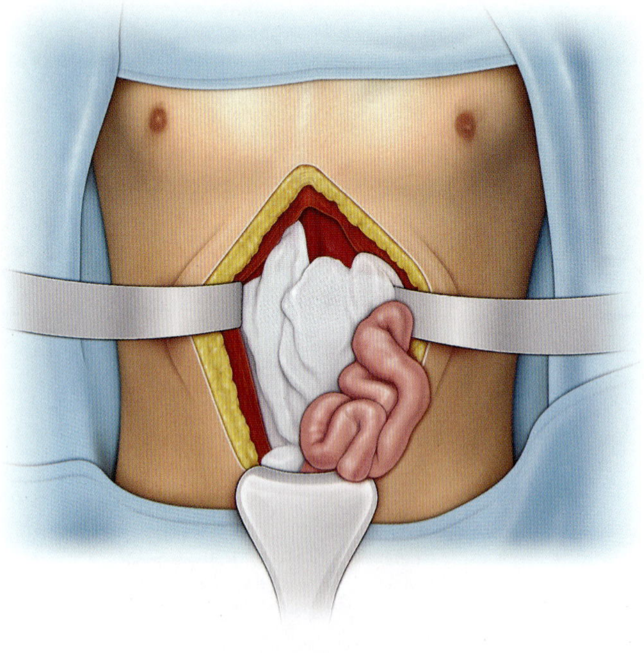

Figure 15-2

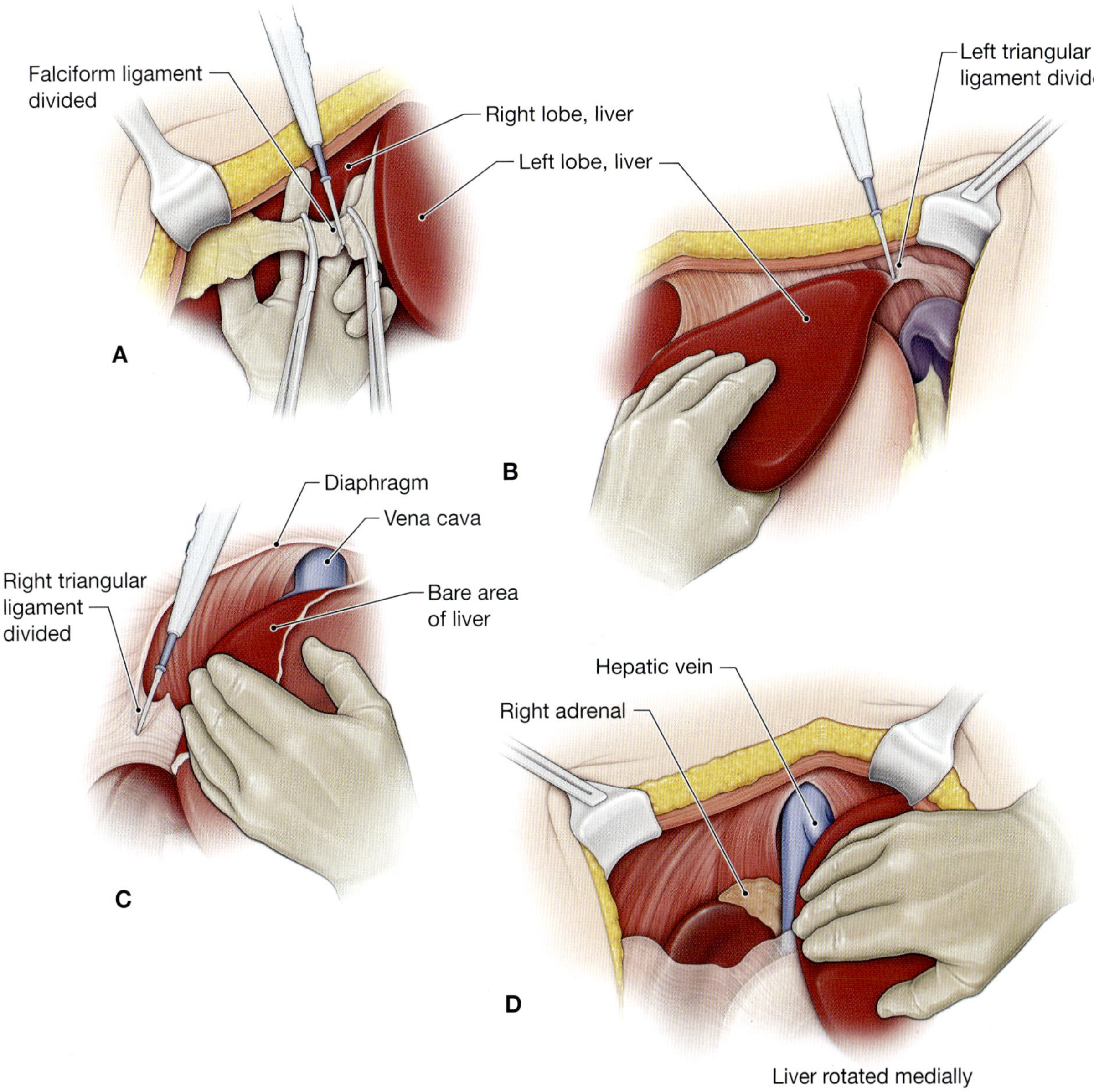

Figure 15-3 A-D

This maneuver can be applied for a maximum of an hour without risk of ischemia or reperfusion injury. Failure to control hemorrhage with this technique suggests bleeding from the hepatic veins, retrohepatic vena cava, or aberrant anatomy.

Hemorrhage Control

Multiple modalities for hemostasis exist and are employed based on the extent of the injury. For superficial bleeding, hemorrhage control can be achieved using electrocautery, direct suture-ligation or clipping of major bleeders, perihepatic packing, or application of hemostatic agents. For deeper liver lacerations, deep, figure-of-eight, tension-free sutures using 0-chromic on a large blunt-tip liver needle can be employed (Figure 15-5). Omentum can be used

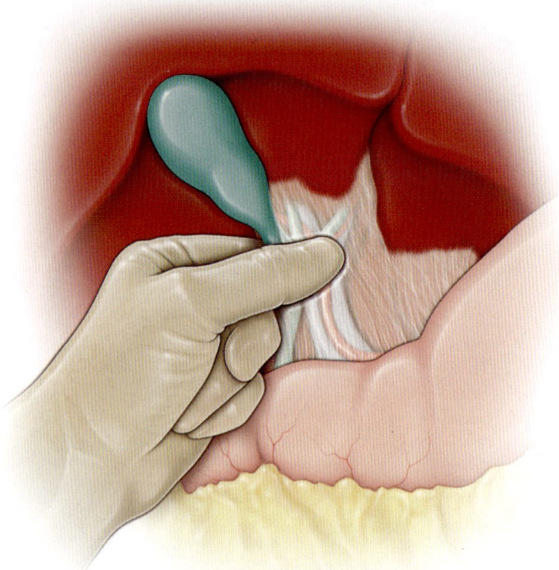

Porta hepatis pinched between thumb and index finger

Figure 15-4

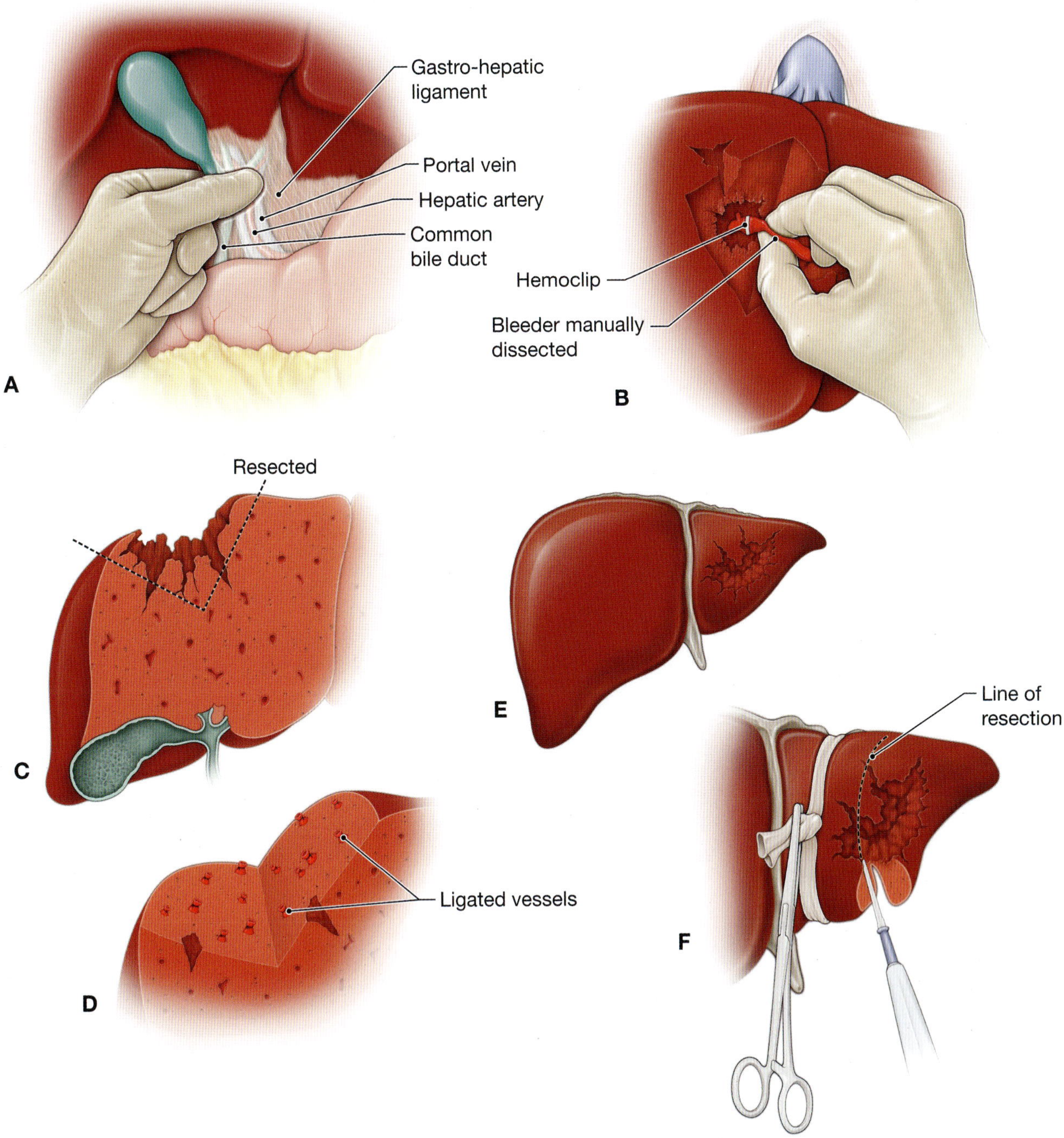
Gastro-hepatic ligament
Portal vein
Hepatic artery
Common bile duct
A
Hemoclip
Bleeder manually dissected
B
Resected
C
E
Ligated vessels
D
Line of resection
F

Figure 15-5

to fill large defects (Figure 15-6). If unable to control deeper bleeding with these techniques in penetrating trauma, tractotomy with a linear stapler or electrocautery and subsequent balloon tamponade can be used. If tractotomy is not feasible due to the depth of the injury through normal parenchyma, balloon tamponade can be utilized alone. High-velocity penetrating or severe blunt trauma may result in extensive parenchymal damage requiring nonanatomical liver resection, selective hepatic artery ligation, total vascular liver isolation (Figure 15-7A, B), or atriocaval shunting. If the patient remains hemodynamically compromised, early perihepatic packing and damage control should be employed.

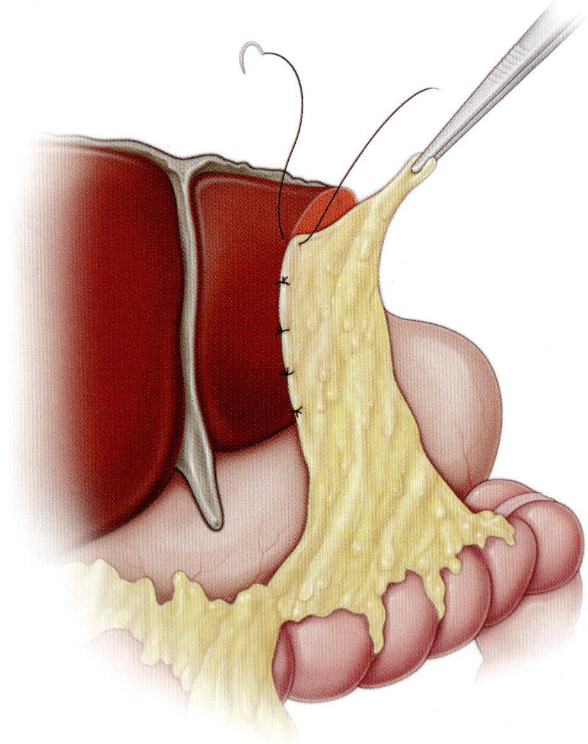

Figure 15-6

Hepatic Vascular Exclusion

When perihepatic packing is ineffective in controlling the bleeding, vascular isolation of the liver can be achieved by clamping the supraceliac aorta below the diaphragm, the suprahepatic and infrahepatic IVC, and the porta hepatis via the above-described Pringle maneuver. If access to the suprahepatic IVC is difficult due to hematoma and bleeding, access to the intrapericardial IVC can be achieved via a lower limited sternotomy. Total isolation can be achieved by placing a femoral vein to left internal jugular shunt connected to a hemoperfusion pump. During this procedure, the portal venous system may require decompression using the inferior mesenteric vein. Retrohepatic venous bleeding can be reduced by atriocaval shunting. To complete this, the laparotomy incision is extended into a median

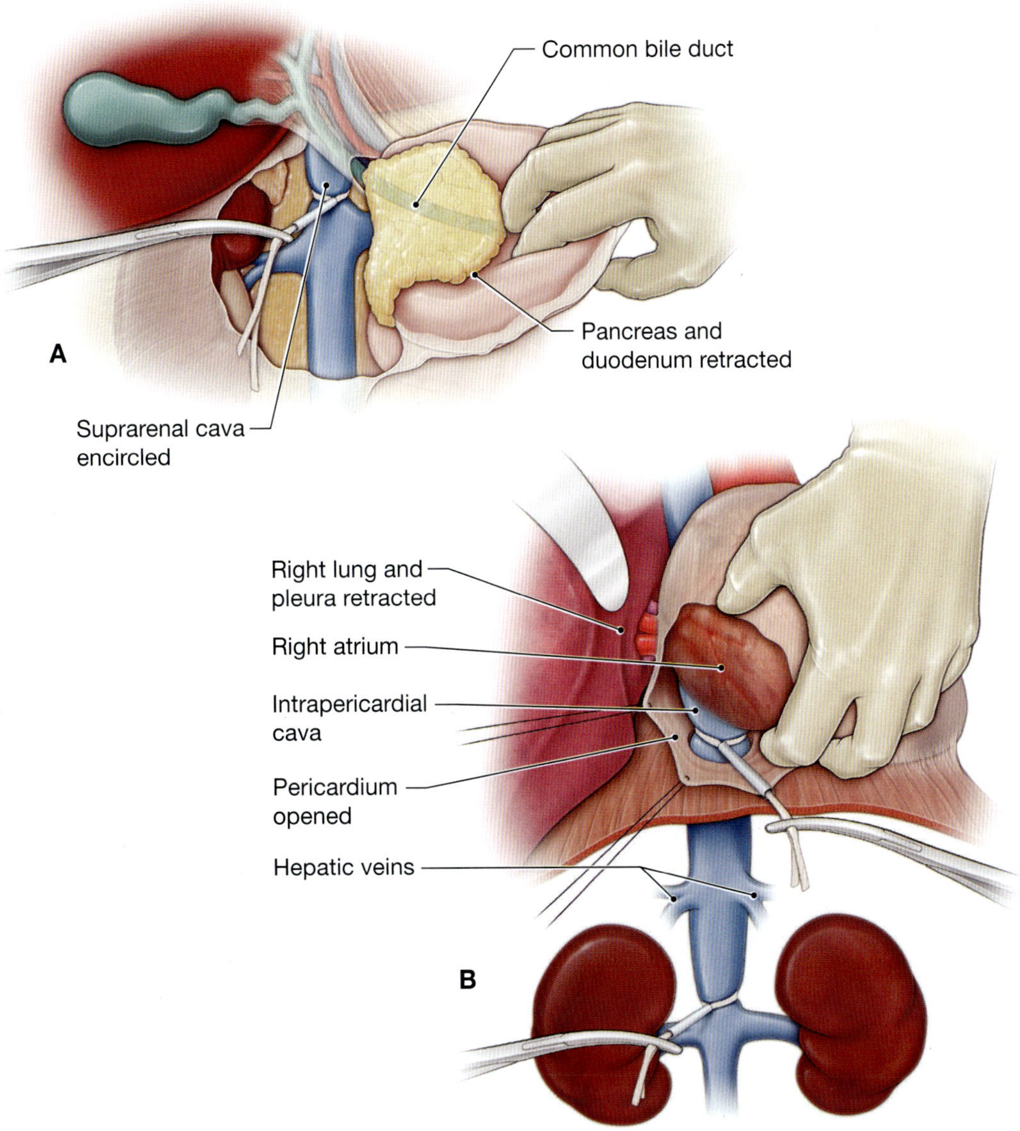

Figure 15-7 A, B

sternotomy and the pericardium is opened. An umbilical tape tourniquet or vessel loop is placed around the intrapericardial IVC. The right atrial appendage is then occluded with a vascular clamp, and a purse-string silk suture is placed. A side hole is then cut into a size 8 endotracheal tube (ETT) 8 to 10 cm from the clamped proximal end and is inserted into the purse string and guided into the IVC. The balloon of the ETT is inflated just above the renal veins, and the tape or vessel loop tourniquet is tightened. This can also be completed with a 36-Fr chest tube inserted so the fenestrated holes are within the right atrium (Figure 15-8A, B). Both of these exclusion procedures allow time for exploration and repair of any noted hepatic vascular injuries.

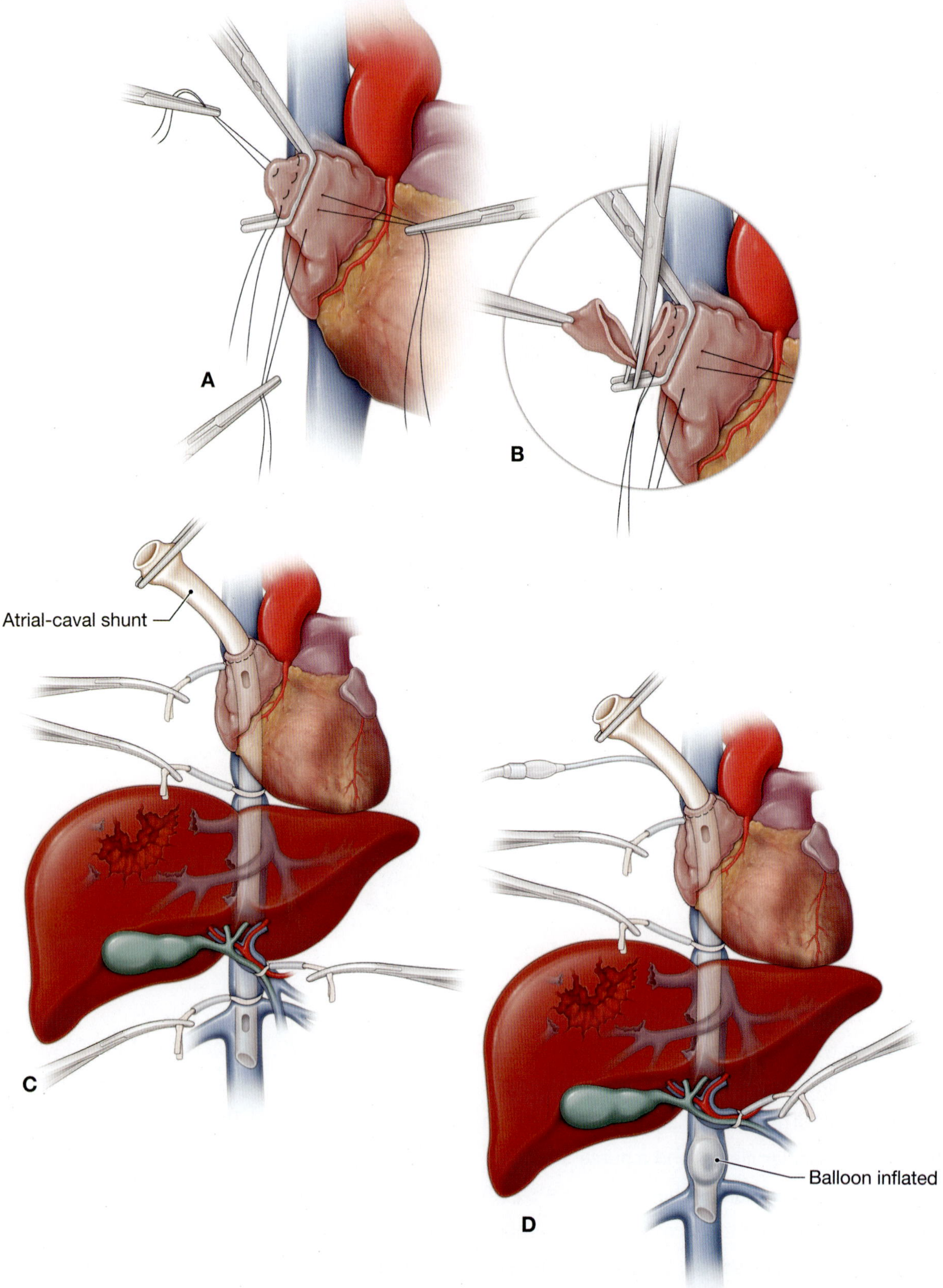

Figure 15-8 A-D

Bile Duct Injury Management

Injuries to the gallbladder can be treated with cholecystectomy alone or insertion of a Malecot tube for decompression (Figure 15-9A-D). Injuries to the common bile duct (CBD) are more difficult to repair due to the small duct size. The type of ductal repair depends

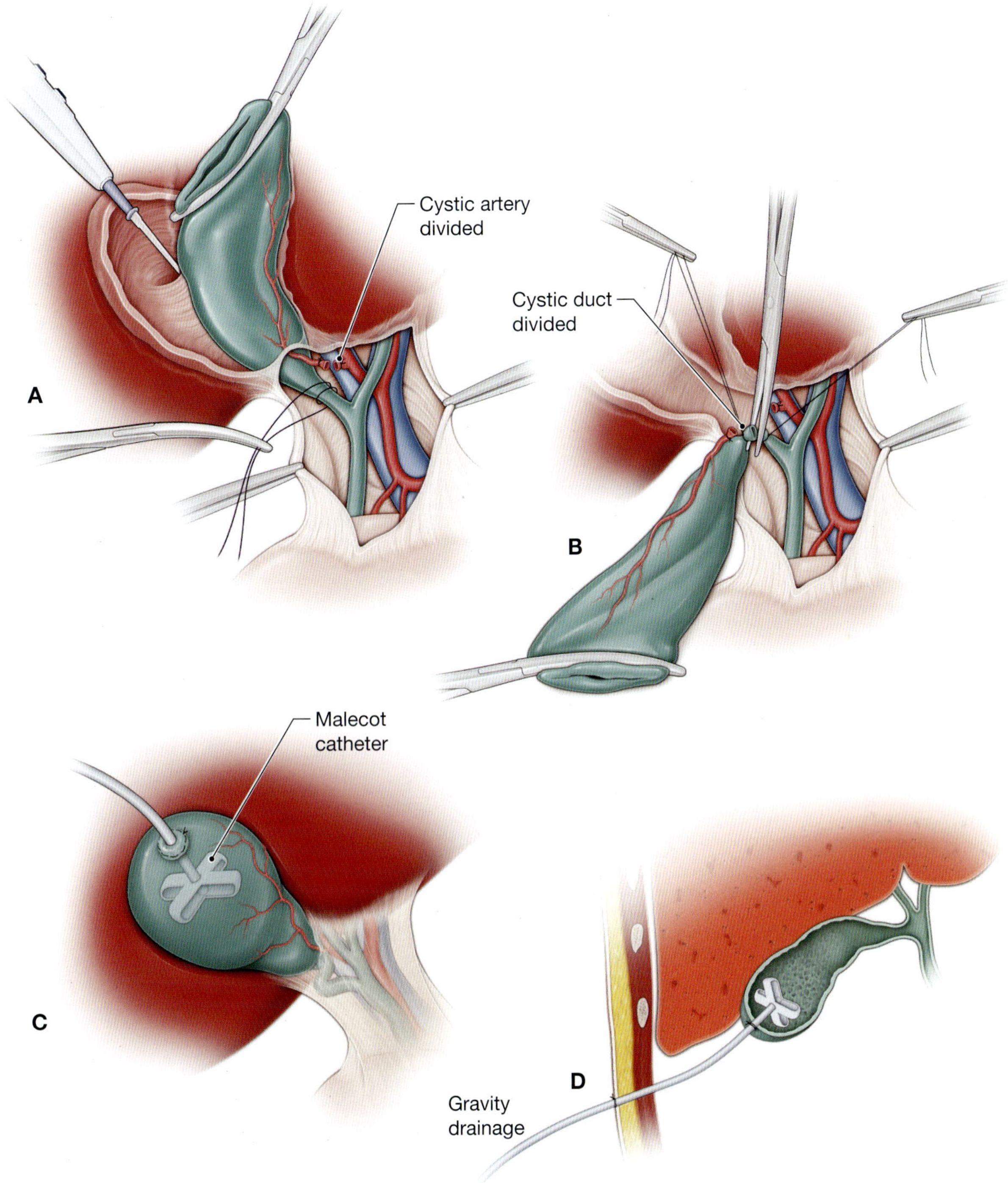

Figure 15-9 A-D

on the extent of injury. Complete transection requires reconstruction with a Roux-en-Y hepaticojejunostomy (Figures 15-10A, B and 15-11A-C). Incomplete transection involving <50% of the ductal circumference can be repaired primarily over a T-tube placed through a separate ductotomy (Figure 15-12A-E).

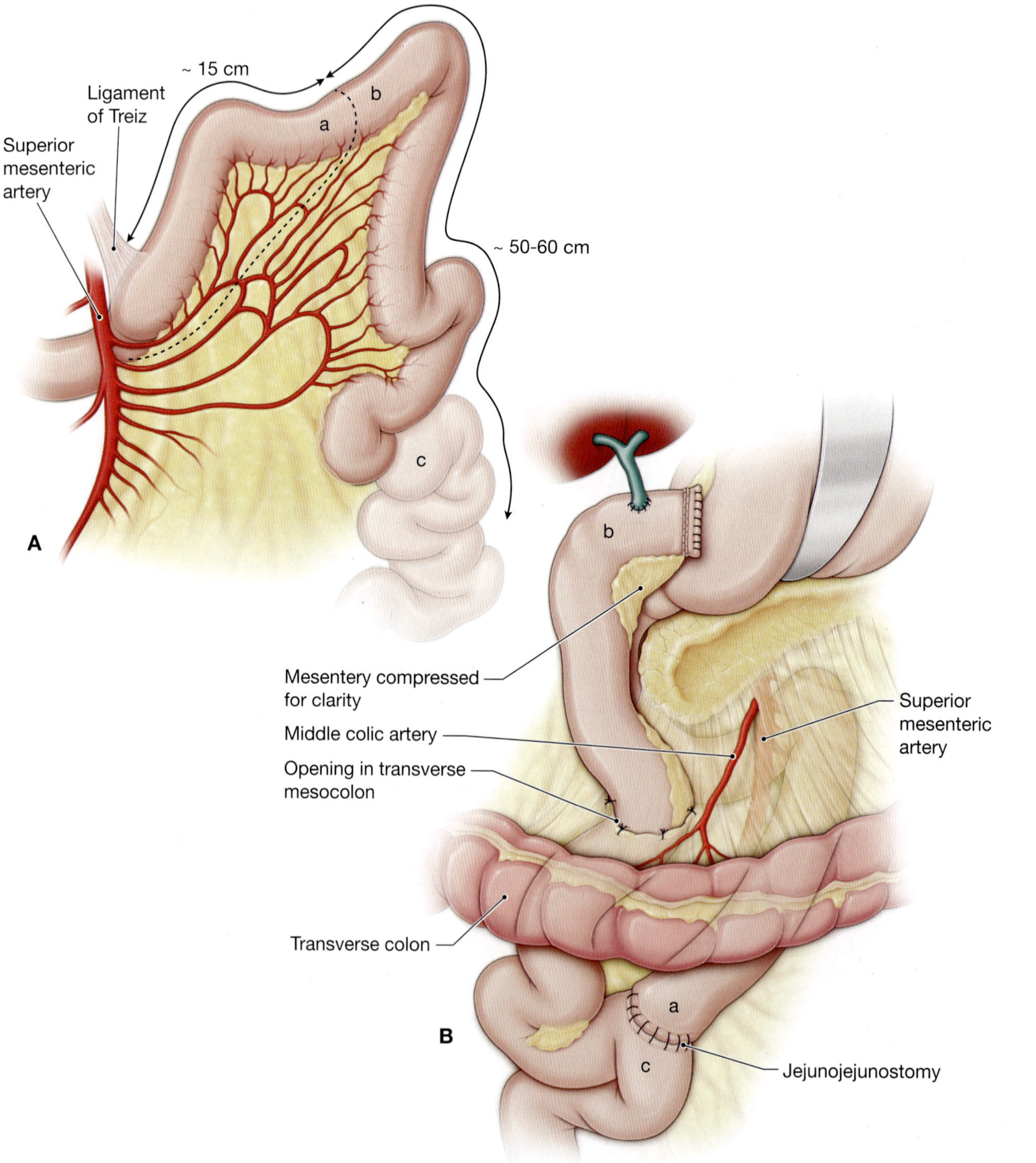

Figure 15-10 A, B

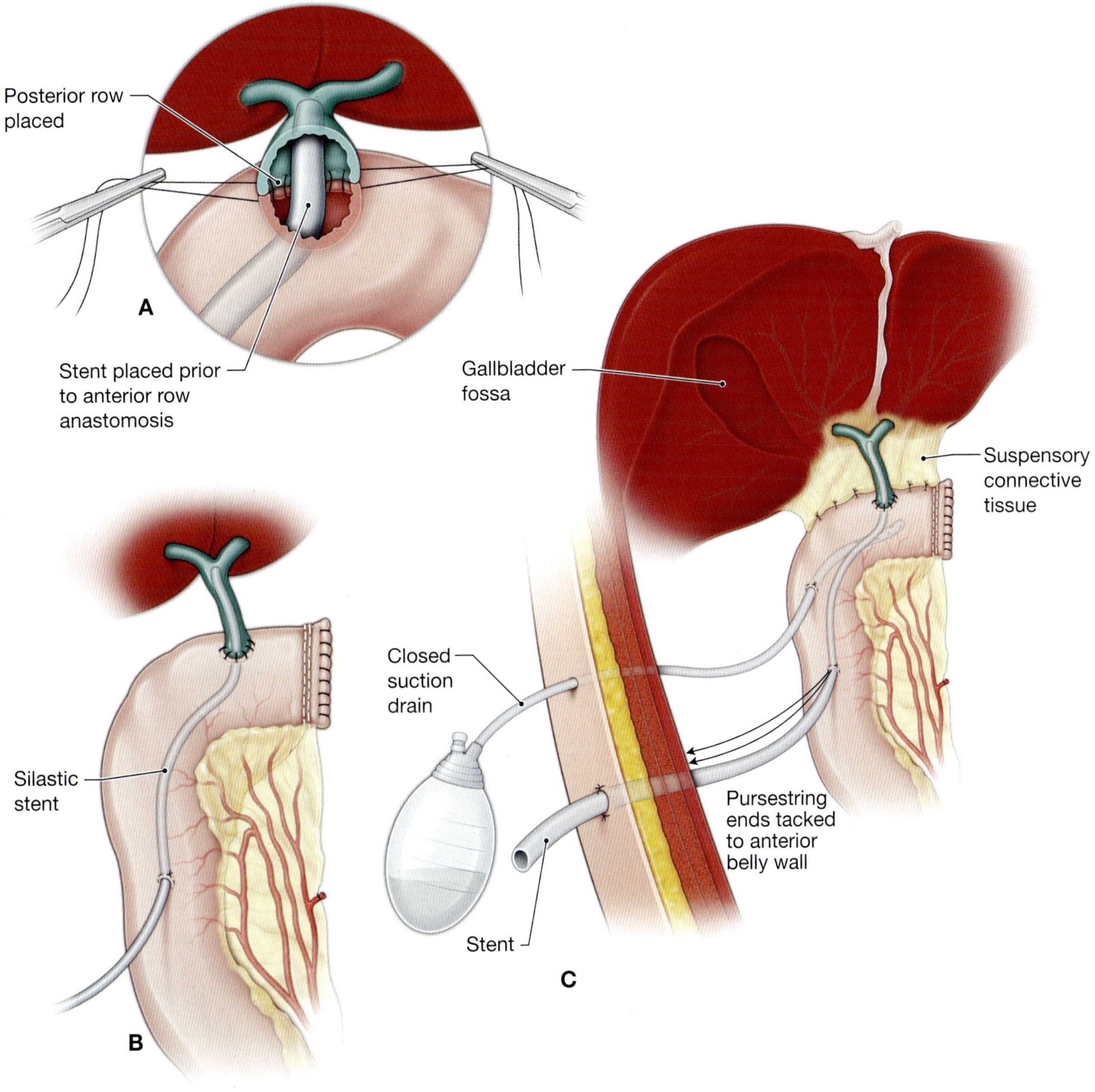

Figure 15-11 A-C

Reconstruction should not be attempted during damage control procedures. If the patient is unstable, the CBD can be ligated or externally drained with reconstruction completed at a later date.

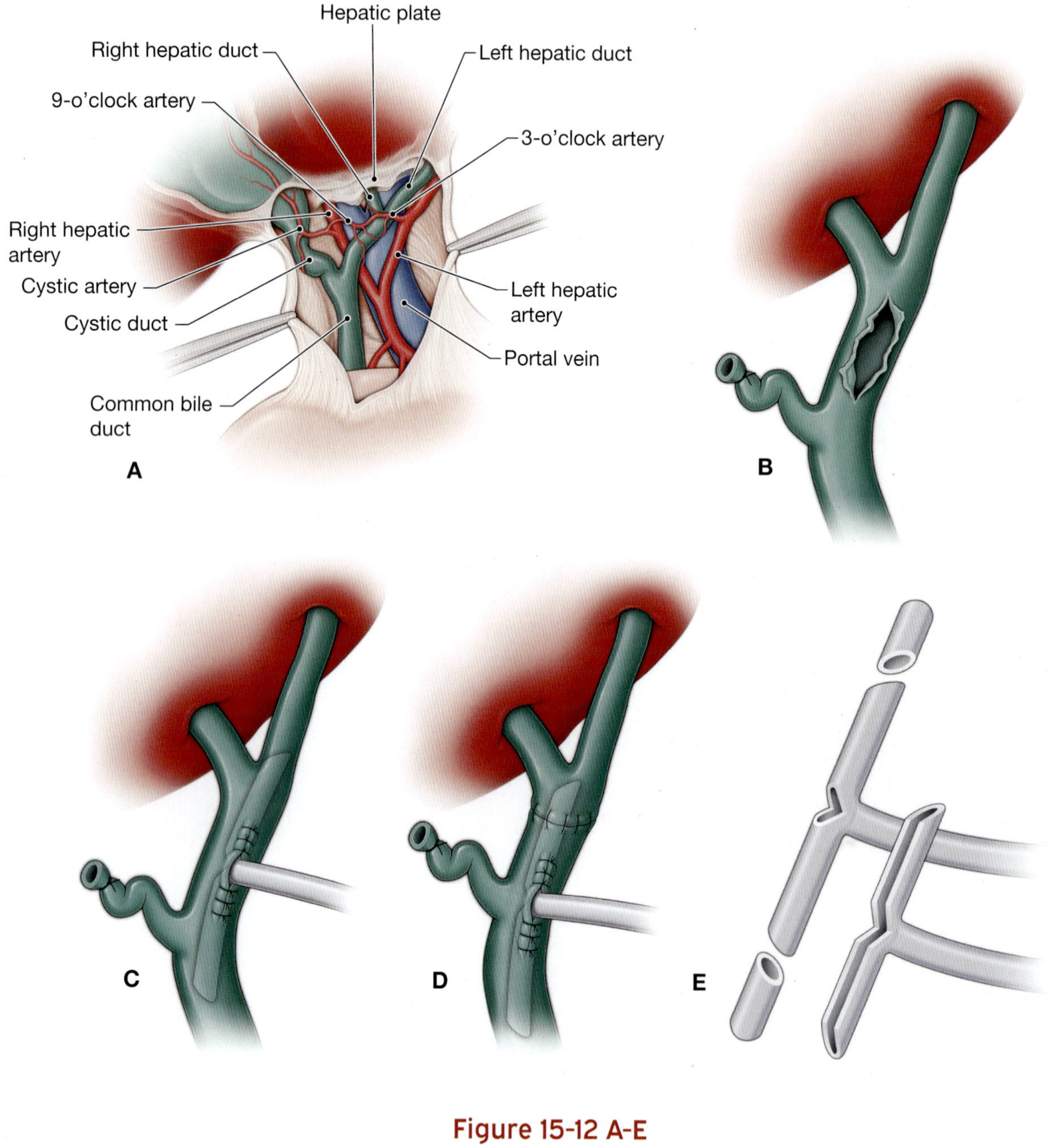

Figure 15-12 A-E

Complications

Complications are common and can manifest days to months after liver injury. These complications can include hemorrhage, necrosis, abscess, biloma, biliary fistula, pseudoaneurysm, arteriovenous fistula, hemobilia, and intrahepatic biliary strictures. Many of these complications can be asymptomatic initially but subsequently develop into life-threatening problems as time progresses. As many as 50% of patients will suffer from a postinjury complication after liver trauma.

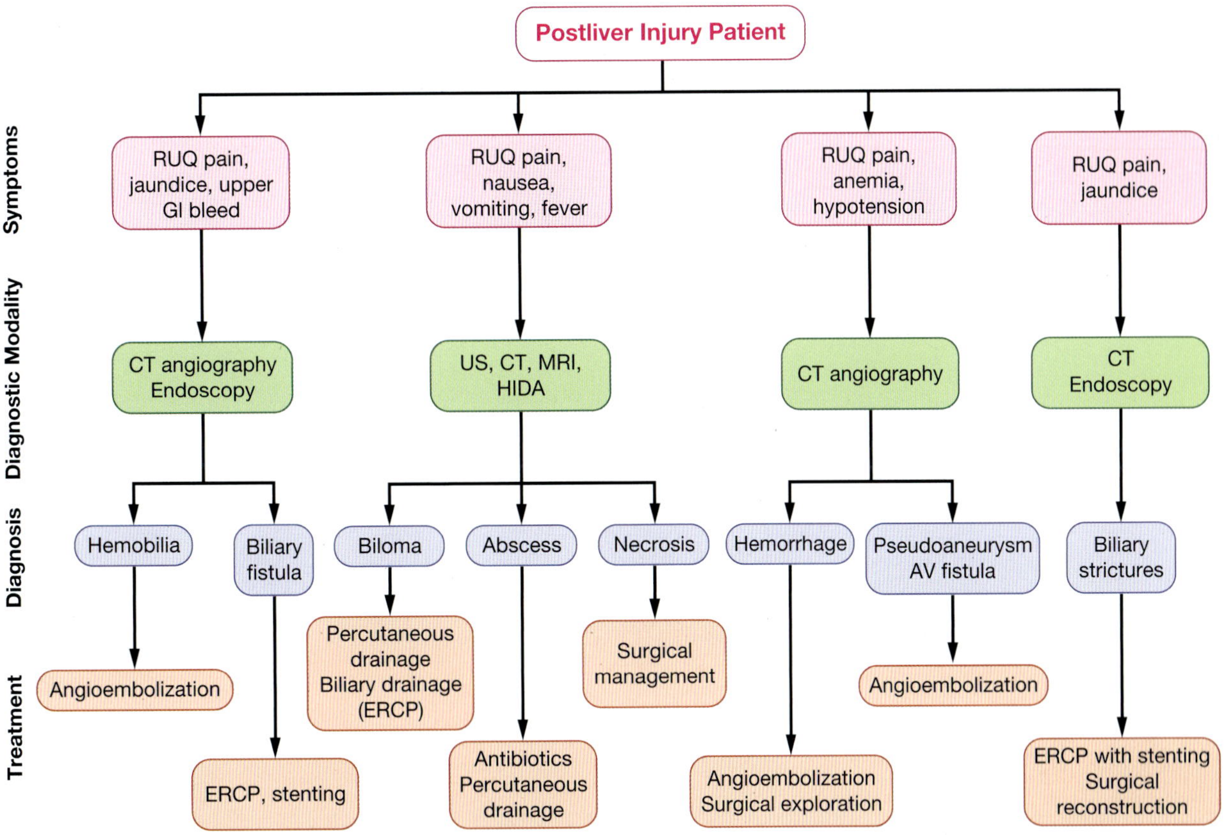

Figure 15-13

16

PANCREAS

Jeffrey Glaser, MD, MBA, MB, FACS

TIPS

1. **Suspicion for pancreatic injuries based on nonspecific computed tomography (CT) images and laboratory work is best evaluated with magnetic resonance cholangiopancreatography (MRCP) or endoscopic retrograde cholangiopancreatography (ERCP) to evaluate pancreatic duct integrity.**
2. **Operative access to the pancreas is often best obtained with entry into the lesser sac via the gastrocolic ligament.**
3. **Major devastating pancreatic injuries are typically best treated with damage control procedures at the initial operation due to the high incidence of concurrent injuries.**

Introduction

While uncommon, traumatic injuries to the pancreas can occur after both blunt and penetrating trauma. They typically occur in the setting of multiorgan trauma and can easily be missed at initial evaluation. Most cases of pancreatic injury result from penetrating trauma in the United States. The incidence of pancreatic trauma is reported to be less than 2% of blunt trauma cases but with a mortality rate of up to 34%. Motor vehicle accidents account for the majority of cases followed by bicycle and motorcycle accidents. The high incidence of associated intra-abdominal injuries is often the cause of laparotomy for patients with pancreatic injuries, and intraoperative evaluation of the pancreas is essential in these cases.

In patients who present without an indication for laparotomy, the diagnosis is much more difficult because clinical exam findings and traditional lab work are unreliable to identify pancreatic trauma. However, delay in diagnosis of pancreatic injuries is associated with high morbidity and mortality, and therefore, a high index of suspicion is required to identify injuries. Amylase and lipase, although frequently elevated in up to 80% of cases, often represent false-positive results. Radiographic findings on the standard computed tomography (CT) obtained to assess for intra-abdominal injury may demonstrate nonspecific findings or no findings at all. In the stable patient with a concern for pancreatic injury, workup should include magnetic resonance cholangiopancreatography (MRCP) or endoscopic retrograde cholangiopancreatography (ERCP) to evaluate the pancreas and pancreatic duct. Operative intervention and intraoperative decision-making are based on patient stability as well as the location of injury and involvement of the main pancreatic duct of Wirsung.

Anatomy

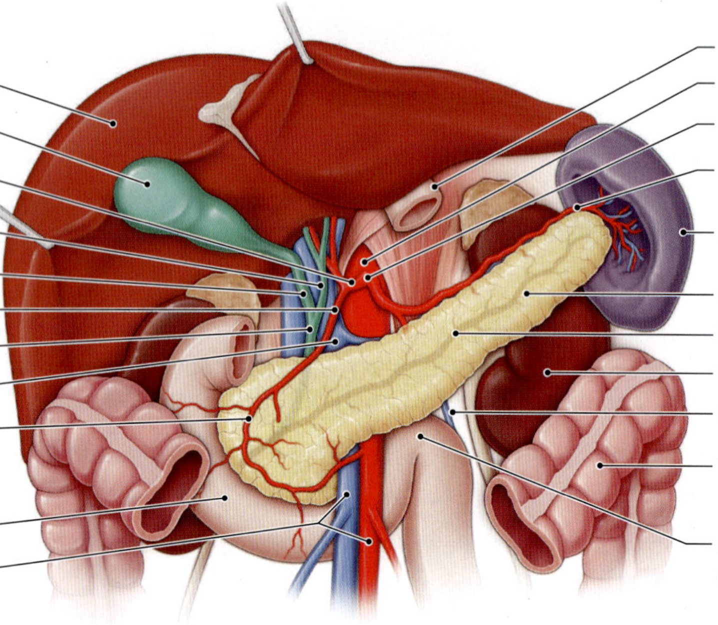

Figure 16-1

Grading

TABLE 16-1. American Association for the Surgery of Trauma (AAST) Grading System: Pancreas Injury Scale

Grading	Injury	Description
Grade I	Hematoma	Minor contusion without duct injury
	Laceration	Superficial laceration without duct injury
Grade II	Hematoma	Major contusion without duct injury or tissue loss
	Laceration	Major laceration without duct injury or tissue loss
Grade III	Laceration	Distal transection or parenchymal injury with duct injury
Grade IV	Laceration	Proximal transection or parenchymal injury involving ampulla
Grade V	Laceration	Massive disruption of pancreatic head

Source: Reproduced with permission from Moore EE, Cogbill TH, Malangoni MA, et al. Organ injury scaling, II: pancreas, duodenum, small bowel, colon, and rectum. *J Trauma.* 1990;30(11):1427-1429.

Grade	AAST Injury Scale - Pancreas	
I	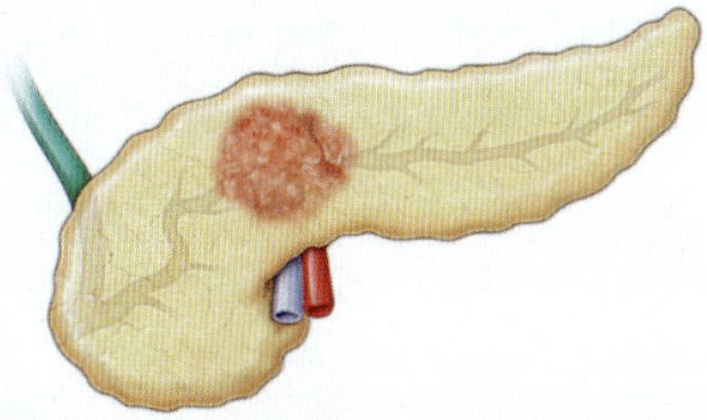	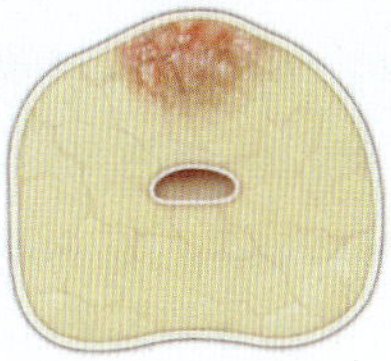
II	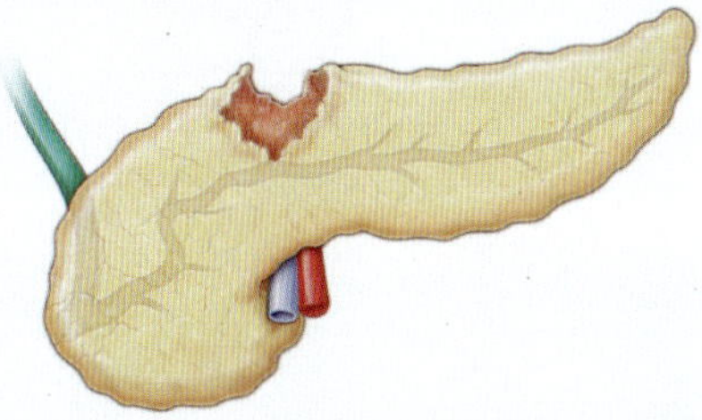	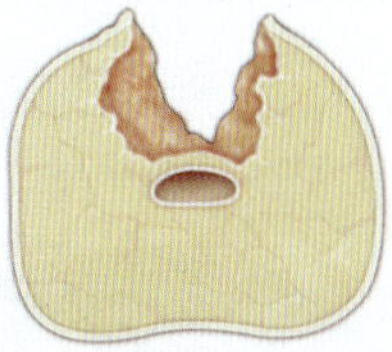
III	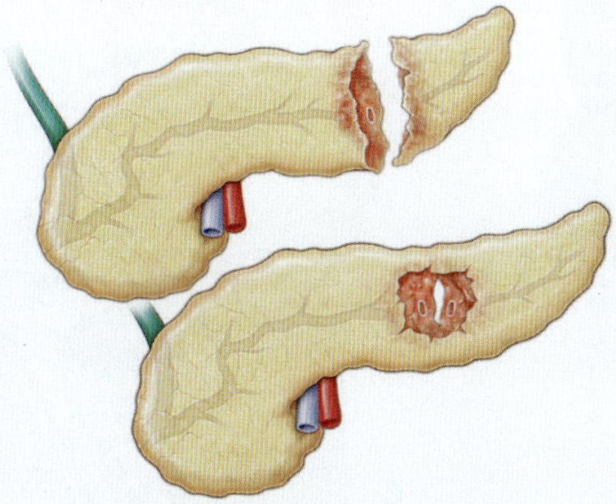	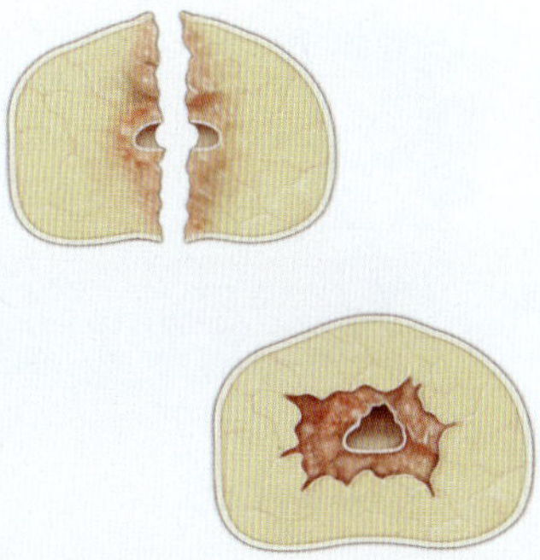
IV	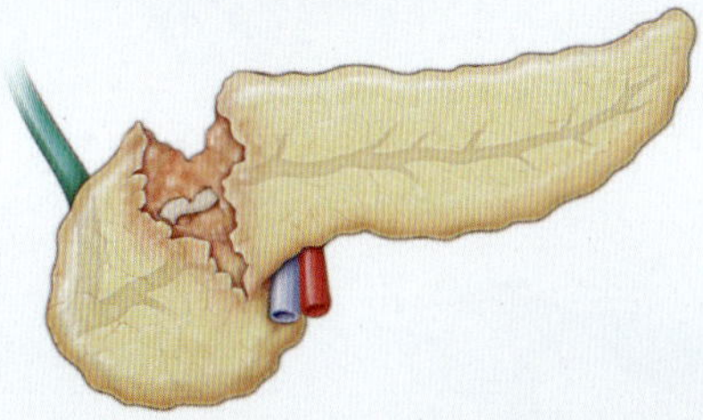	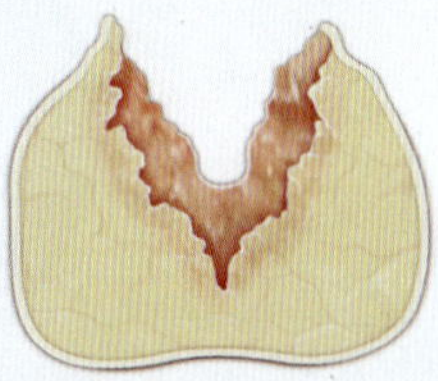
V	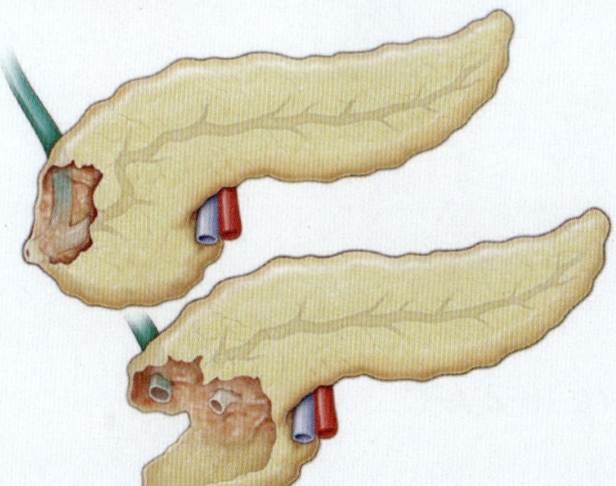	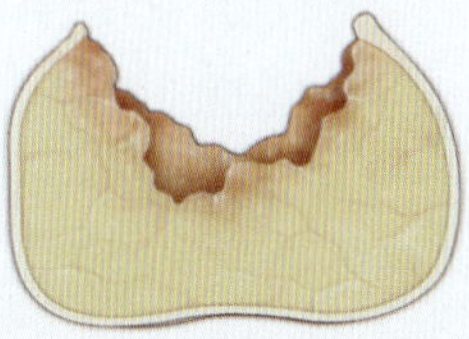

Operative Steps

Exposure of the Pancreas

The first step in the operative management of the injured distal pancreas is access through a midline incision. Then it is necessary to enter into the lesser sac typically though the plane between the greater omentum and transverse mesocolon. Subsequent reflection of the stomach superiorly and anteriorly will allow visualization of the anterior surface of the body of the pancreas. Continue the omental dissection to the left, and mobilize the splenic flexure of the colon and free the lateral peritoneal attachments to the spleen in order to mobilize the spleen and tail of the pancreas to allow palpation and partial visualization of the posterior aspect (Figure 16-2A-C).

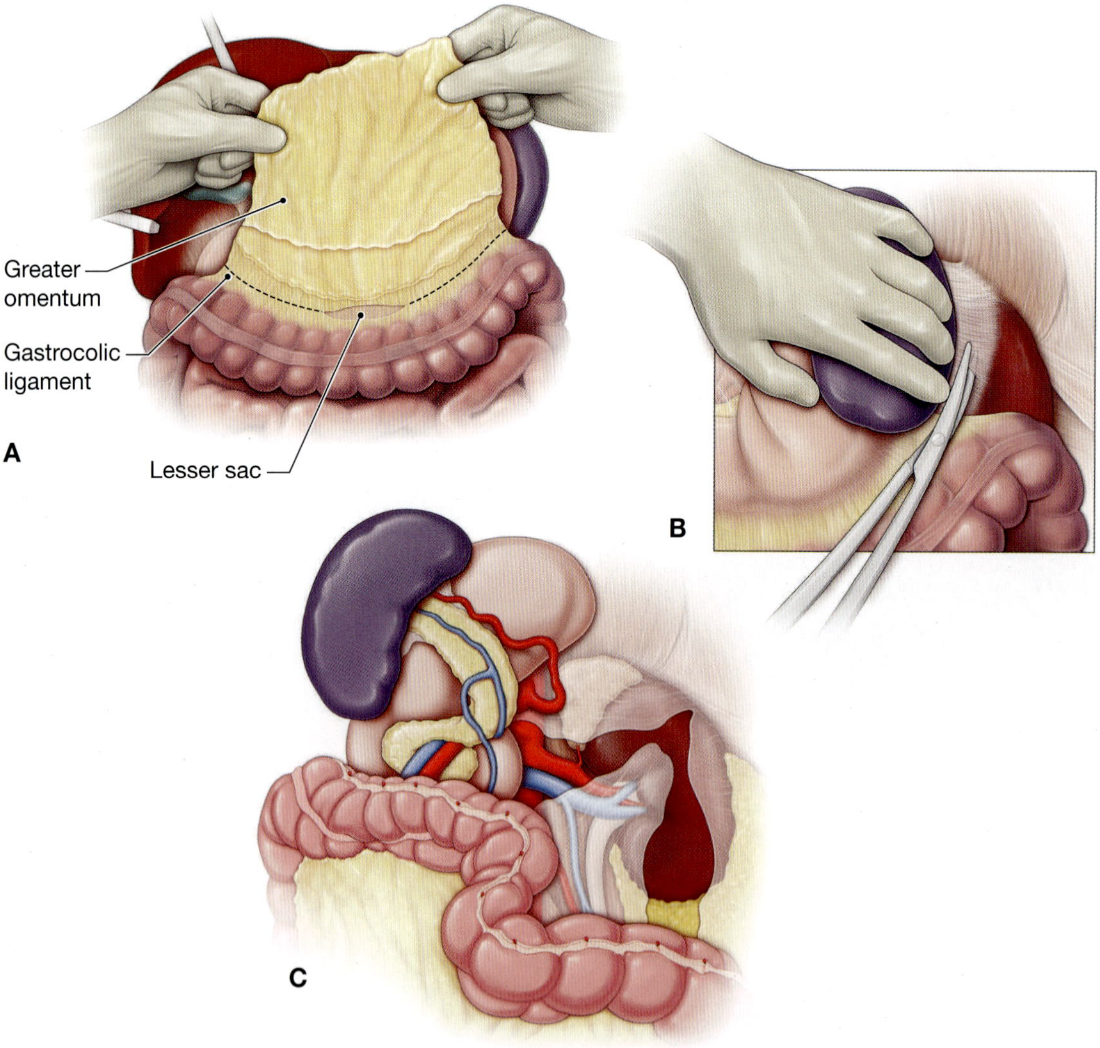

Figure 16-2 A-C

Distal Pancreatectomy

Once the pancreas is exposed as above, take down the short gastric vessels connecting the spleen and stomach and continue to mobilize the spleen and tail of the pancreas off the underlying kidney and adrenals. Gentle finger dissection behind the pancreas should allow the posterior wall to be elevated off the posterior tissue with care taken to avoid injury to the superior mesenteric vessels. Ligate the splenic artery first and then the splenic vein. Staple across the pancreatic parenchyma and remove the distal pancreas and spleen (Figure 16-3A, B).

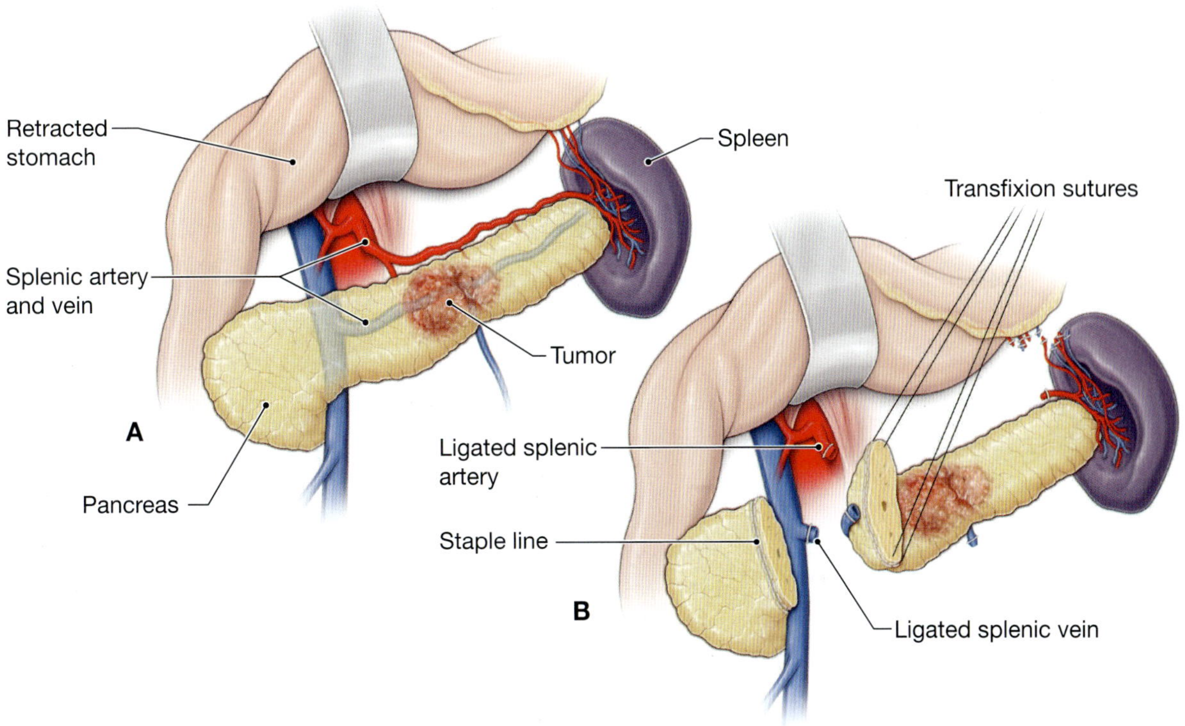

Figure 16-3 A, B

Pancreaticoduodenectomy

While rarely performed for acute trauma, in the case of a devastating injury to the head of the pancreas or disruption of the blood supply to this area, it may be necessary to perform a pancreaticoduodenectomy. The initial step for this procedure is to perform an extended Kocher maneuver to mobilize the duodenum to the ligament of Treitz and mobilize the hepatic flexure of the colon. Entry into the lesser sac is performed as above to expose the body of the pancreas (Figure 16-4A).

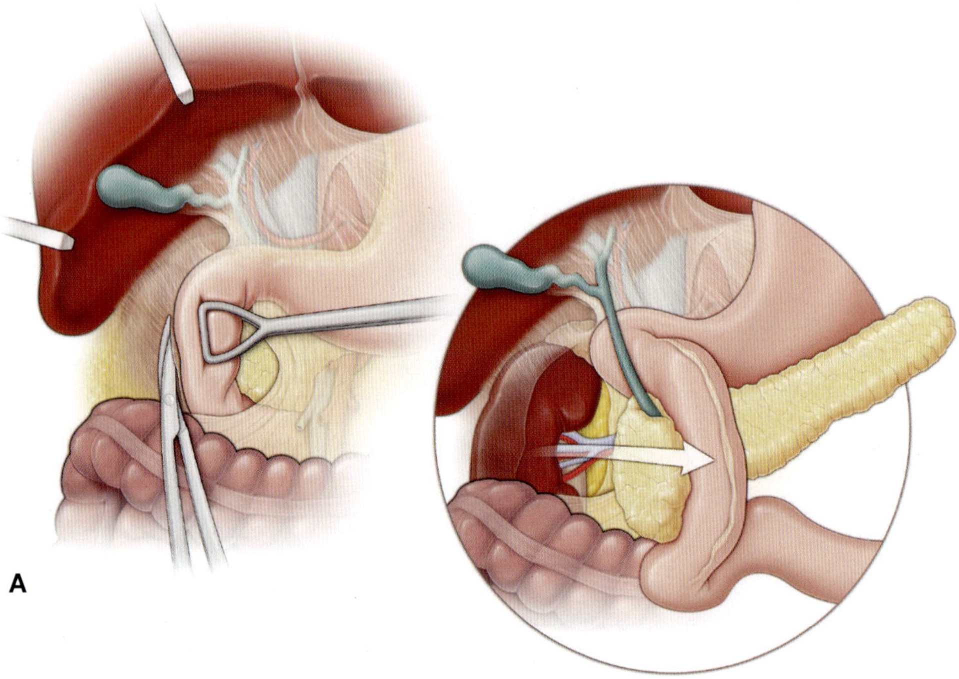

A

Figure 16-4 A

Dissection and mobilization along the inferior aspect of the pancreas beginning around the mid aspect will allow visualization of the superior mesenteric vein. Develop a plain between the pancreatic parenchyma and the superior mesenteric vein and portal vein confluence (Figure 16-4B).

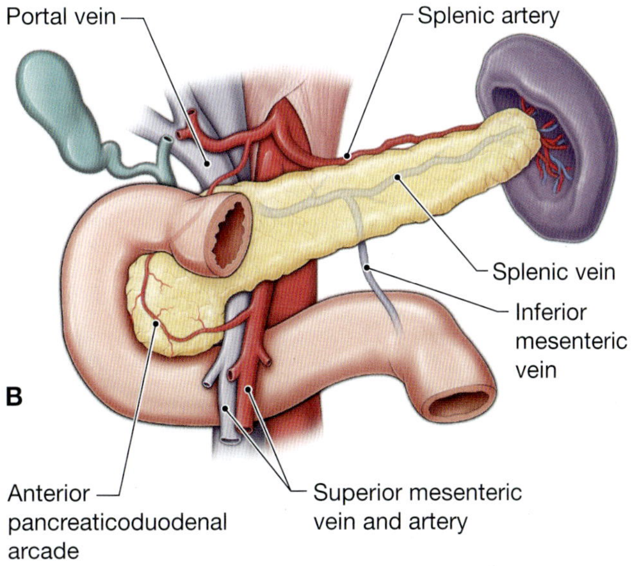

Figure 16-4 B

Incise the peritoneum of the hepatoduodenal ligament and identify and encircle the common bile duct and proper hepatic artery. Behind these structures, identify the portal vein and dissect along the portal vein to connect with the dissection along the superior mesenteric vein (Figure 16-4C).

Dissect the gallbladder free from the liver bed and dissect free the cystic duct and common bile duct confluence. Divide the common hepatic duct just proximal to the insertion of the cystic duct and ligate the gastroduodenal artery (Figure 16-4D).

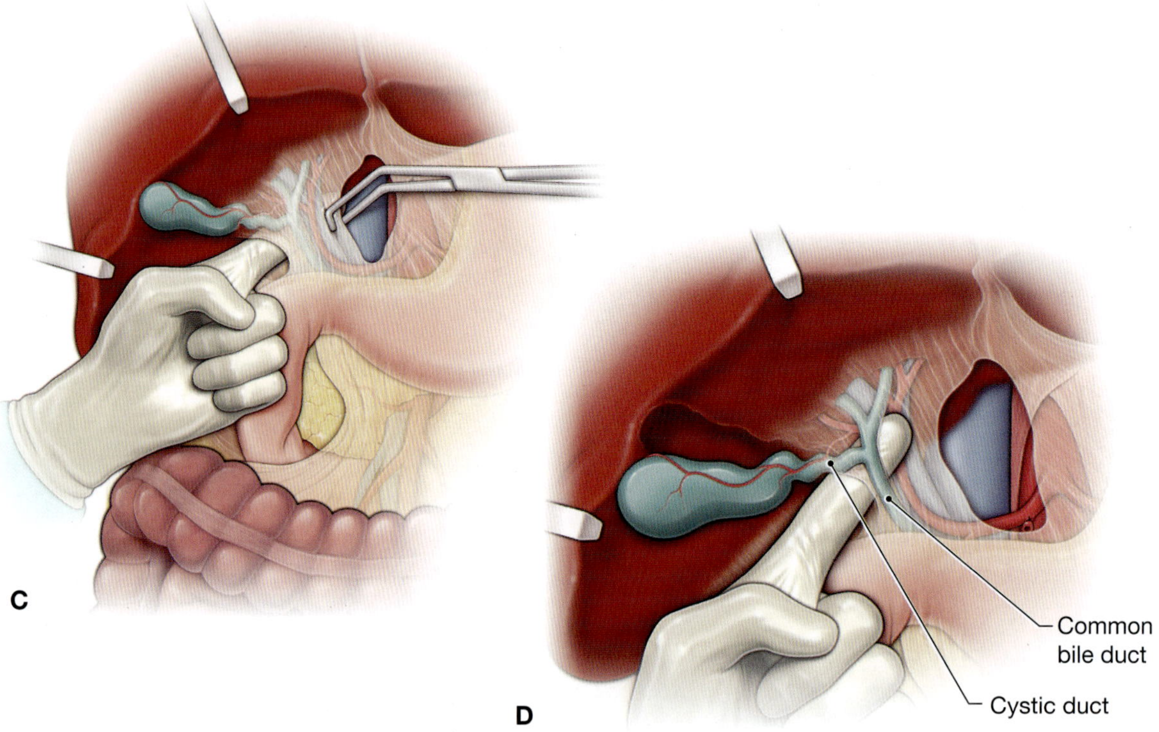

Figure 16-4 C, D

Ligate and divide the right gastric artery and divide the duodenum, and then place stay sutures in the proximal and distal aspects of the pancreatic parenchyma around the anticipated site of transection. Then divide the pancreas with a scalpel. Reflect the body and head of the pancreas to the right and divide the final attachments of the pancreatic parenchyma and the posterior structures including vascular branches off the superior mesenteric artery.

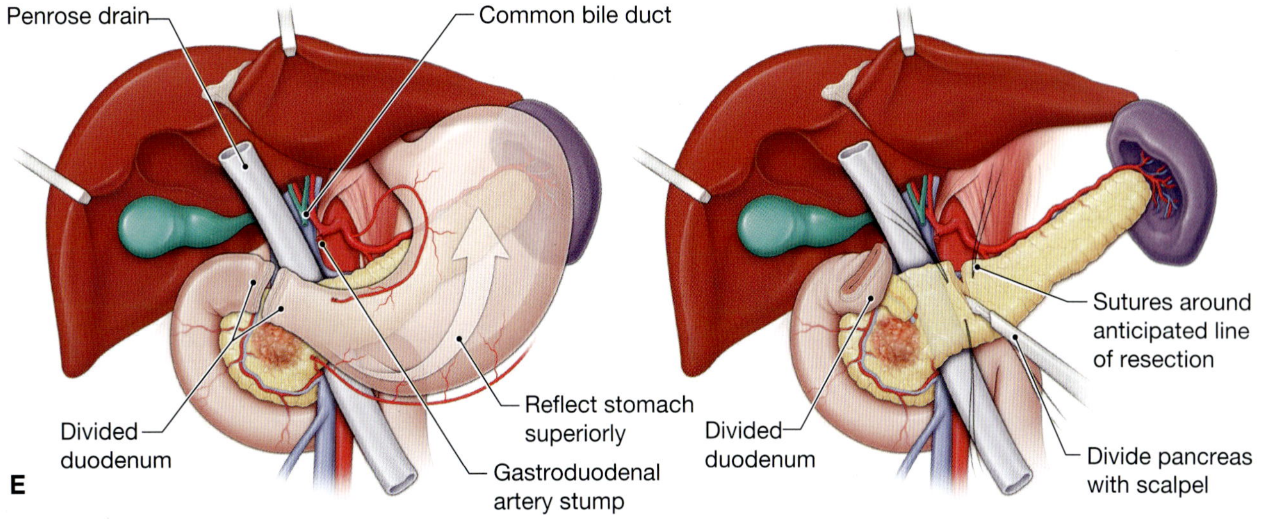

Figure 16-4 E

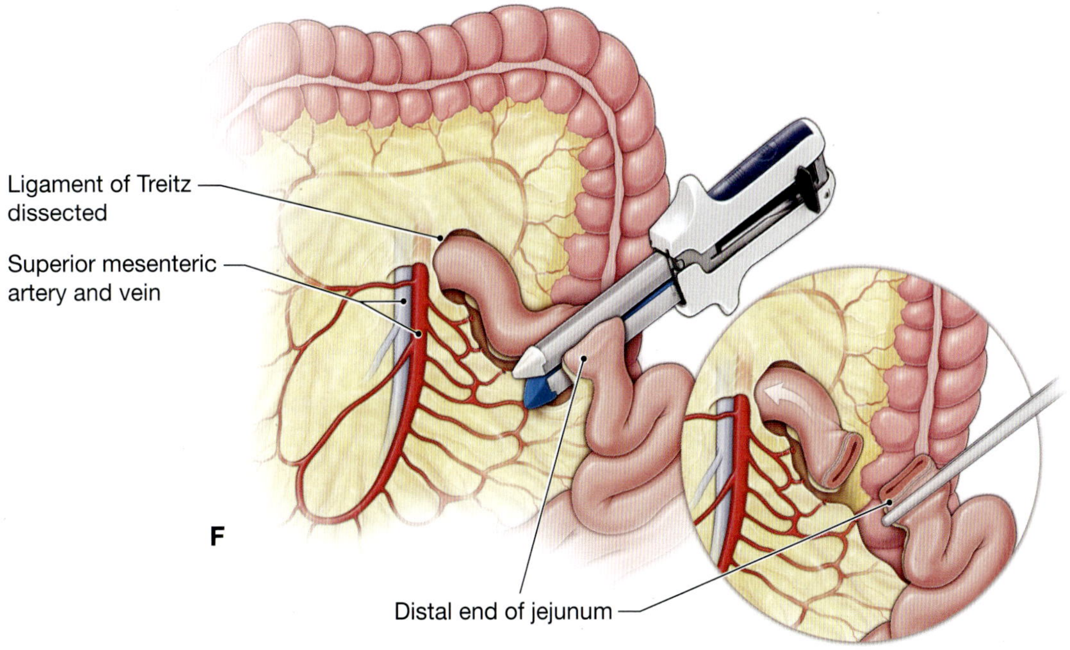

Figure 16-4 F

Divide the mesentery of the jejunum and divide the jejunum distal to the ligament of Treitz to free the specimen and remove it from the field.

Reconstruct the anatomy by performing a pancreaticojejunostomy, hepaticojejunostomy, and duodenojejunostomy.

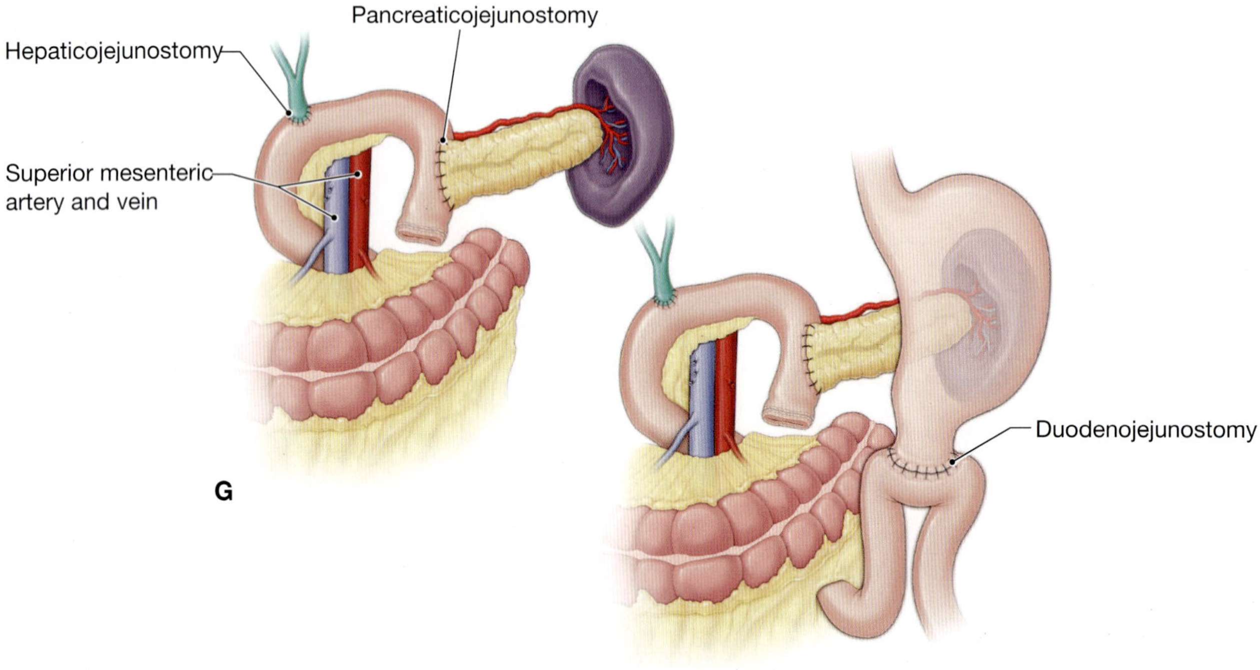

Figure 16-4 G

Pancreaticoenterostomy

In the setting of isolated ductal injuries or mid-pancreatic injuries, pancreaticoenterostomy may be an option for preservation of pancreatic parenchyma. The injured pancreas is exposed as above, and the proximal aspect should be transected and stapled as in the case of a distal pancreatectomy. The distal pancreatic tissue should be examined and the pancreatic duct identified. The ideal form of anastomosis has yet to be truly identified, but typically an end-to-side pancreaticojejunostomy is performed with the pancreatic duct anastomosed to the jejunal mucosa and the pancreatic parenchyma anastomosed to the surrounding jejunum.

Modified forms are performed as well, overlying a drainage tube and without an inner layer of the anastomosis.

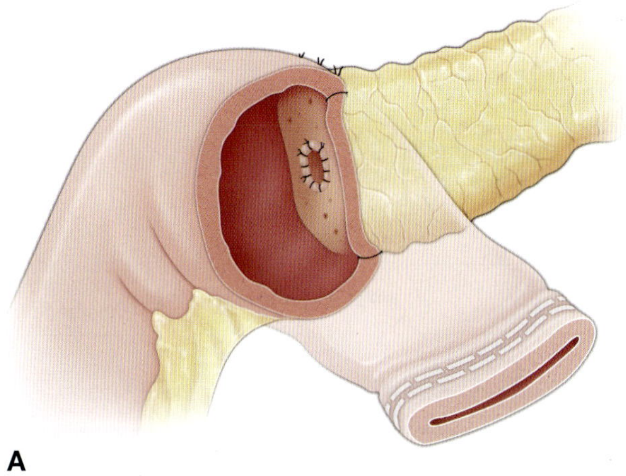

Figure 16-5 A

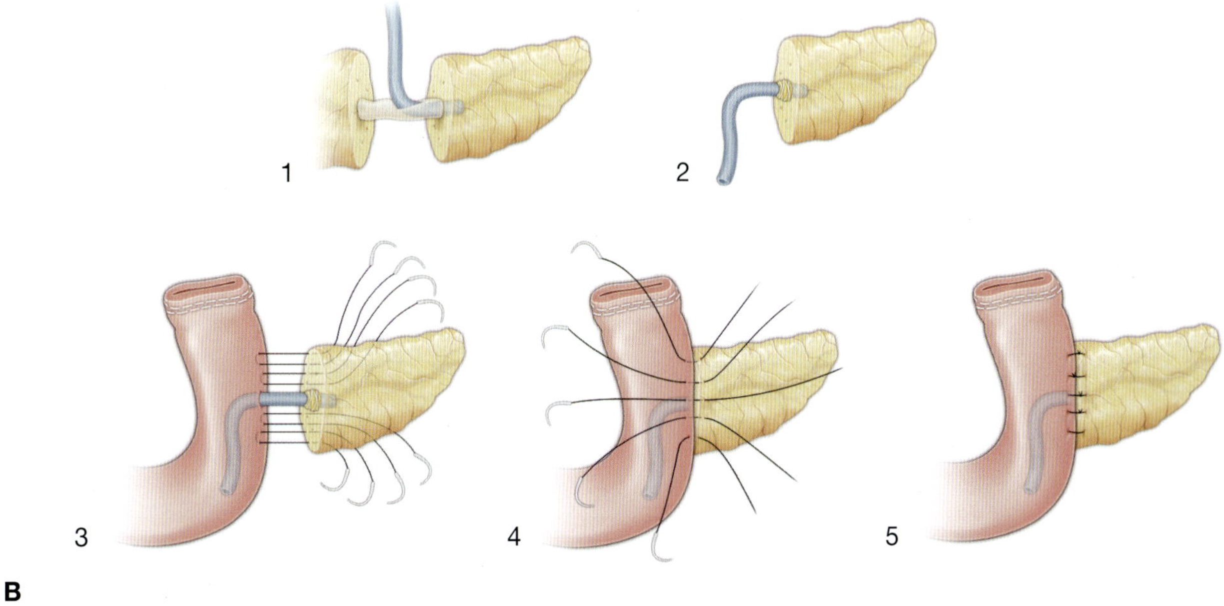

Figure 16-5 B

Complications

Complications from pancreatic trauma are wide ranging. These complications most notably include pancreatitis, pancreatic fistula, pancreatic insufficiency, pancreatic duct stricture, intra-abdominal abscess, and abdominal hemorrhage. Missed pancreatic injuries are at risk for development of pancreatitis or intra-abdominal abscesses with pancreatic fistulas, leading to a significant increase in morbidity and mortality for these patients. Devascularization and damage to a large portion of pancreatic parenchyma can lead to pancreatic insufficiency with both endocrine and exocrine issues. Longer-term complications such as pancreatic duct strictures can lead to the need for additional procedures down the line for patients. Higher-grade injuries are more likely to result in need for intervention as well as in increased risk of complications.

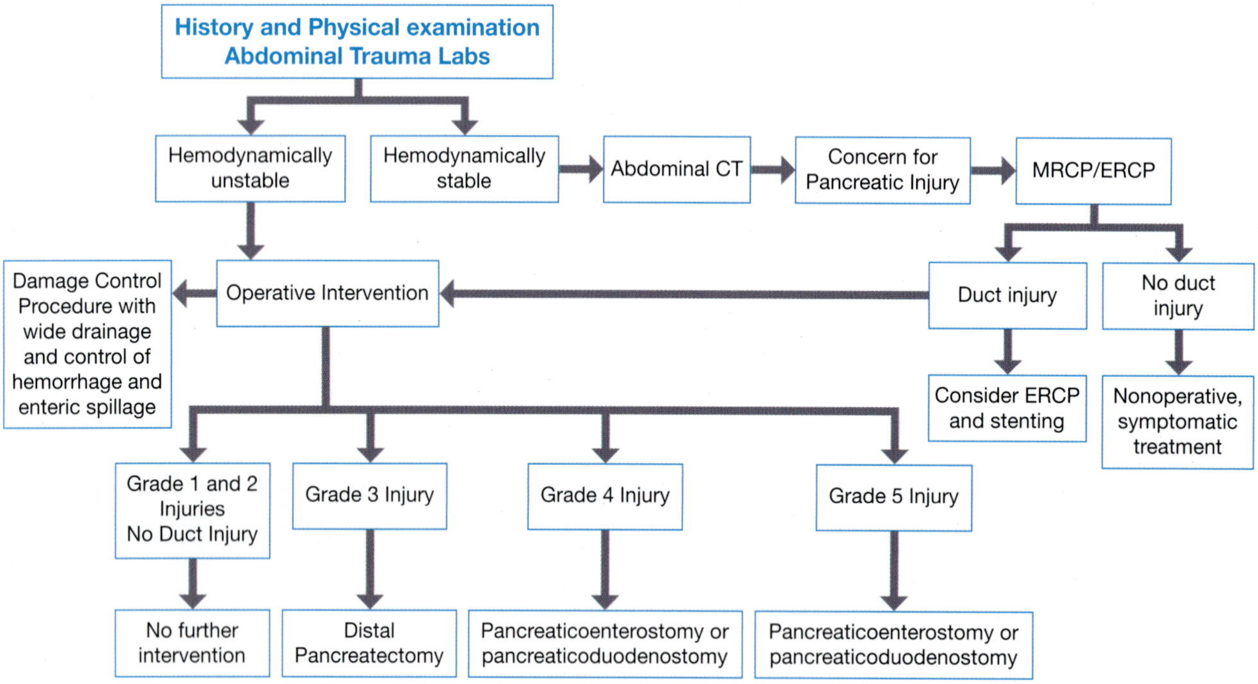

Figure 16-6

17

SMALL BOWEL TRAUMA

Matthew D. Painter, MD, FACS
Mark Cipolle, MD, PhD, FACS, FCCM

TIPS

1. **Diagnosis of bowel injury is often made during laparotomy for penetrating injury or on computed tomography imaging for blunt injury, which may show free air or intra-abdominal fluid. Full-thickness injury requires operative repair.**
2. **Mesenteric injury can lead to devascularization, which may require resection of the affected bowel.**
3. **Delay in diagnosis of bowel injury is associated with increased mortality after only 8 hours, mandating early definitive management of full-thickness bowel injury.**

Introduction

Injury to the small bowel or mesentery must be differentiated by mechanism. Injury to the small bowel or mesentery in penetrating injury occurs at an incidence of approximately 90% in gunshot wounds. In stab wounds, this incidence drops to 25% to 30%. In penetrating trauma, it is the most likely organ to be injured. However, for blunt trauma, it is the third most likely organ to be injured (behind the liver and spleen), with a cited incidence of 1% to 3%.

In penetrating trauma, the most common method for diagnosis is intraoperative. However, with a growing body of literature suggesting selective nonoperative management for penetrating trauma, computed tomography (CT) imaging may be used to make the diagnosis of a full-thickness small bowel injury. In blunt abdominal trauma, injuries may be noted incidentally at laparotomy for management of other injuries or on CT imaging as well. Intraoperatively, succus is the main indicator of a small bowel injury; on CT imaging, full-thickness injury is suggested by intra-abdominal fluid or free air.

Mortality rate after blunt small bowel injury is 10%, whereas mortalities in penetrating trauma are typically due to associated injuries. Missed hollow viscus injury accounts for an increased mortality in trauma patients, with increased mortality noted after only 8 hours of delay to operation; as such, care should be taken in the diagnostic workup of these injuries to definitively exclude them.

Anatomy

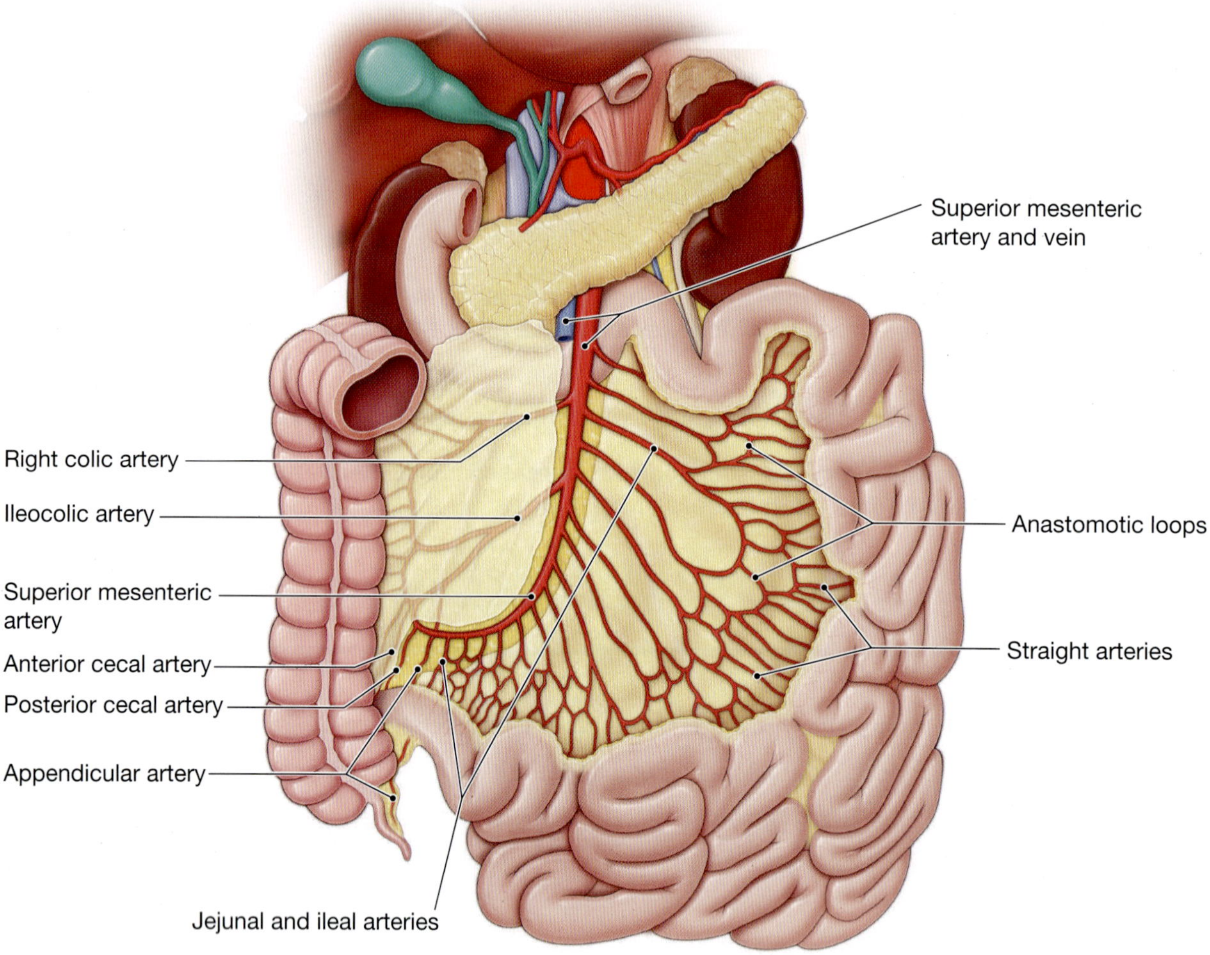

Figure 17-1

TABLE 17-1. American Association for the Surgery of Trauma (AAST) Injury Grade: Small Bowel Injury Scale

Grade	Type of Injury	Description
I 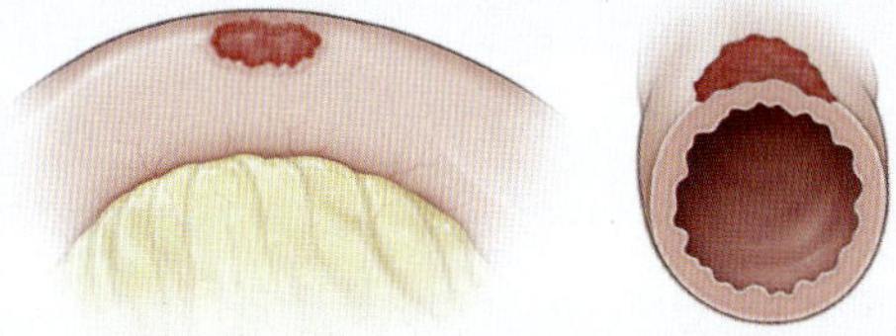	Hematoma Laceration	Contusion or hematoma without devascularization Partial thickness, no perforation
II 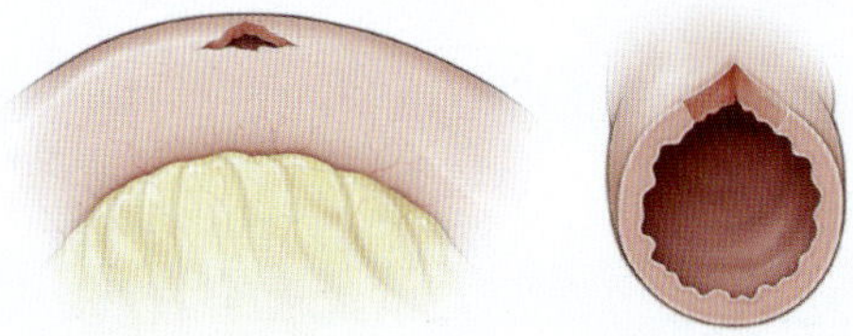	Laceration	Laceration <50% circumference
III 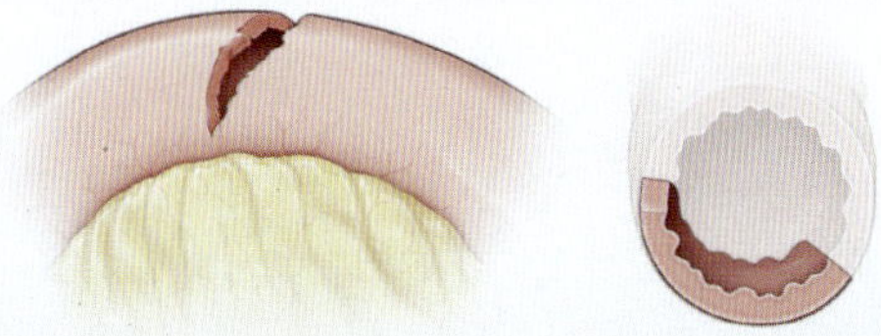	Laceration	Laceration ≥50% circumference
IV 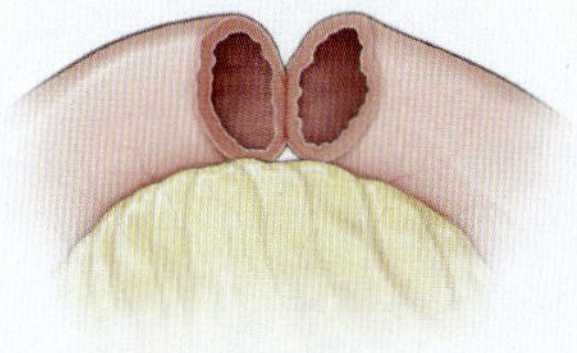	Laceration	Transection of the small bowel
V 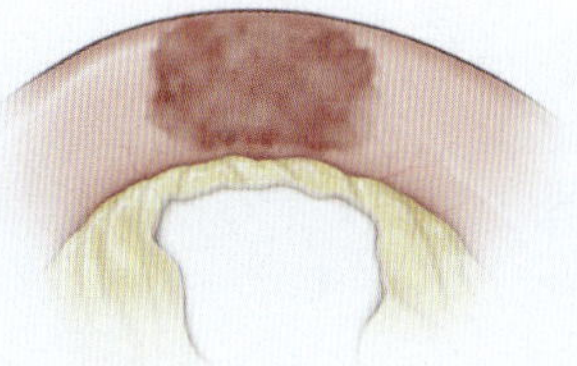	Laceration Vascular	Transection of the small bowel with segmental tissue loss Devascularized segment

Source: Reproduced with permission from Moore EE, Cogbill TH, Malangoni MA, et al. Organ injury scaling, II: Pancreas, duodenum, small bowel, colon, and rectum. *J Trauma*. 1990;30(11):1427-1429.

Operative Steps

Small Bowel Repair

1. Access via midline laparotomy incision
2. Debridement of nonviable tissue
3. Full-thickness suture closure of defect
4. May add second layer of seromuscular sutures for imbrication

Access is by midline laparotomy incision. Partial-thickness injuries should have seromuscular imbricating sutures placed to cover exposed muscle/submucosa. Full-thickness injuries should have debridement of devitalized tissue and suture repair in either one or two layers. Ensure repair does not stricture the bowel lumen (Figure 17-2).

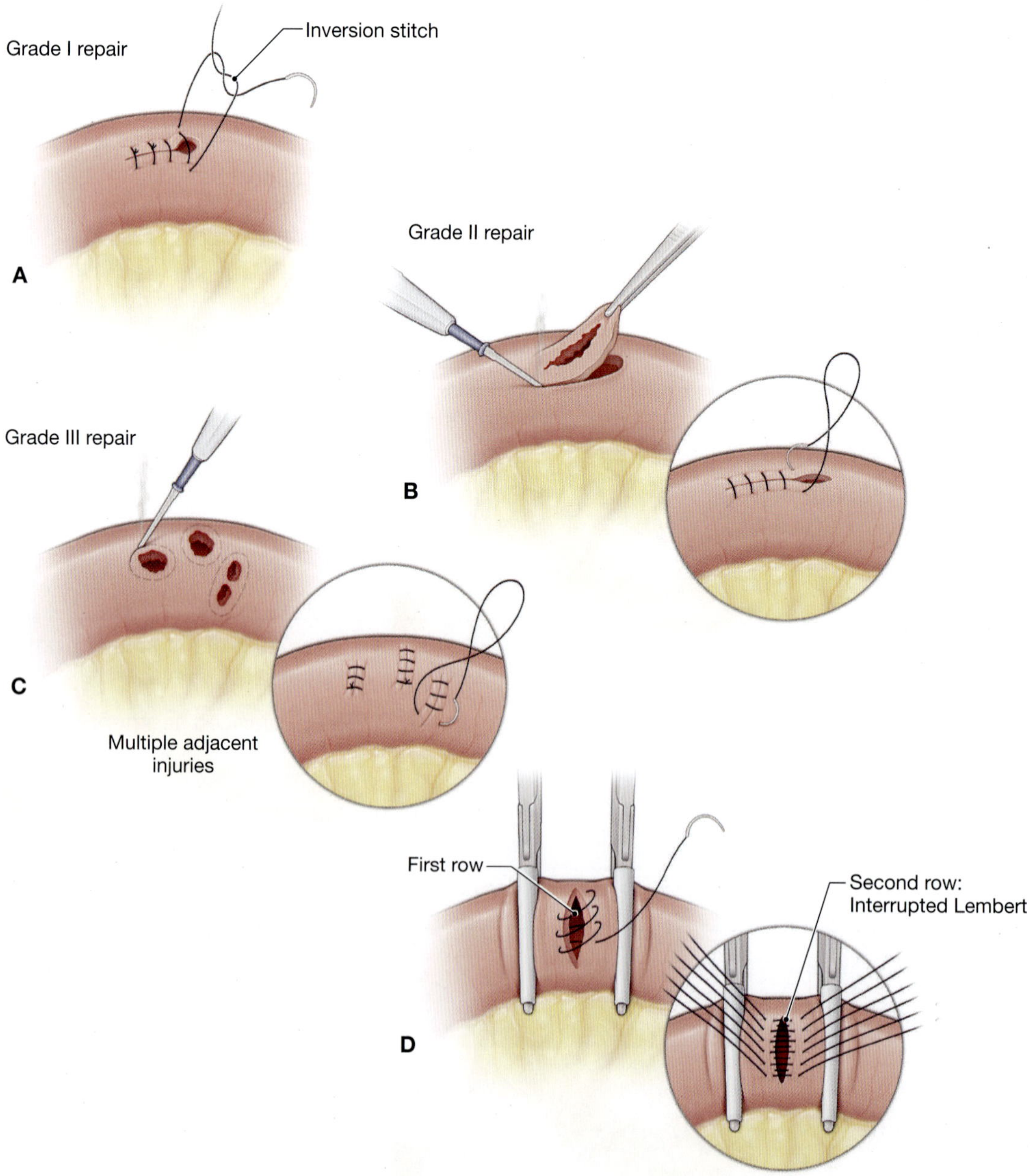

Figure 17-2

Enteroenterostomy

1. Access via midline laparotomy
2. Resection of nonviable or multiply injured segment of bowel
3. Ligation of mesentery with clamps/ties or energy device
4. Handsewn or stapled anastomosis
   i. Handsewn
      a. Stay sutures at 3 o'clock and 9 o'clock
      b. Full-thickness sutures to posterior wall of anastomosis
      c. Full-thickness sutures to anterior wall of anastomosis
      d. May add second layer of seromuscular sutures both posteriorly and anteriorly for imbrication
   ii. Stapled
      a. GIA stapler device inserted into lumens of proximal/distal bowel and creation of common channel of anastomosis
      b. Closure of back of anastomosis with either GIA or TA stapler
      c. Tension-relieving stitch at "crotch" of anastomosis
5. Closure of mesenteric defect

Resection should be considered for >50% circumferential injury, devascularized/devitalized segments, or multiply injured segments of bowel.

Handsewn (End to End) Place bowel clamps proximally/distally to avoid spillage of succus. Resect bowel with knife or scissors and ligate mesentery with serial clamps or energy device. Stay sutures will help to maintain orientation. Full-thickness sutures of the posterior wall should be accomplished first, followed by the anterior wall. Interrupted or running techniques using absorbable or permanent sutures can be used. A second layer of seromuscular sutures may also be used to imbricate the anastomosis. Close the mesenteric defect to prevent internal hernia with sutures (Figure 17–3).

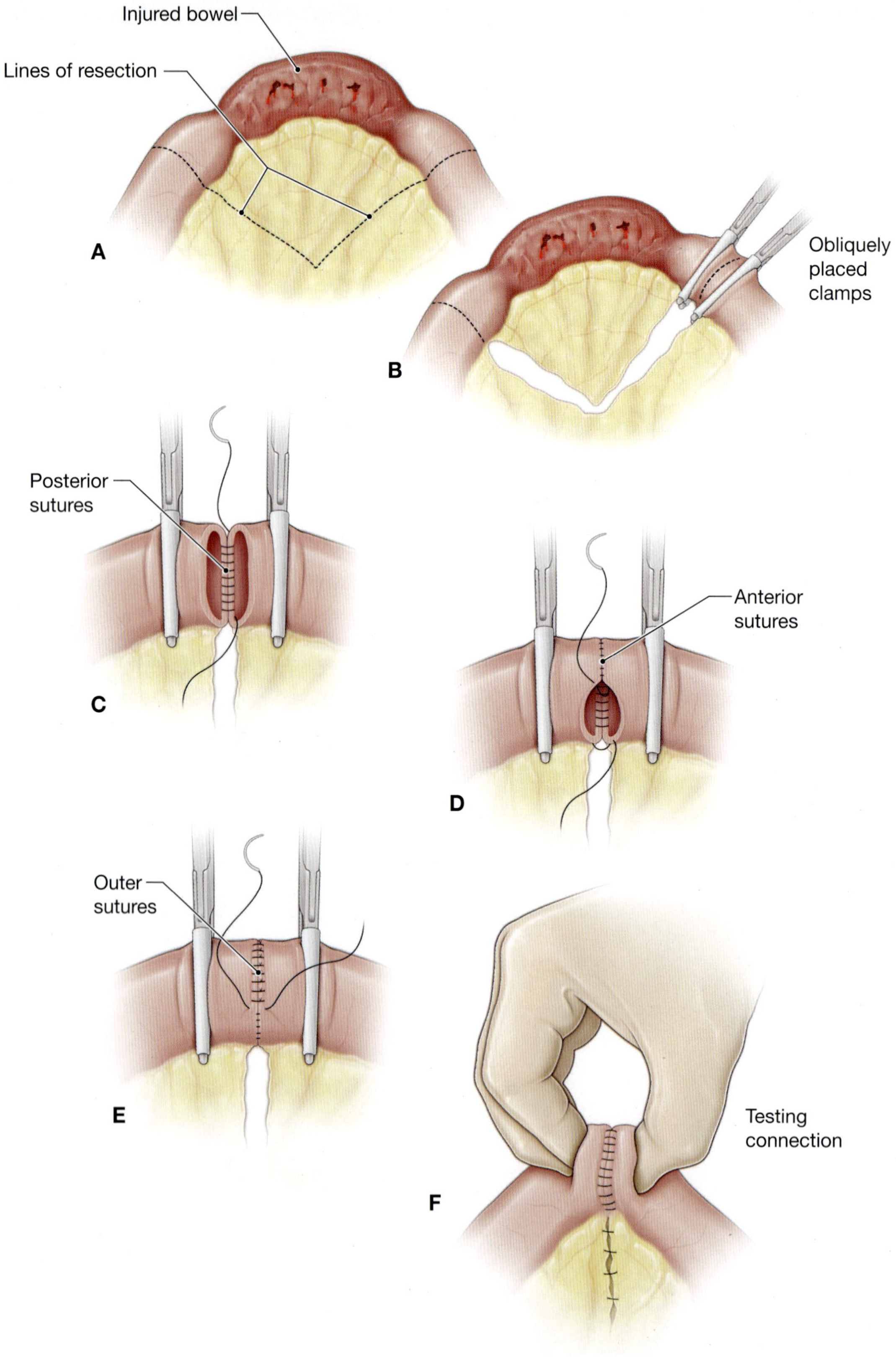

Figure 17-3 A-F

Stapled (Side to Side) Create mesenteric windows proximally and distally to injured segment and use a GIA stapler device to resect the injured bowel. Ligate mesentery with serial clamps or energy device. The stapler device is then inserted into the proximal and distal segments with creation of the enteroenterostomy. The back of the anastomosis can be closed with another firing of the GIA stapler or a TA stapler. Close the mesenteric defect to prevent internal hernia with sutures (Figure 17–4).

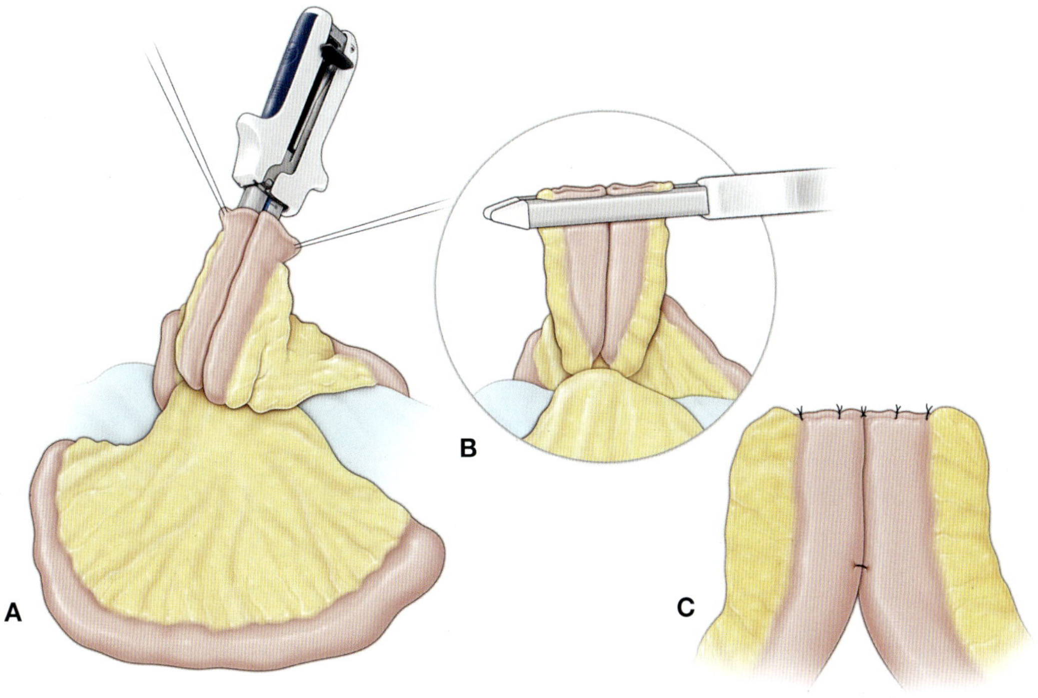

Figure 17-4 A-C

Ileostomy

1. Access via midline laparotomy
2. Resection of nonviable or multiple injured segments of bowel
3. Excision of 5-cm circular skin below umbilicus within body of right rectus muscle
4. Cruciate incision of anterior rectus sheath and splitting of rectus muscle
5. Incision of posterior rectus sheath/peritoneum in linear fashion
6. Dilation to two to three fingerbreadths and delivery of ileum
7. Maturation of ostomy in Brooke fashion with four cardinal sutures at 3, 6, 9, and 12 o'clock

If anastomosis cannot be performed after resection (either due to hemodynamic or anatomic considerations), ileostomy can be created. Ileostomy should be placed within the body of the rectus muscle, away from the umbilicus, costal margin, and anterior superior iliac spine of the iliac bone.

Excise skin overlying the rectus muscle and divide the anterior rectus sheath in a cruciate fashion, followed by linear incision of the posterior rectus sheath. Dilation of the fascial incision should be performed to two to three fingerbreadths. Brooke ileostomy should be performed to allow for stoma elevation above skin of at least 2 to 3 cm to improve appliance adherence and maintain ileostomy output off the surrounding skin (Figure 17–5).

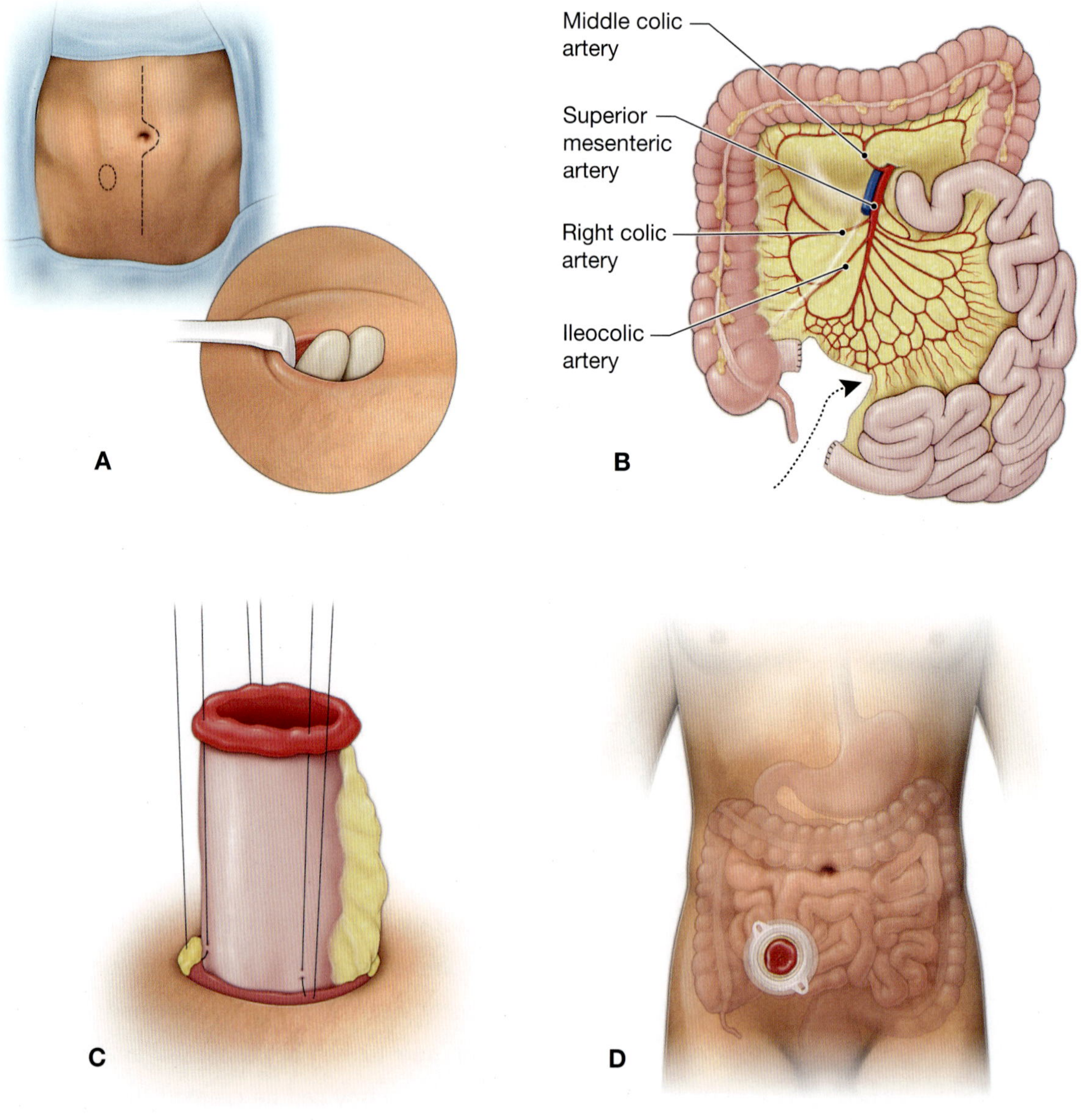

Figure 17-5 A-D

Complications

Morbidity and mortality are increased in small bowel injury when diagnosis is delayed. There is noted to be an increased incidence of wound infection, wound dehiscence, intra-abdominal abscess, acute respiratory distress syndrome, and sepsis with isolated small bowel perforations. Complications of resection or repair of injury are uncommon but include leak, enterocutaneous fistula, and intra-abdominal abscess. Patients undergoing damage control techniques are at higher risk of these complications.

Occasionally, patients will suffer partial-thickness injury of the bowel or ischemia due to mesenteric injury, which can present with delayed bowel obstruction from adhesions or ischemic structure. Symptoms are variable, from vague abdominal pain to obstruction, and can present in delayed fashion after initial injury but typically within 6 weeks.

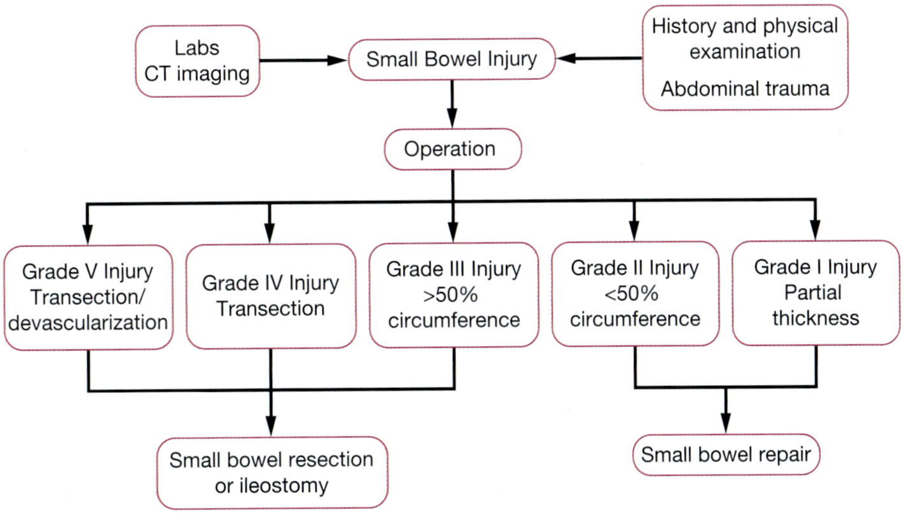

Figure 17-6

18

COLORECTAL TRAUMA

Grant Woodruff, DO
Anthony Dakwar, MD, FACS, FASCRS

TIPS

1. **Contamination control is a priority, but hemorrhage control still comes first.**
2. **Have a high index of suspicion for postoperative infection and other complications following colorectal trauma.**
3. **Proximal fecal diversion is the gold standard for destructive rectal trauma where primary repair is not feasible.**

Introduction

The colon is the second most commonly injured organ in penetrating abdominal trauma.

Patients with penetrating abdominal trauma who present with hemodynamic instability and/or peritonitis and/or evisceration should undergo emergent laparotomy. In the stable patient, the imaging modality of choice is a computed tomography (CT) scan. Penetrating abdominal wounds to the flank can raise suspicion for associated colonic trauma. The flank is defined as the anatomic area between the anterior and posterior axillary lines extending from the sixth intercostal space superiorly to the iliac crest laterally. Historically, triple-contrast (intravenous, oral, and rectal) CT imaging was the conventional study of choice to identify intraperitoneal violation and colon injury with a high sensitivity and specificity. However, due to the more expeditious nature of single contrast scans and the fact that the most sensitive indicator for emergency exploration was extension of the wound track to or near a hollow viscus, not merely extravasation of enteral contrast, many centers have abandoned triple-contrast imaging.

Whereas the incidence of blunt colonic injuries is less than 5% of blunt abdominal trauma, when present, these are commonly associated with high-grade solid organ injuries. The diagnosis of colorectal injuries in stable patients begins with a physical exam with frequent serial reexamination to avoid delay in diagnosis. Blunt injuries to the pelvis, high-riding prostates, and gross blood per rectum raise suspicion for associated rectal trauma, and in these cases, single-contrast CT imaging remains the diagnostic modality of choice to screen for other associated injuries in stable patients.

Operative management of colonic injuries with primary repair or resection with anastomosis is preferred. Exceptions include the hemodynamically unstable trauma patient and patients with extensive medical comorbidities or high-grade, destructive colonic injuries that would require diversion. Occasionally, abbreviated damage control laparotomy with control of contamination, resection, and leaving the patient in discontinuity and temporary closure with definitive repair at a later date following resuscitation and restoration of physiology may be necessary. With improved resuscitation strategies, this approach is now used less frequently.

Intraperitoneal rectal injuries are treated as left-sided colonic injuries. Management of extraperitoneal rectal trauma with proximal diversion (typically with a sigmoid loop colostomy) remains the gold standard for management for those injuries not amenable to primary repair. The "4 Ds" of rectal trauma (**d**iversion, **d**ebridement, presacral **d**rainage, and **d**istal rectal washout) are mentioned for historical purposes, neither of the latter two are necessary.

Missed injuries following colorectal trauma can lead to intra-abdominal sepsis and multisystem organ failure. Late complications of colorectal trauma include intra-abdominal abscesses, anastomotic leak, and fistula formation. One should have a high index of suspicion for postoperative infections following colorectal trauma, with a low threshold for postoperative imaging where percutaneous drainage is diagnostic and the usual treatment of choice.

Anatomy

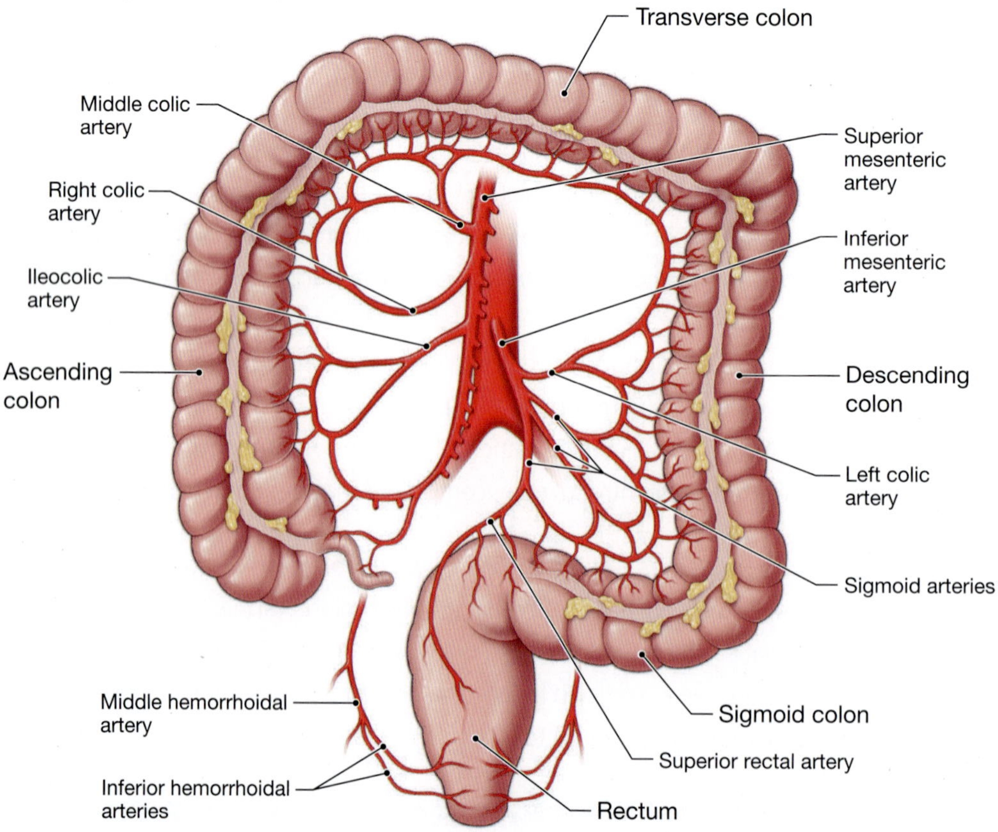

Figure 18-1

TABLE 18-1. American Association for the Surgery of Trauma (AAST) Grade Injury: Colon Injury Scale

Grade*	Type of Injury	Description of Injury	ICD-9	AIS-90
I	Hematoma	Contusion or hematoma without devascularization	863.40-863.44	2
	Laceration	Partial thickness, no perforation	863.40-863.44	2
II	Laceration	Laceration <50% of circumference	863.50-863.54	3
III	Laceration	Laceration ≥50% of circumference without transection	863.50-863.54	3
IV	Laceration	Transection of the colon	863.50-863.54	4
V	Laceration	Transection of the colon with segmental tissue loss	863.50-863.54	4
	Vascular	Devascularized segment	863.50-863.54	4

*Advance one grade for multiple injuries up to grade III. *863.41,863.51-ascending;863.42, 863.52-transverse;863.45,863.53-descending; 863.44,863.54-rectum.

Source: Reproduced with permission from Moore EE, Cogbill TH, Malangoni MA, et al. Organ injury scaling, II: Pancreas, duodenum, small bowel, colon, and rectum. *J Trauma.* 1990;30(11):1427-1429.

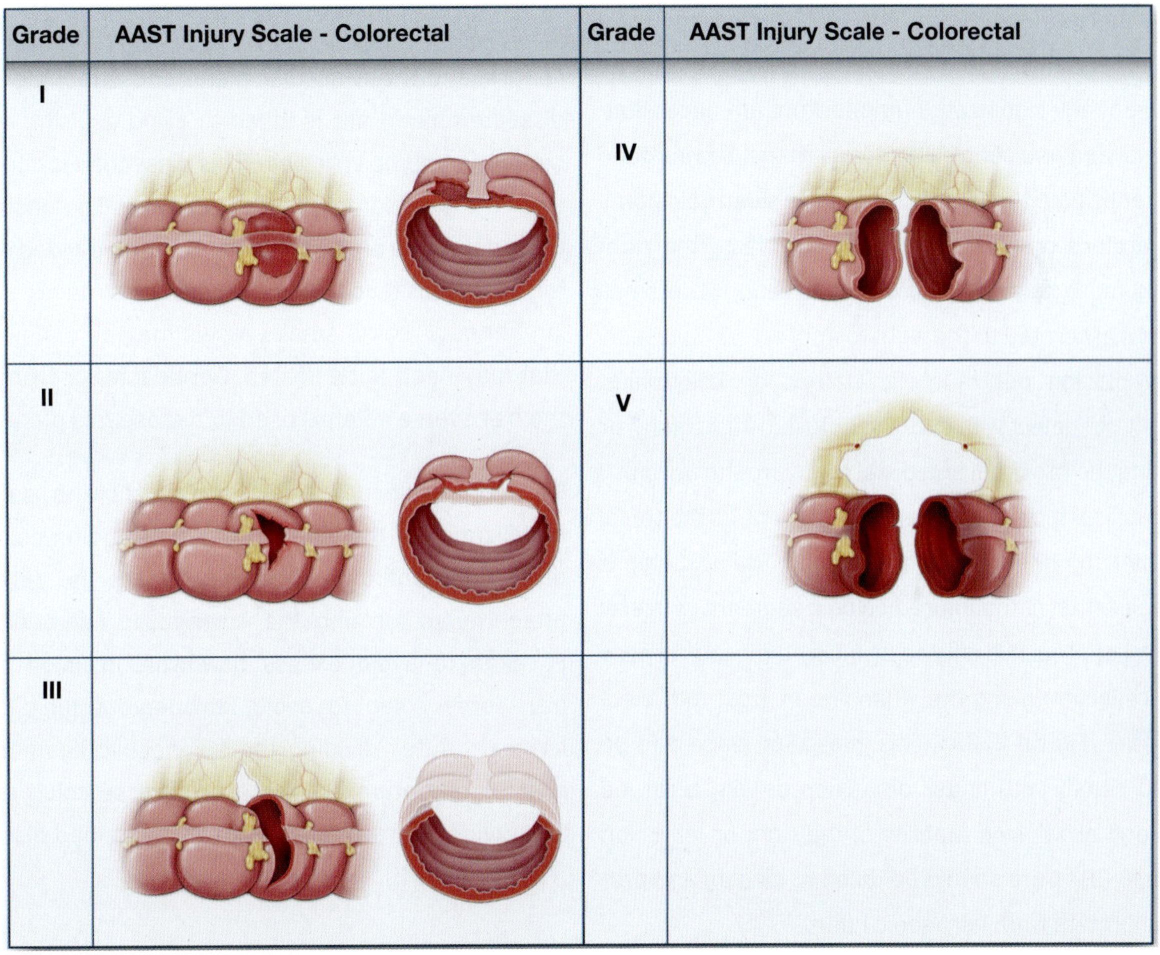

TABLE 18-2. American Association for the Surgery of Trauma (AAST) Grade Injury: Rectum Injury Scale

Grade*	Type of Injury	Description of Injury	ICD-9	AIS-90
I	Hematoma	Contusion or hematoma without devascularization	863.45	2
	Laceration	Partial-thickness laceration	863.45	2
II	Laceration	Laceration <50% of circumference	863.55	3
III	Laceration	Laceration ≥50% of circumference	863.55	4
IV	Laceration	Full-thickness laceration with extension into the perineum	863.55	5
V	Vascular	Devascularized segment	863.55	5

*Advance one grade for multiple injuries up to grade III.

Source: Reproduced with permission from Moore EE, Cogbill TH, Malangoni MA, et al. Organ injury scaling, II: Pancreas, duodenum, small bowel, colon, and rectum. *J Trauma.* 1990;30(11):1427-1429.

Operative Steps

Colon Mobilization

After a midline laparotomy, the first step in operative management of colonic injuries is to control contamination absent any significant hemoperitoneum necessitating identifying and controlling hemorrhage. The surgeon should anticipate the possibility of a left-sided colostomy and therefore make the umbilical swerve to the right to leave more room for colostomy creation. The small bowel is eviscerated to the right to improve visualization. Rapidly placing nontraumatic clamps on colotomies, securing the defect with running suture (whip-stitch), or encircling the proximal and distal colon around an injury with umbilical tape can all serve to prevent further fecal contamination within the operative field. The next step is full mobilization of the injured colonic segment. A lateral to medial approach is utilized by incising the lateral peritoneal reflection along the white line of Toldt with electrocautery (Figure 18-2A). This avascular plane can be entered bluntly with finger dissection or with a curved clamp and allows free mobility of the right or left colon (Figure 18-2B). Care should be taken to identify and protect the ureters from iatrogenic injury.

For hepatic flexure mobilization, the plane of dissection continues superiorly following adequate mobilization of the cecum and ascending colon. Gentle traction is placed on the transverse colon to expose the hepatic flexure, and the avascular plane and attachments are dissected free. Care is taken to avoid avulsing the origin of the middle colic vein. This dissection is continued toward the proximal transverse colon. The gastrocolic ligament will be encountered and can be divided to allow further mobilization. This attachment is mainly avascular, although some small vessels may be encountered that may need to be ligated. Gentle inferior traction on the transverse colon is used to expose this plane.

For splenic flexure mobilization, following sufficient mobilization of the sigmoid and descending colon, the dissection continues superiorly toward the peritoneal attachments forming the splenocolic ligament. Care is taken to avoid excess downward traction on the transverse colon to avoid iatrogenic splenic capsular tears. After dividing the splenocolic ligament, the greater omentum off of the transverse colon is lifted and divided toward the previously described dissection (Figure 18-2C-E).

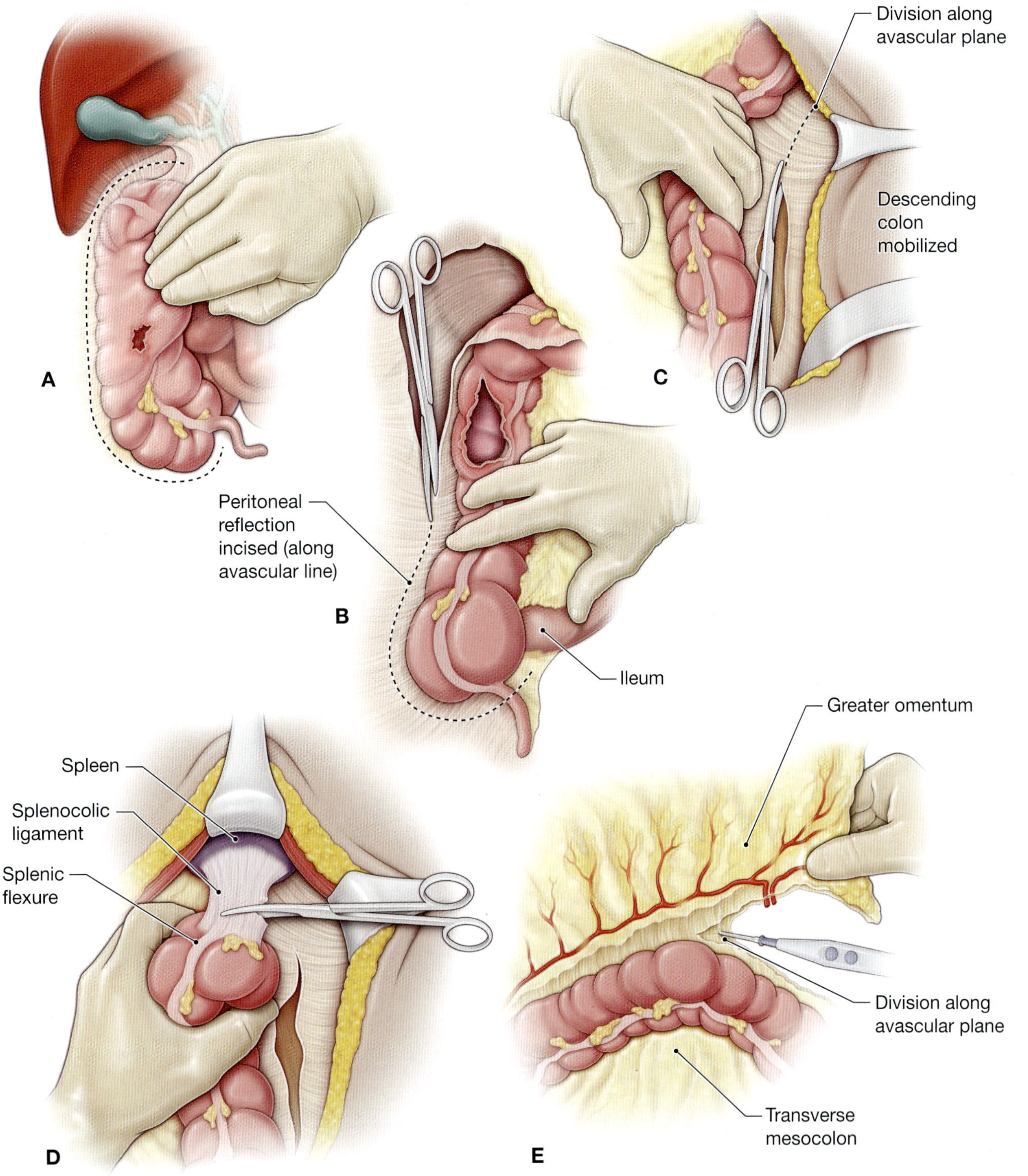

Figure 18-2 A-E

Primary Repair

If a full-thickness injury is identified, primary suture repair is a feasible option in injuries involving less than 50% circumference of the bowel wall and if there is no vascular compromise to the bowel (Figure 18-3A). The first step in the primary repair is to debride the edges of the injury until healthy tissue is encountered (Figure 18-3B).

A single-layer approach may then be used to approximate the bowel by simply throwing multiple single interrupted sutures or a continuous stitch across the injured bowel (Figure 18-3C). Full-thickness bites of bowel to have mucosal and submucosal approximation is crucial. Depending on surgeon preference, a double-layer technique may be used to include a second layer of Lembert sutures to buttress the repair. These are seromuscular bites that imbricate the repair suture line (Figure 18-3D).

Colocolostomy

In injuries with >50% bowel wall compromise and/or with vascular compromise (eg, a mesenteric bucket handle injury with intact bowel), segmental colon resection is performed with primary anastomosis. This can also

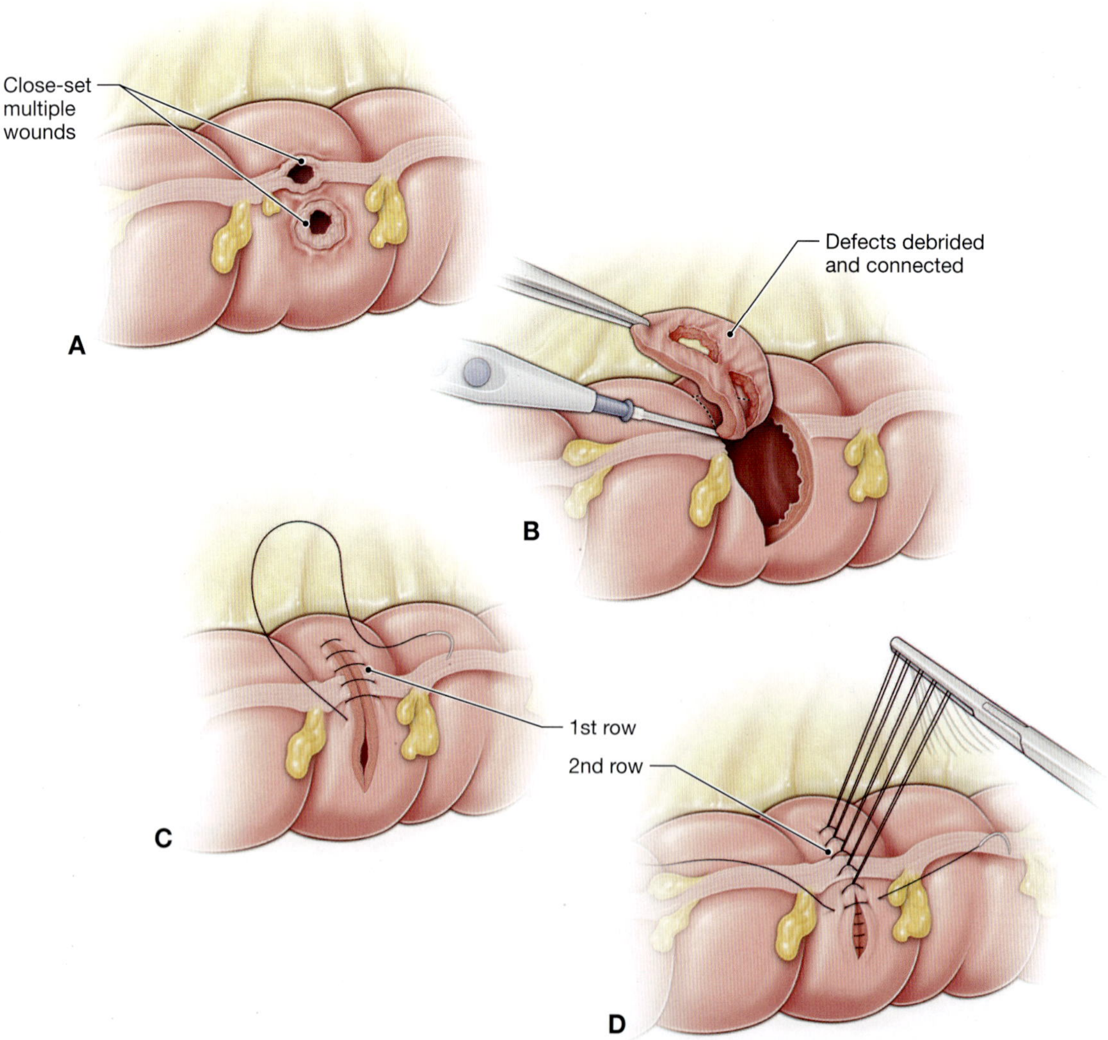

Figure 18-3 A-D

be performed after a damage control laparotomy to restore gastrointestinal continuity. This is an acceptable approach that portends favorable outcomes should it be done at the first take-back operation. Otherwise, exteriorization and ostomy creation are selected to avoid complications of anastomotic dehiscence.

Anastomosis can be handsewn or stapled based on surgeon preference. With a handsewn technique, an end-to-end, side-to-side, or end-to-side technique can be employed. The first step is to approximate the bowel and place stay sutures in each of the corners to aid in approximation of the bowel edges and prevent kinking. A row of interrupted 3-0 silk Lembert sutures is then placed along the posterior layer. After completion, two 3-0 absorbable sutures are placed in the center of the posterior wall, and this suture is run in each direction. Full-thickness bites along the inner layer are performed for mucosal opposition. This is continued anteriorly as a continuous Connell suture (out-to-in, in-to-out technique) for the inner closure in each direction until the sutures can be secured in the middle. Finally, a final layer of 3-0 silk Lembert sutures is placed over the anterior anastomosis to bolster the repair. Some surgeons may employ a single-layer anastomosis in either a running or interrupted fashion using a circumferential layer of full-thickness 3-0 silk sutures (Figures 18-4A-D and 18-5A-D).

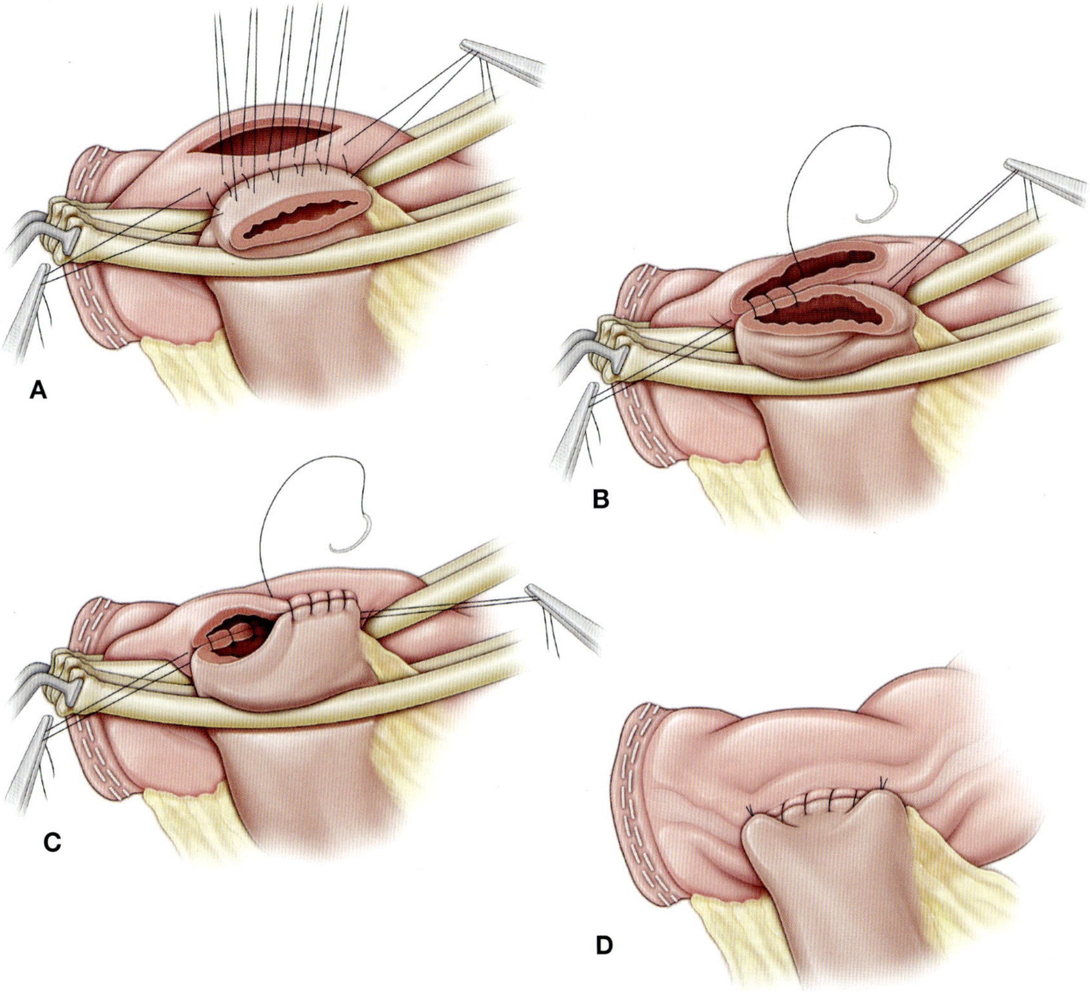

Figure 18-4 A-D. End to side.

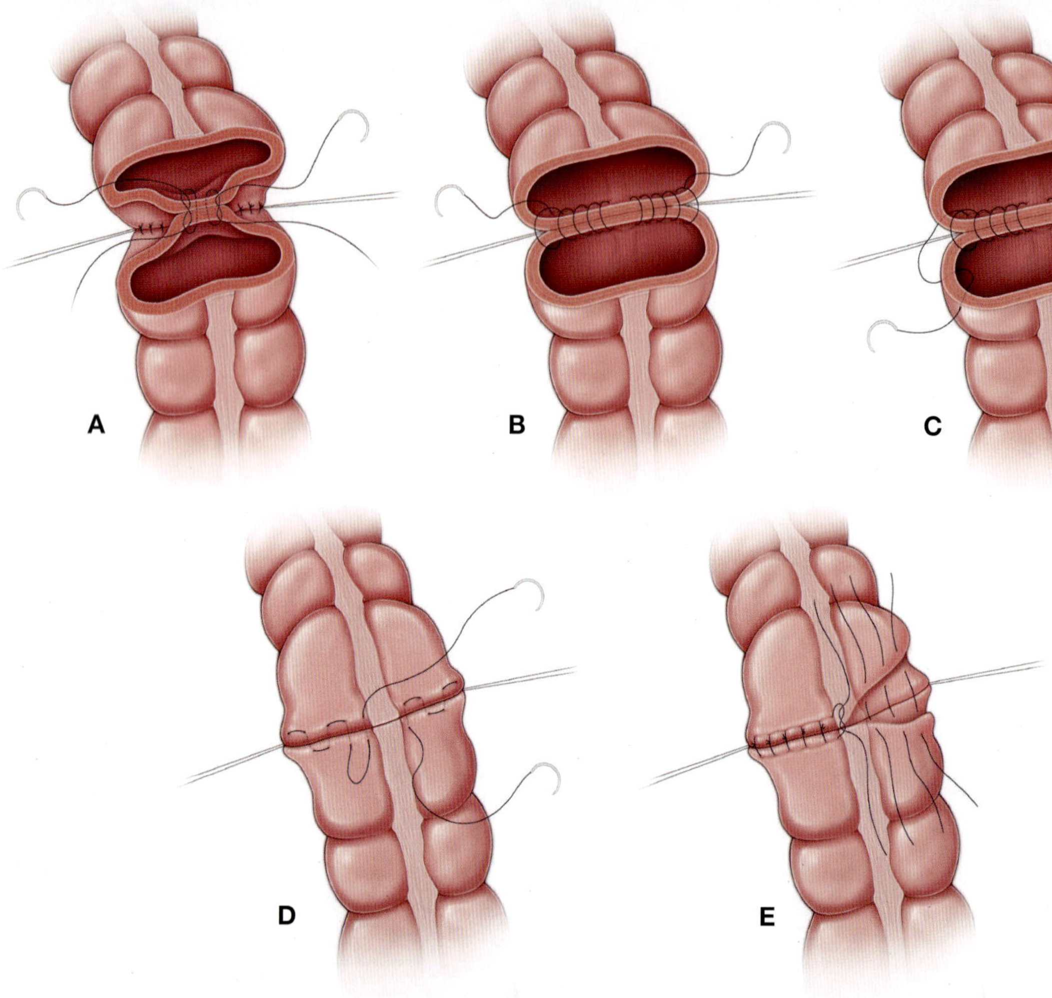

Figure 18-5 A-D. End to end.

A stapled anastomosis is also a standard anastomotic technique. After resection, the first step is identifying the mesenteric and antimesenteric borders. A 1-cm incision is then made along the antimesenteric border, a linear cutting stapler device is introduced into each of the bowel lumens, and the stapler is closed. Prior to stapling, it is essential to ensure the bowel mesentery is free from the staple device. Once cleared, a 4- to 6-cm common channel is created, preferably by one firing of a 60-mm stapler. The staple line is inspected for hemostasis. Allis clamps are placed on the open common channel to offset the staple lines, and this is then closed with another firing of the linear cutting stapler. Depending on surgeon preference, Lembert sutures can be placed across the common channel staple line to bury the staple line, although that is not necessary. A "crotch stitch" can also be placed at the apex of the common channel to help prevent any tension on the anastomosis. If omentum is available, this can also be placed over the anastomosis (Figure 18-6A-C).

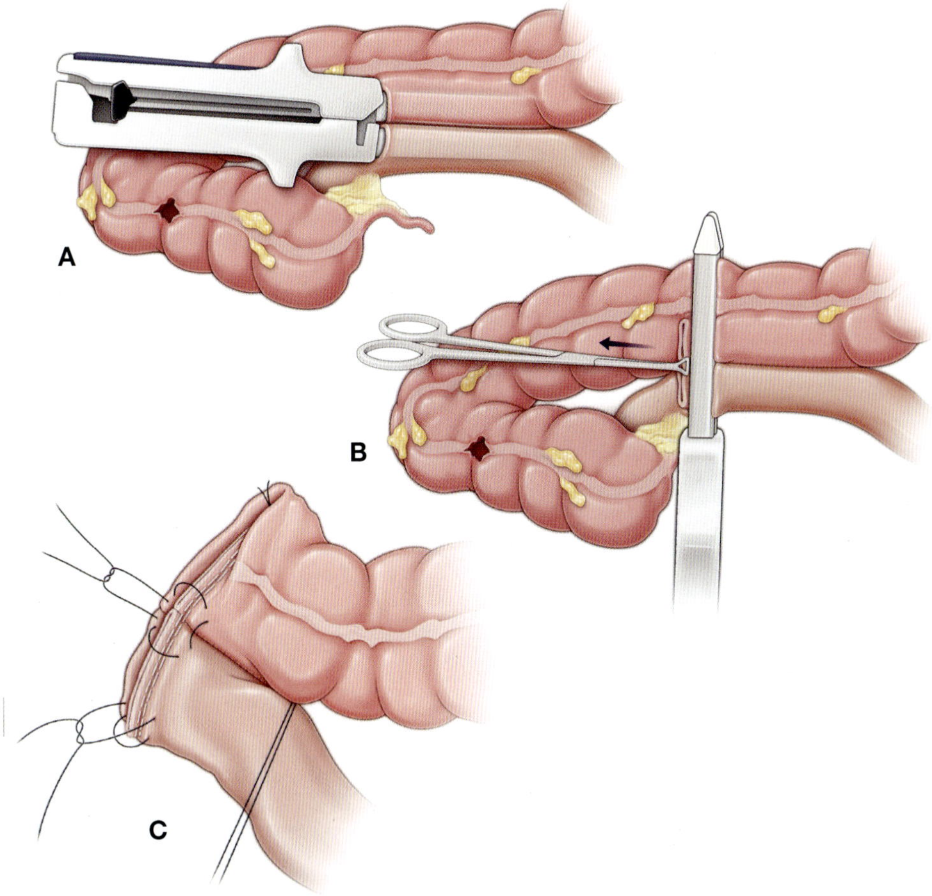

Figure 18-6 A-C

Colorectal Anastomosis (Figure 18-7)

For injuries that involve the sigmoid colon or intraperitoneal rectum, a colorectal anastomosis is employed in the hemodynamically stable trauma patient. After debridement to healthy viable tissue, the first step is to ensure a tension-free anastomosis by allowing adequate mobilization of the sigmoid and descending colon. In some case, further mobilizing the splenic flexure is required to ensure a tension-free anastomosis. A circular stapled technique is the preferred anastomosis of choice for a colorectal anastomosis (typically 29-31 mm). The proximal bowel staple line is removed, and the anvil is inserted into the bowel lumen. A pursestring suture is then placed around the open lumen to fit snug around the shaft of the anvil. Next the circular stapler is passed transanally, opened so the trocar pierces through the end of the stapled edge of the rectum, and then connected to the anvil. Once engaged and closed down, the stapler is fired, and a leak test is performed by covering the anastomosis with saline irrigation, insufflating the rectum with air while watching for the presence of bubbles in the pelvis. This can be done using a flexible or rigid proctoscopy.

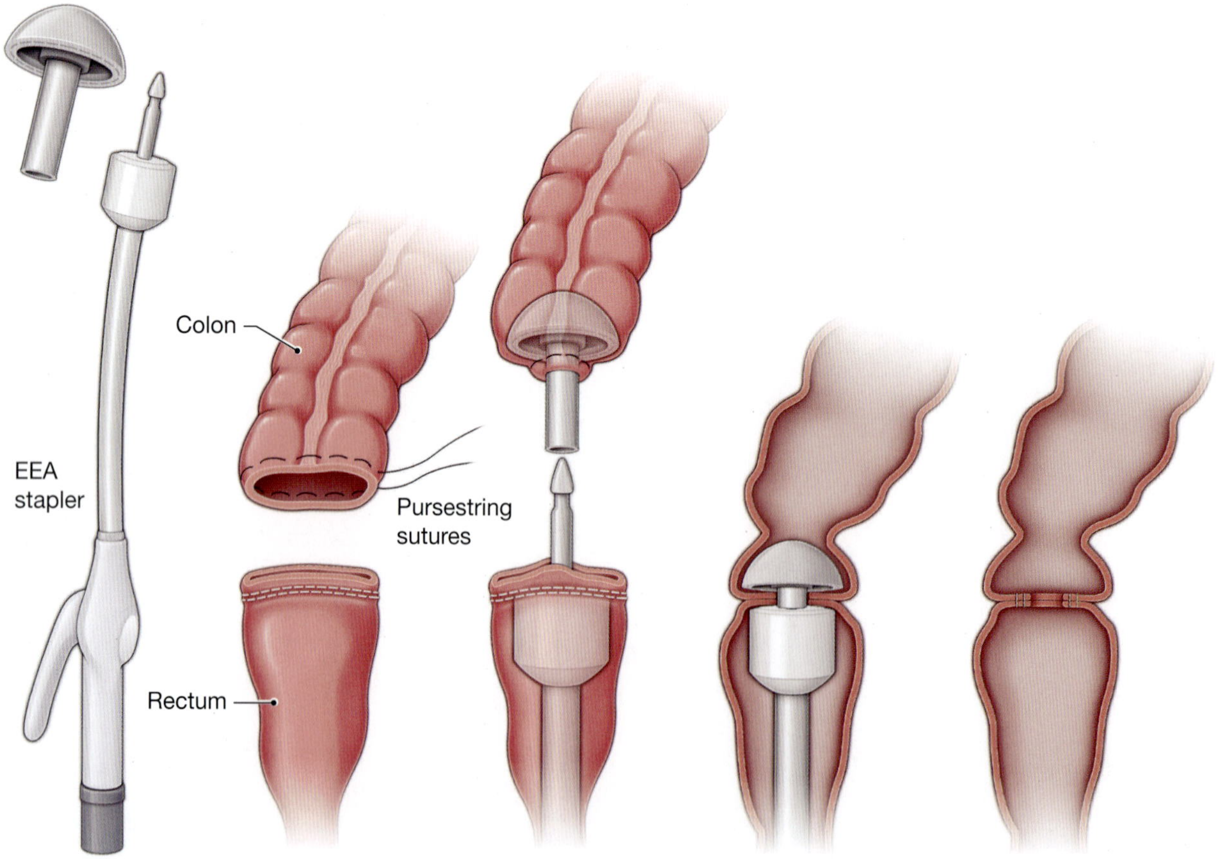

Figure 18-7

Colostomy

In trauma patients with hemodynamic instability or highly destructive injuries that would preclude primary repair or anastomosis, a colostomy for diversion is the treatment of choice. After a thorough exploration, a colostomy site is chosen in either the left or right lower quadrants depending on injury location. The colon is then adequately mobilized so that no tension is placed near the selected stoma location. Over the stoma location, a circular incision is made down to the anterior rectus fascia. A cruciate incision is made over the anterior fascia exposing the rectus musculature. "Coring" of subcutaneous tissue is not necessary. A muscle-sparing technique is employed by splitting the anterior and posterior rectus muscles parallel along its fibers. A cruciate incision is then made along the posterior rectus fascia, and the peritoneum is then entered. The stomal opening should allow passage of two fingers without difficulty. Using a Babcock clamp, the colon is then grasped and delivered through the abdominal wall. Approximately 2 cm of colon should protrude above the level of the abdominal wall. Depending on the clinical scenario, a loop or end colostomy can be performed. If a loop is chosen, a longitudinal incision is made along the taeniae coli exposing both lumens of colon. Next, the colostomy is matured using 3-0 absorbable sutures with full-thickness bites circumferentially around the ostomy to the dermis. Seromuscular tacking sutures of 3-0 silk can be placed between the colon and the posterior fascia. Although the colostomy can be flush with the skin as the effluent is not corrosive to the surrounding skin, some surgeons prefer to mature it in Brooke fashion similar to maturing ileostomies. This entails using four quadrant stitches that go through the bowel wall, followed by a tacking seromuscular bite, and finally through the dermis and held taut using a hemostat. One or two sutures between the four-quadrant everting stiches are placed from the bowel wall to the dermis and secured.

End Colostomy

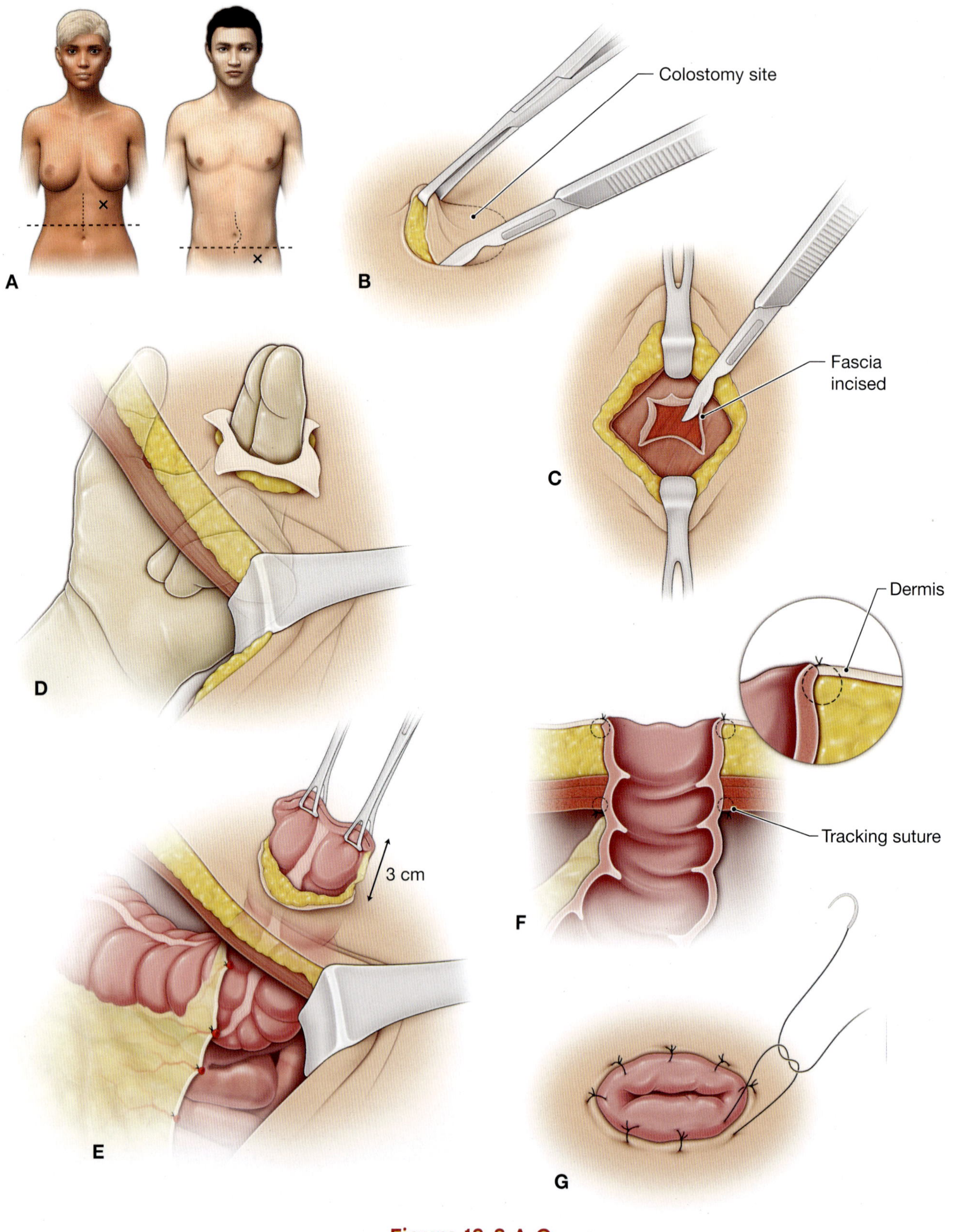

Figure 18-8 A-G

Loop Colostomy

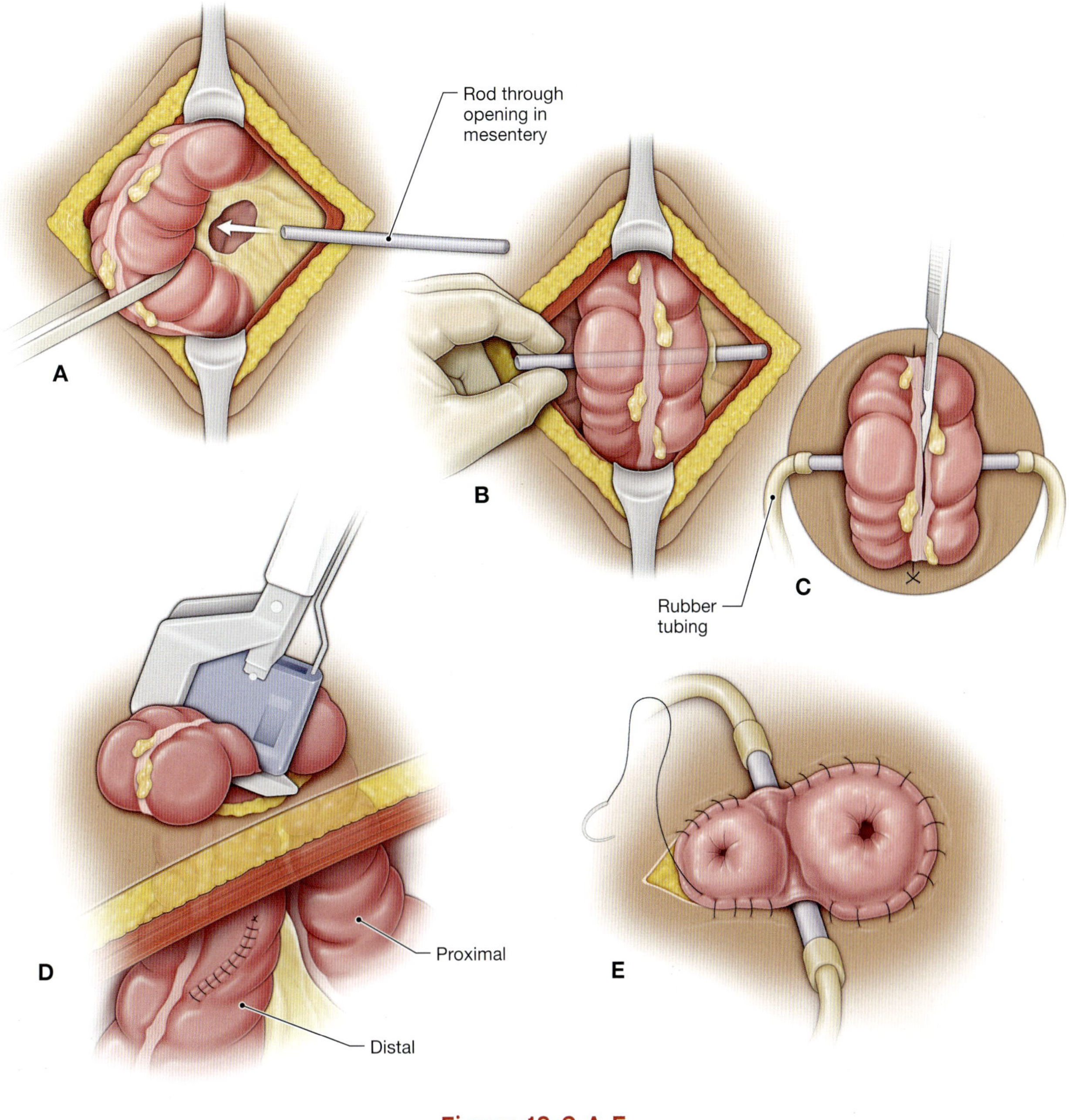

Figure 18-9 A-E

Rectal Trauma

Rectal repair depends on injury location. Intraperitoneal rectal injuries are managed like distal colon injuries. The primary repair of extraperitoneal rectal injuries is performed much like that for colon injuries and can be performed when technically feasible. Use of intraoperative flexible sigmoidoscopy is a helpful adjunct in the identification of rectal injury. Rectal injuries that are not easily accessible for repair or with large rectal wall defects will require proximal diversion. Presacral drainage can be omitted in the vast majority of cases.

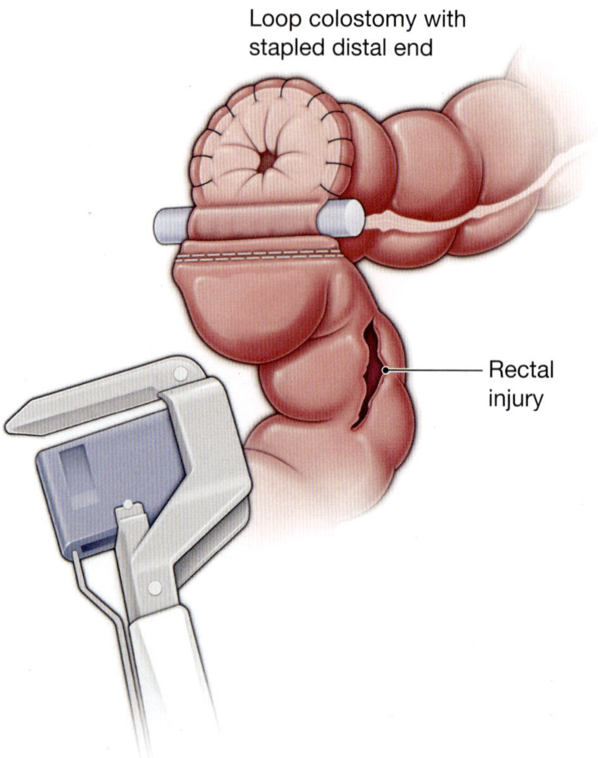

Figure 18-10

Perineum

The focus of perineum and anal trauma is early debridement of all nonviable tissue and proper wound care in the postoperative period to prevent sepsis. Multiple trips to the operating room for further exploration and debridement may be required. Minor injuries can be repaired primarily; however, more extensive injuries will require proper wound care and possible fecal diversion. Once the perineum is healed of injury, assessment of anal sphincter tone and definitive management can be addressed.

Complications

Early mortality following colorectal trauma is usually associated with hemorrhage from mesenteric bleeding. Missed colonic injury can lead to multisystem organ failure from intra-abdominal sepsis. Common complications related to colorectal trauma include anastomotic leak, fistulas, and intra-abdominal abscess formation. The primary cause of fistula and intra-abdominal abscess formation is usually from associated anastomotic leak, although gross contamination preoperatively also places patients at higher risk for intra-abdominal abscess formation. Patients with high transfusion requirements, hemodynamic instability, and multiple medical comorbidities are at higher risk of anastomotic leak. Surgeons may elect for either damage control laparotomy and/or fecal diversion at the time of laparotomy depending on patient selection.

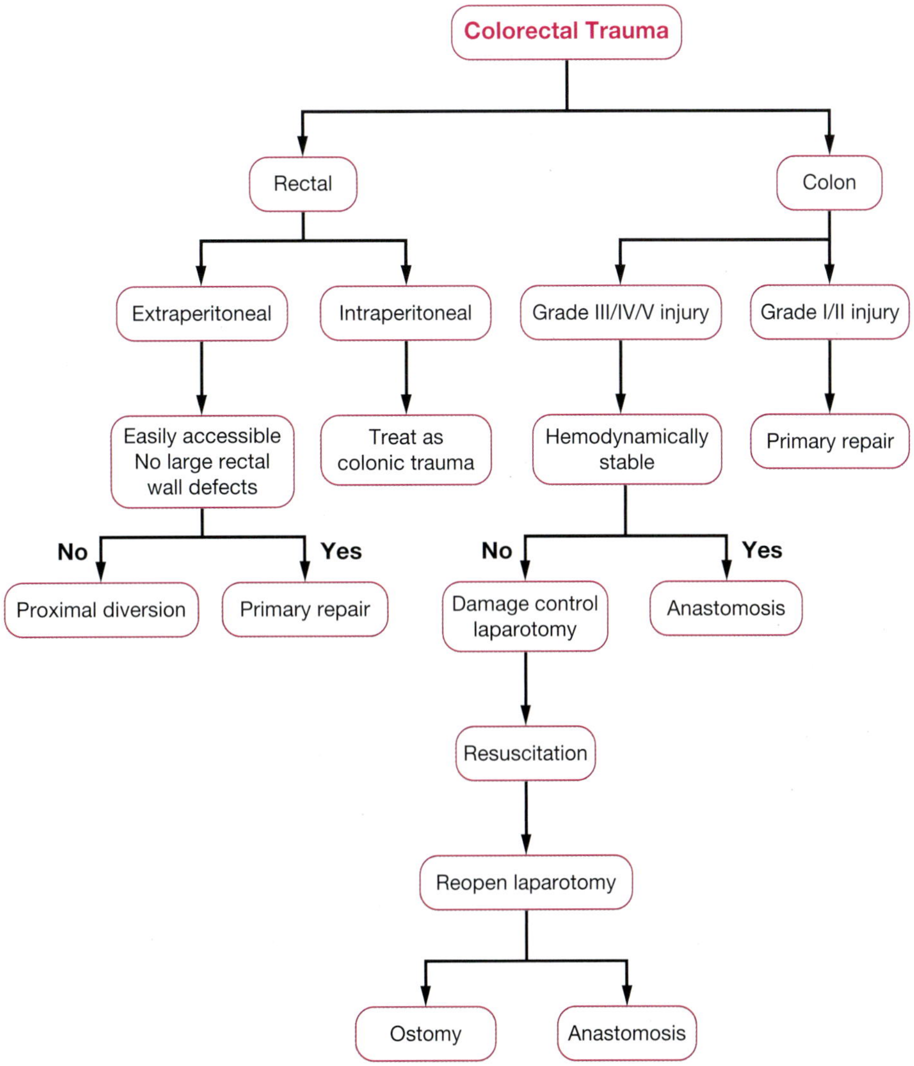

Figure 18-11

19 RENAL TRAUMA

Michael Coburn, MD
Shyam Sukumar, MBBS

TIPS

1. **The treatment of most renal injuries in hemodynamically stable patients is expectant, nonoperative management.**

2. **For hemodynamically unstable patients, especially in patients with adverse radiographic findings (high-grade injuries, large perirenal hematomas, or vascular contrast extravasation), earlier intervention should be considered.**

Introduction

Renal injuries are the most common form of urologic trauma from an external source. Most blunt injuries and many penetrating injuries can be managed with conservative management. Appropriate monitoring and prompt operative management of patients who fail conservative management or have complications are critical.

Contrast-enhanced computed tomography (CT) scans are the mainstay of urologic imaging in the setting of renal trauma. Delayed-phase imaging is important to identify collecting system and ureteral injuries. Imaging should be obtained for the following types of injuries: penetrating trauma, blunt trauma with suggestive mechanism, blunt trauma with gross hematuria, blunt trauma with microhematuria and hypotension, and all pediatric patients with >5 red blood cells/high-power field on urinalysis.

The imaging phenotypes that portend more significant injuries include the following: large perirenal hematomas (>3.5 cm), extravasation of vascular contrast, medial renal lacerations, and medial urinary extravasation suggesting a renal pelvic or ureteropelvic junction injury.

For patients who are hemodynamically unstable, especially in the context of adverse radiographic findings, earlier intervention with either angioembolization or surgical exploration should be considered.

Anatomy

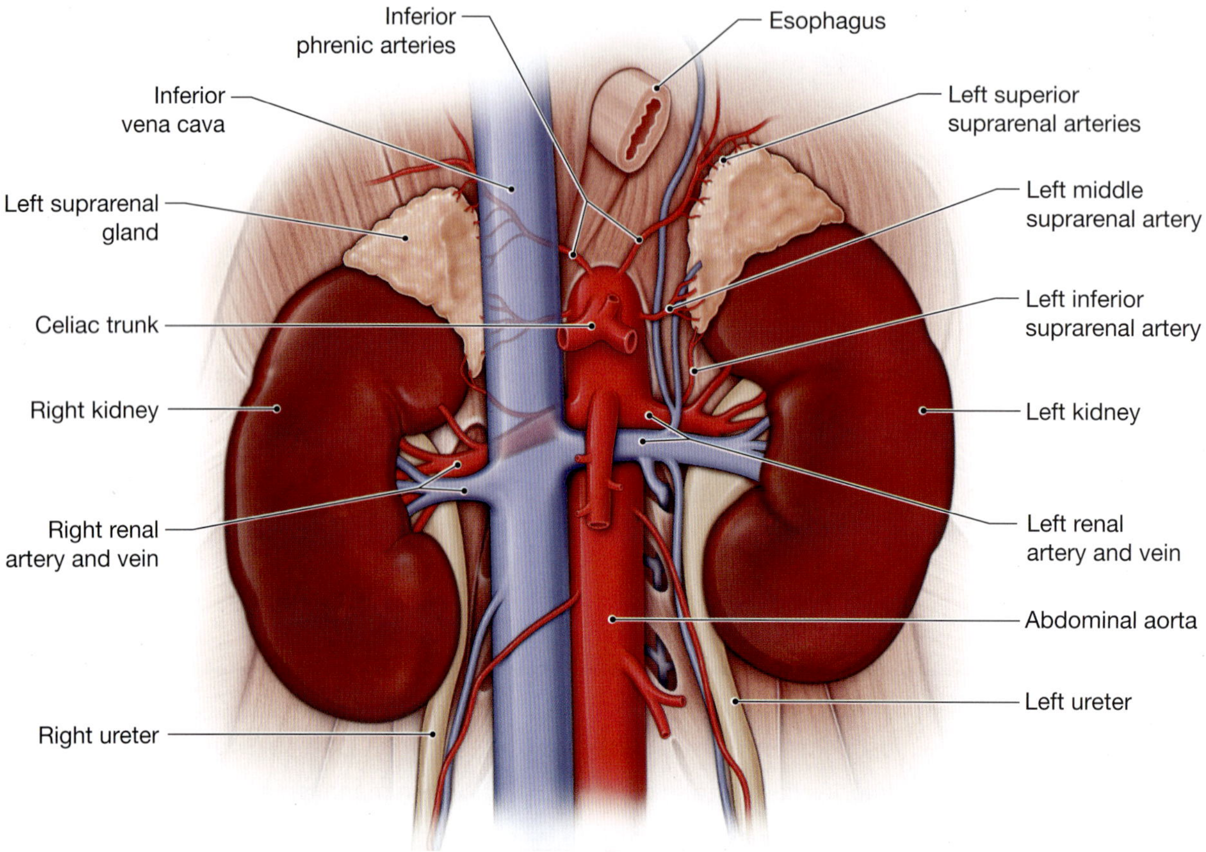

Figure 19-1

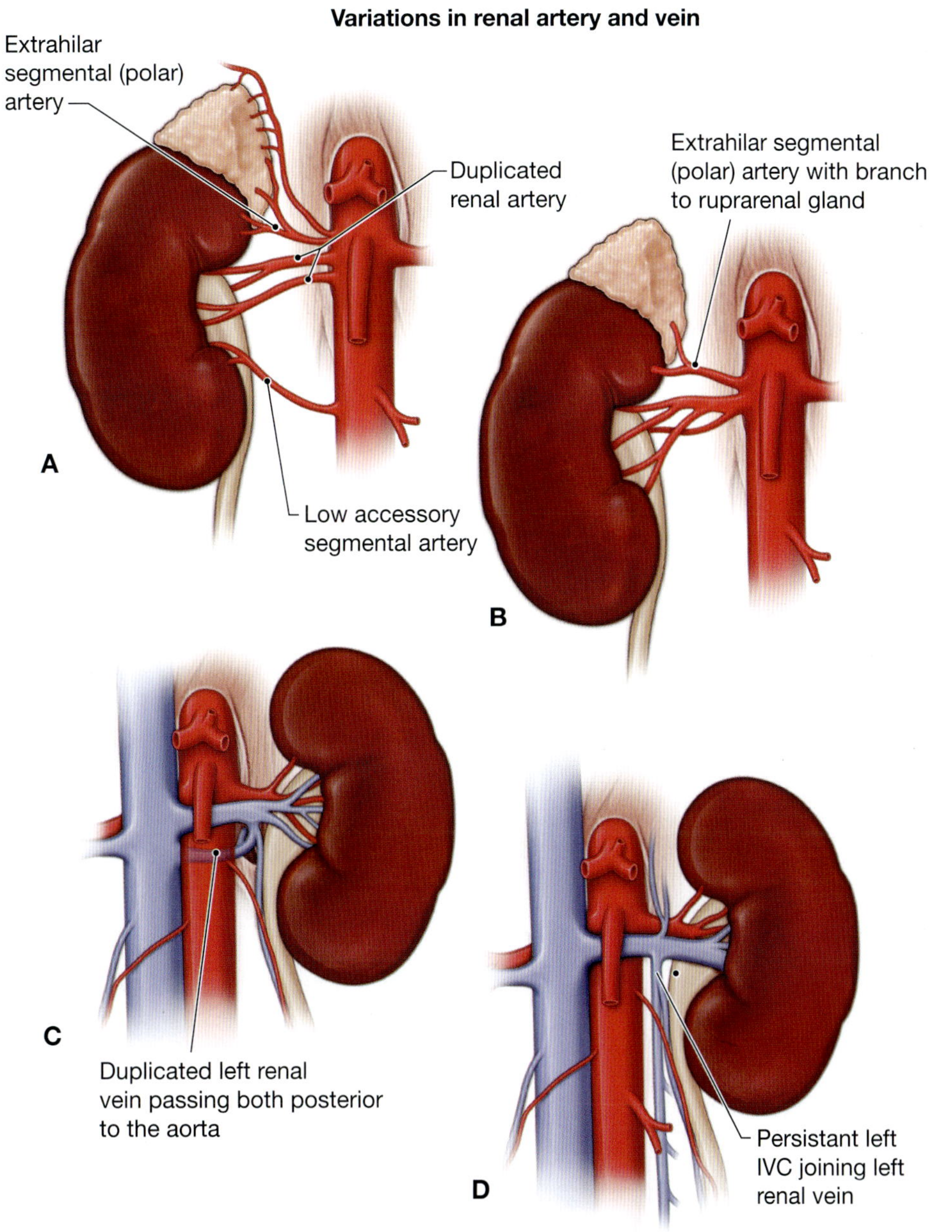
Variations in renal artery and vein
Extrahilar segmental (polar) artery
Duplicated renal artery
Low accessory segmental artery
A
Extrahilar segmental (polar) artery with branch to ruprarenal gland
B
C
Duplicated left renal vein passing both posterior to the aorta
D
Persistant left IVC joining left renal vein

Figure 19-2

19 RENAL TRAUMA

TABLE 19-1. American Association for the Surgery of Trauma (AAST) Organ Injury Scale

Grade	AAST Injury Scale - Renal

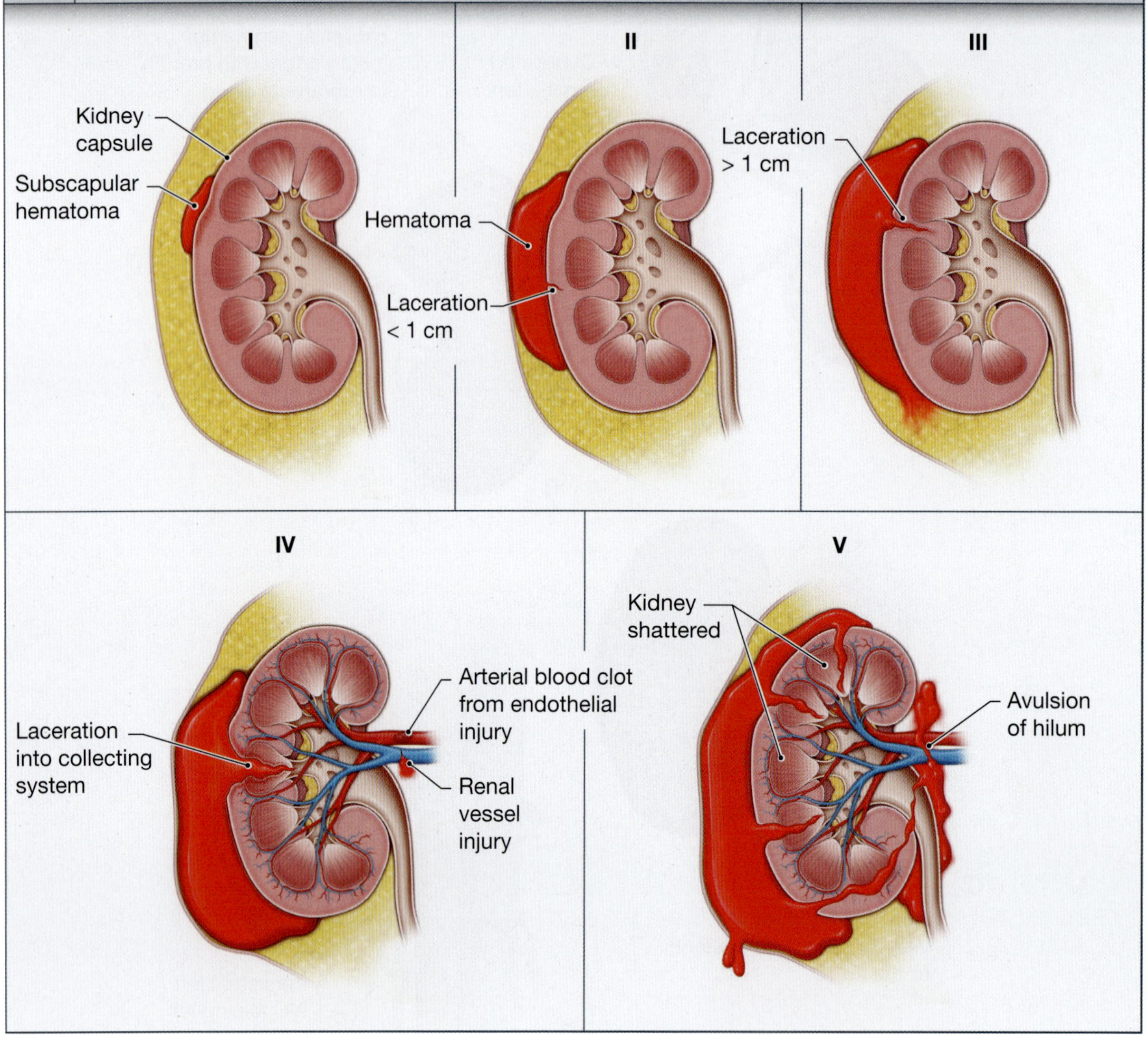

Operative Steps

Exposure and Early Vascular Control

A midline transperitoneal incision is used for abdominal access. The transverse colon is lifted superiorly, and the small bowel is exteriorized to expose the posterior peritoneum overlying the retroperitoneal structures. Early vascular control is a controversial issue. However, to obtain early vascular control, a longitudinal incision is made over the aorta and immediately medial to the inferior mesenteric vein. The inferior mesenteric vein is a good landmark in challenging cases with a very large hematoma. The right and left renal veins and the underlying renal arteries can then be identified and isolated. Alternatively, early vascular control can be avoided and direct control of the hilum can be obtained.

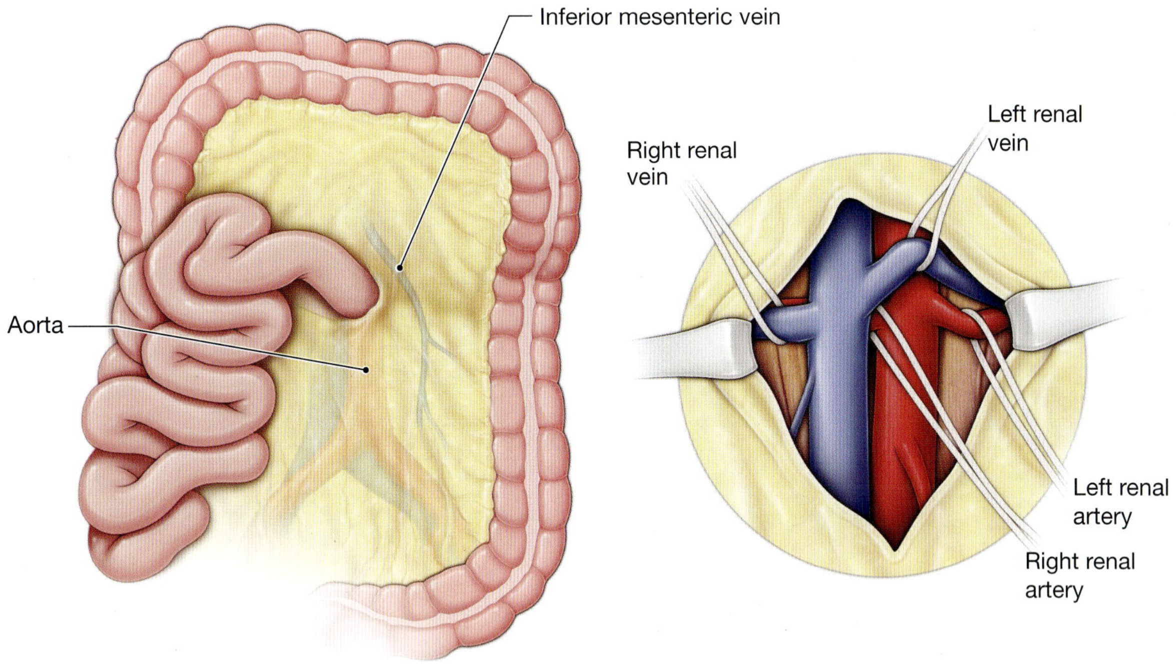

Figure 19-3

Renal Exposure

Once vascular control has been obtained, the colon is mobilized medially using an incision along the line of Toldt. On the right, it is important to carefully mobilize the duodenum using a generous Kocher maneuver. The renal and vascular anatomies are then examined.

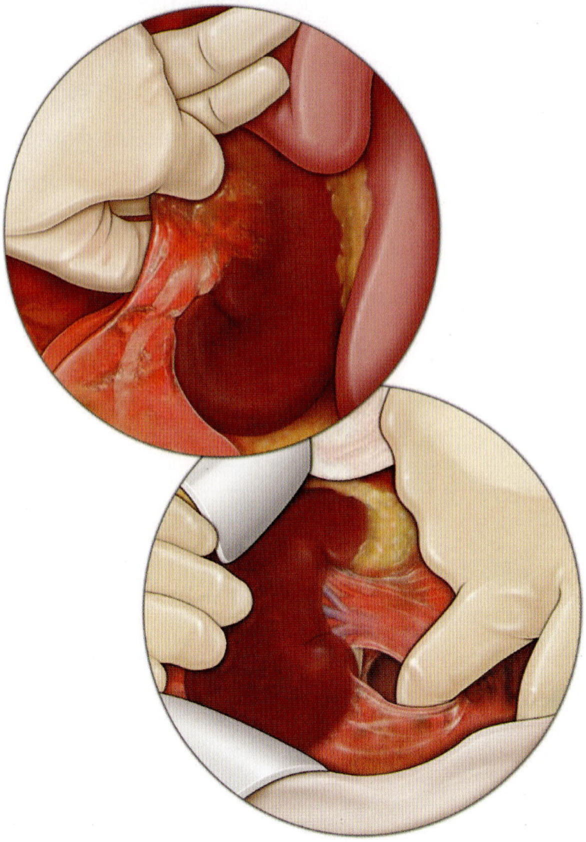

Figure 19-4

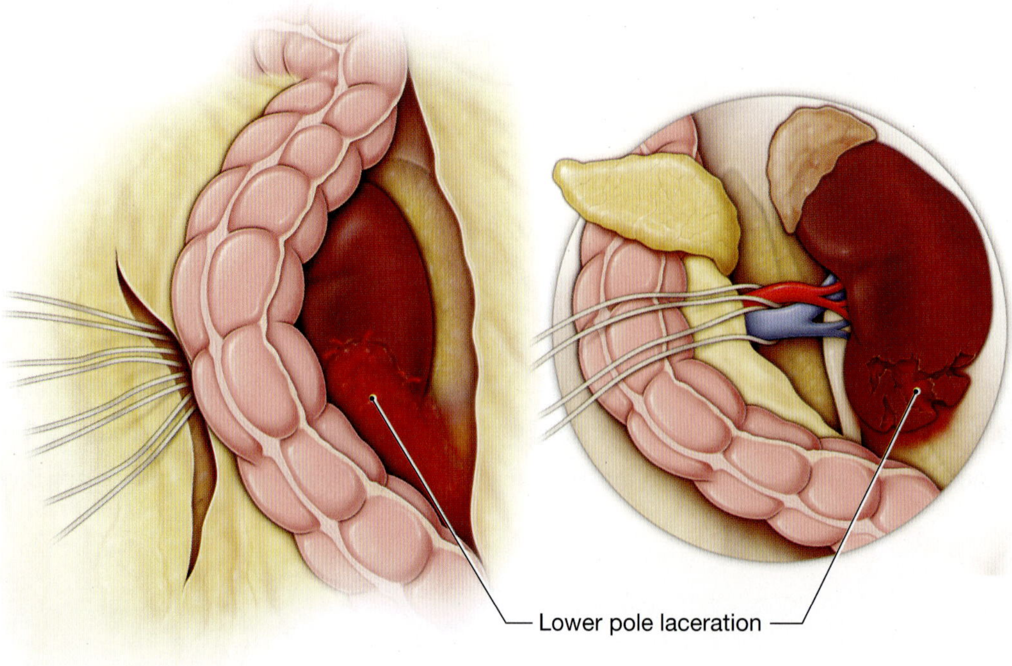

Figure 19-5

Renorrhaphy and Vascular Repair

The injury is identified and nonviable tissue debrided. Significant polar lacerations are managed using partial nephrectomy. Individual bleeders are managed using figure-of-eight ligature of 4-0 chromic or Monocryl sutures. It is important to identify and close collecting system injuries. The capsule can be closed over bolsters of hemostatic agents. Partial lacerations to the main renal artery or vein can be managed using interrupted 5-0 Prolene sutures after vascular control has been obtained.

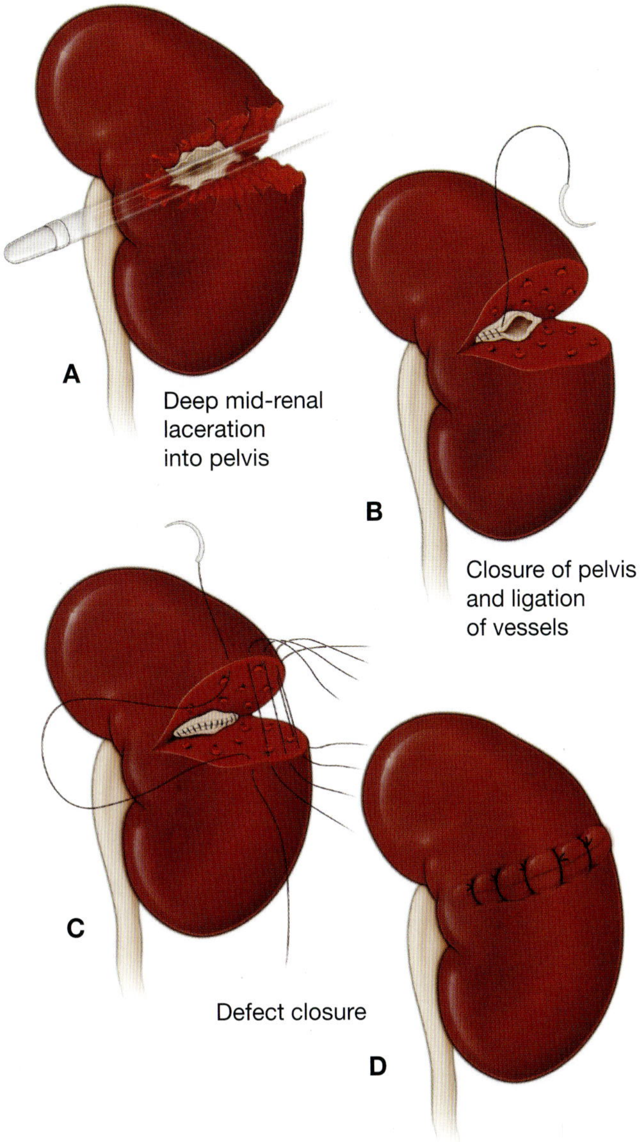

Figure 19-6

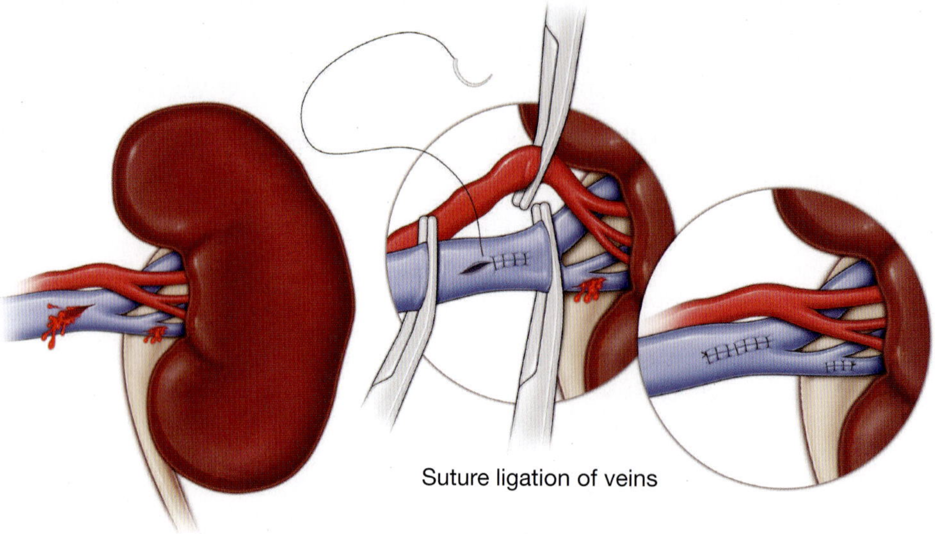

Figure 19-7

Complications

Complications of renal trauma and repair include delayed bleeding, urinary leak, abscess formation, urinary sepsis, fistulization, and delayed onset of hypertension. Close monitoring of urine output, blood pressure, and hemoglobin/hematocrit is important. Drain fluid can be evaluated for creatinine if there is concern for a urinary leak.

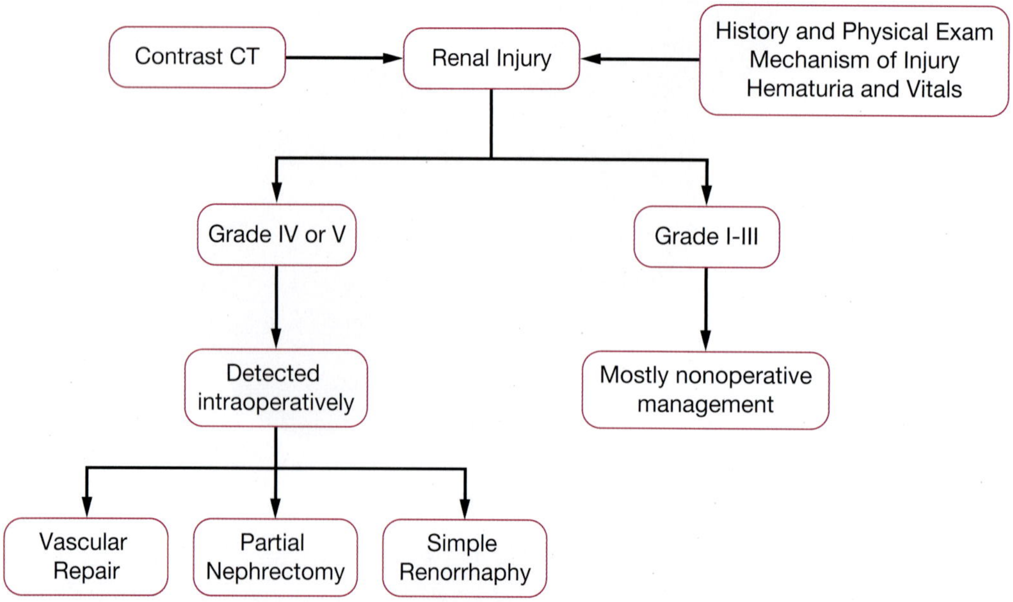

Figure 19-8

URETER AND BLADDER

20

Michael Coburn, MD
Shyam Sukumar, MBBS

TIPS

1. **Upper and mid ureteral injuries are best managed by primary sutured repair—a pyeloplasty or ureteroureterostomy.**
2. **Lower ureteral injuries are best managed with reimplantation, with the possible use of adjunct maneuvers like a psoas hitch or a Boari flap.**

URETER

Introduction

Ureteral trauma from an external source is rare and constitutes <1% of all genitourinary trauma. The ureter is well ensconced in the retroperitoneal location, and so ureteral injuries are usually accompanied by multiple visceral injuries. Penetrating trauma is more common, especially from iatrogenic injuries. It is important to maintain a high index of suspicion and to specifically rule out the presence of ureteral injuries in the setting of iatrogenic bladder trauma.

Contrast-enhanced computed tomography (CT) scans can help diagnose a ureteral injury, but it is critical to obtain delayed-phase imaging. Retrograde pyelograms can be more sensitive for ureteral injuries and can help determine the exact location of injury. Finally, direct intraoperative inspection of the ureter to assess the presence of injury and quality of the tissue is critical. Intravenous use of methylene blue or indigo carmine (10 mL) can help assist in this endeavor by inspecting the pelvis for any extravasation of dye.

20 URETER AND BLADDER

Anatomy

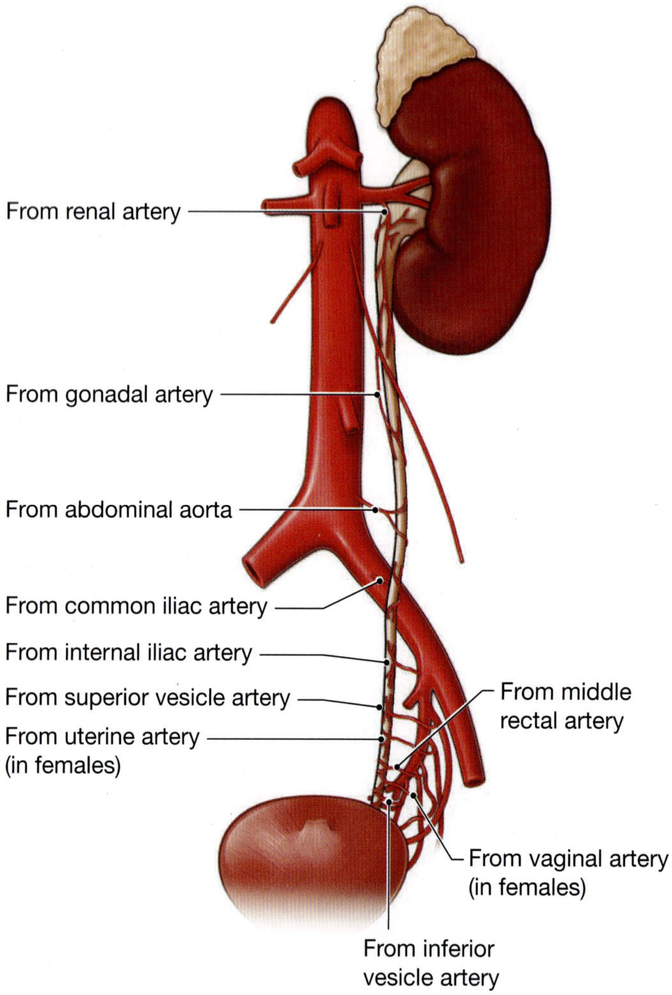

Figure 20-1

TABLE 20-1. American Association for the Surgery of Trauma (AAST) Injury Scale: Ureter

Grade	Type of Injury	Description of Injury
I	Hematoma	Contusion or hematoma without devascularization
II	Laceration	<50% transection
III	Laceration	≥50% transection
IV	Laceration	Complete transection with <2 cm devascularization
V	Laceration	Avulsion with >2 cm of devascularization

Source: Reproduced with permission from Moore EE, Cogbill TH, Jurkovich GJ, et al. Organ injury scaling. III: Chest wall, abdominal vascular, ureter, bladder, and urethra. *J Trauma.* 1992;33(3):337-339.

Operative Steps

Management of Ureteral Trauma Based on Level of Injury

Primary sutured repair remains the mainstay of treatment for upper and mid ureteral injuries. Injuries to the lower ureter are best managed with reimplantation. Ancillary maneuvers like a psoas hitch or a Boari flap are sometimes required to achieve reimplantation in a tension-free manner. Delayed repair of upper or mid ureteral injuries can be achieved using buccal graft ureteroplasty, which is especially useful to manage longer injuries.

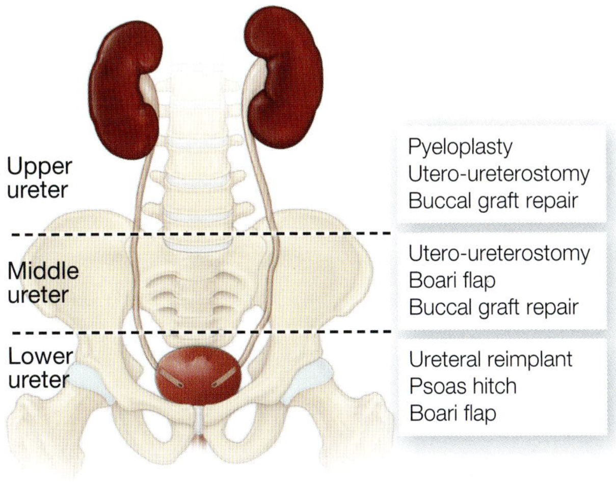

Figure 20-2

Uretero-ureterostomy

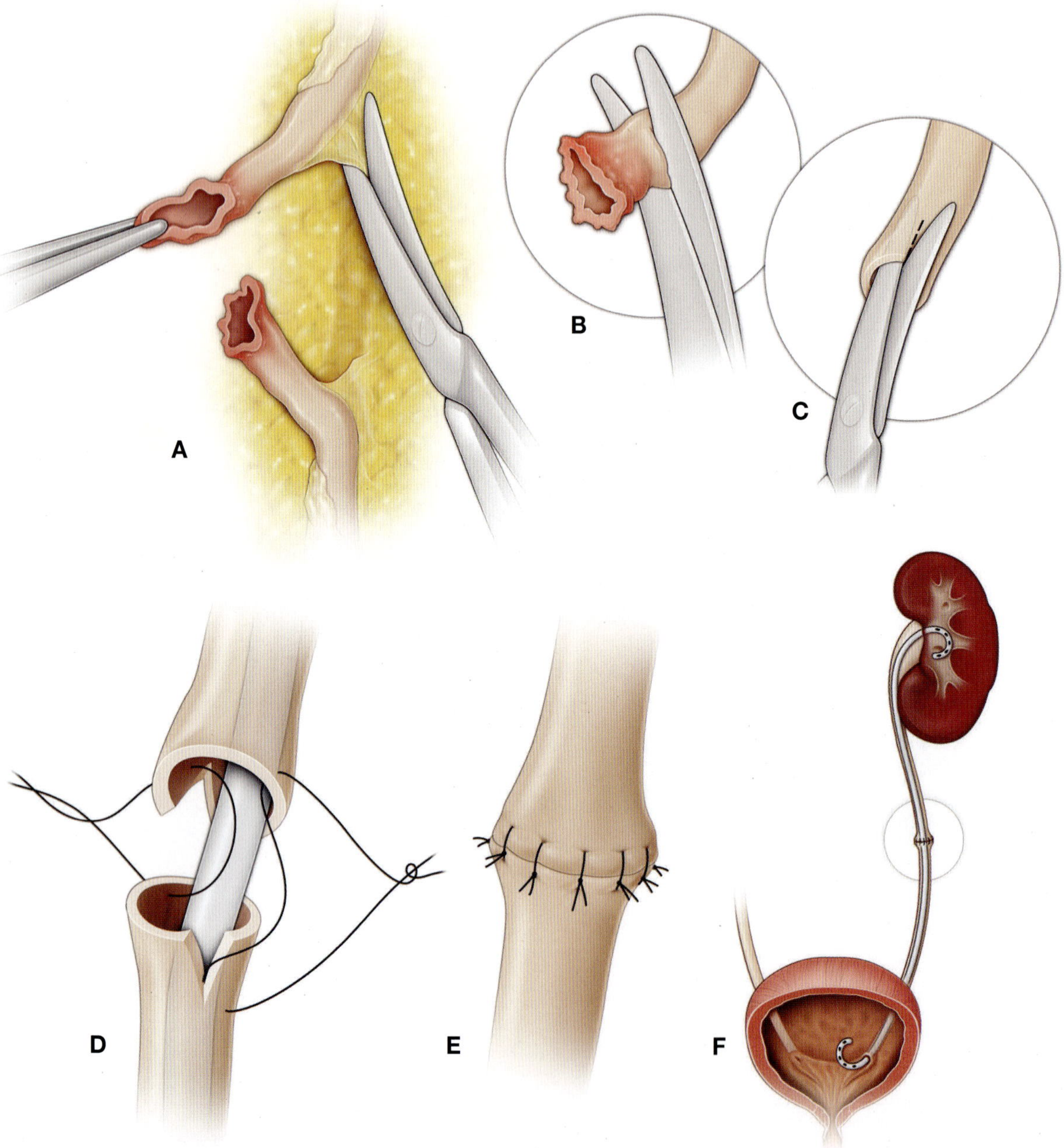

Figure 20-3 A-F

Uretero-ureterostomy is indicated for short injuries of the proximal or mid ureter. The principles of ureteral repair include debridement of nonviable tissue, an elliptical anastomosis with wide spatulation, and a tension-free repair over a ureteral stent using absorbable monofilament suture in an interrupted fashion (Figure 20-3A-F).

Psoas Hitch and Ureteral Reimplantation

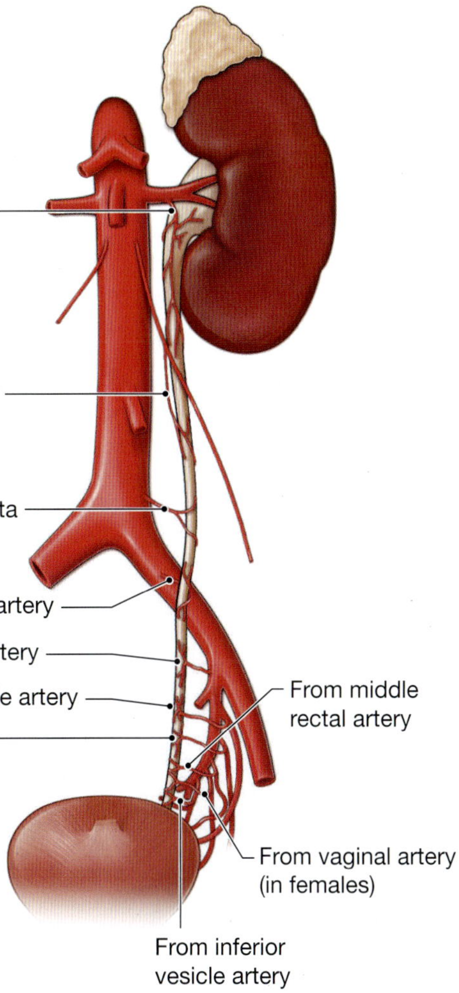

Figure 20-4

The vascular anatomy of the ureter is such that injuries to the distal ureter caudal to the pelvic inlet result in a poorly vascularized distal segment (Figure 20-5). These injuries are best managed using a ureteral reimplantation. Additional maneuvers like a psoas hitch or a Boari flap may be required to achieve a tension-free reconstruction. A psoas hitch involves mobilizing the bladder and anchoring it to the psoas minor muscle using absorbable sutures. Avoiding injury to the genitofemoral and femoral nerves is important. A tunneled technique of reimplantation is optional but not necessary (Figure 20-5A-D).

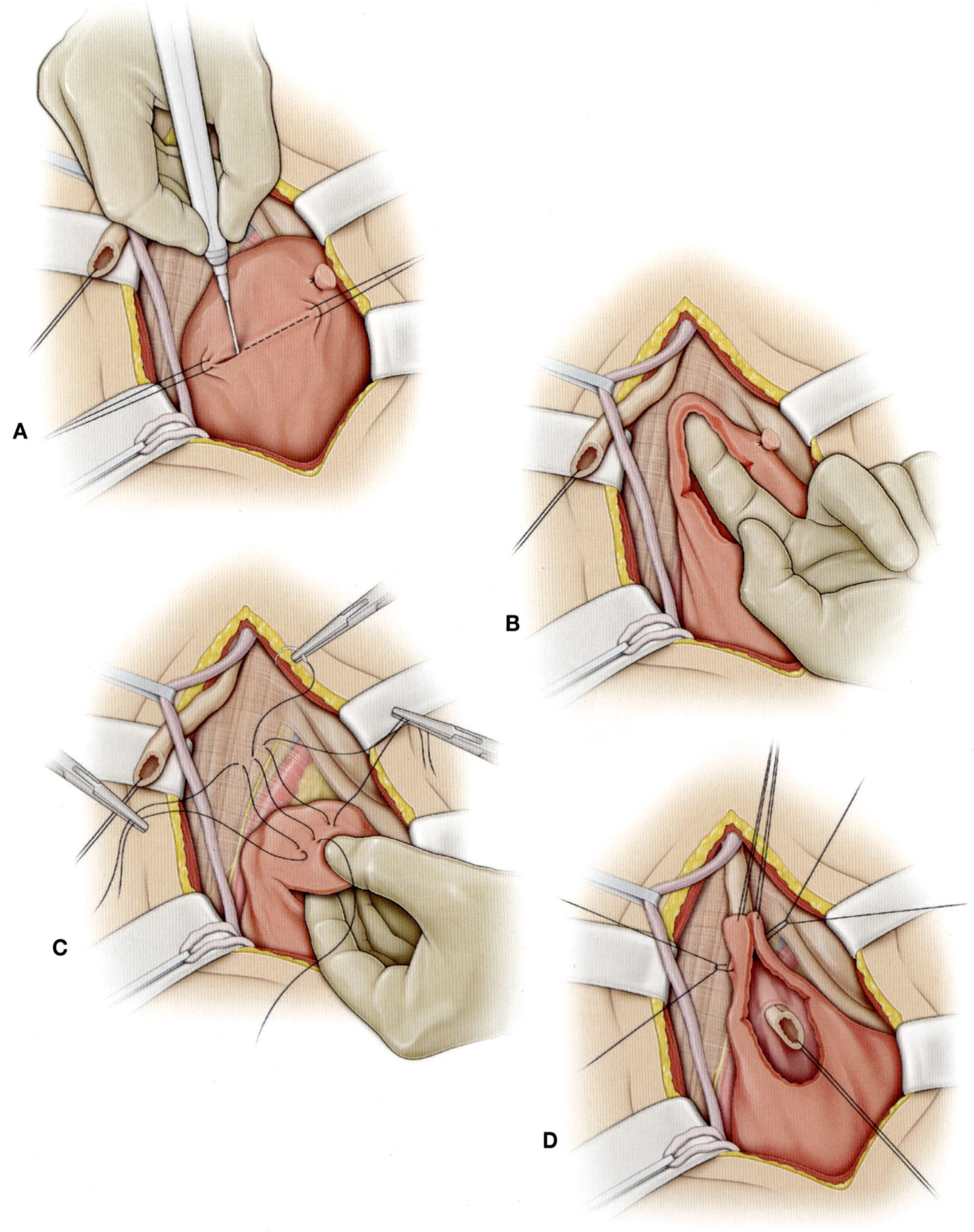

Figure 20-5 A-D

Boari Flap and Ureteral Reimplantation

If a psoas hitch maneuver does not provide enough length for a tension-free repair, then a Boari flap is the next option. A posterior-based flap of bladder is created with attention paid to making the base of the flap wide enough to prevent devascularization. The flap can be hitched to the psoas muscle and tubularized (Figure 20-6A-D). Again, a tunneled reimplantation is optional.

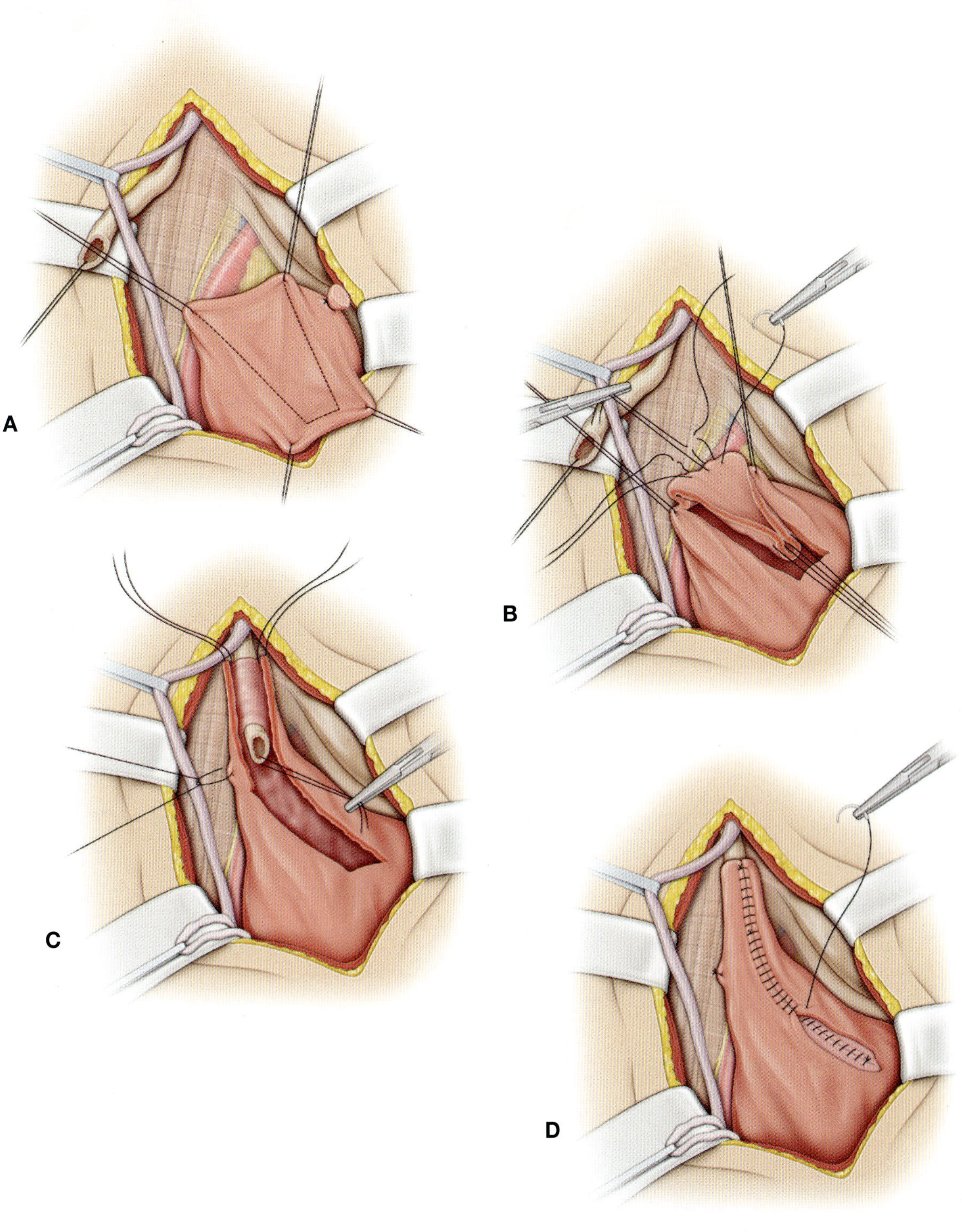

Figure 20-6 A-D

Complications

Complications of ureteral trauma include short-term complications like a urinoma/leak, bleeding, and sequelae of injury to neurovascular structures in the vicinity of the repair. Long-term complications include stricture formation and fistula formation, both of which usually require reconstruction.

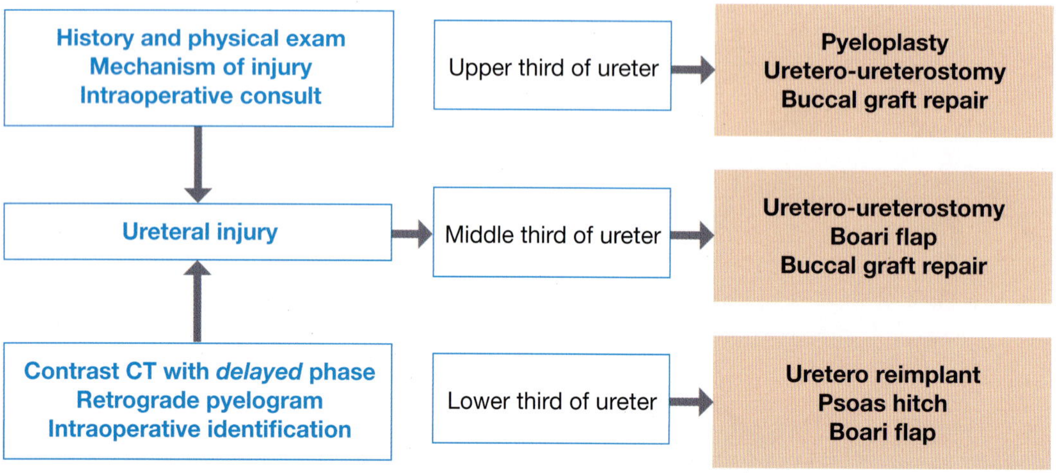

Figure 20-7

TIPS

1. Bladder injury is most commonly associated with a pelvic fracture, but penetrating and iatrogenic injuries are also possible.
2. An important point of decision-making is to determine the type of bladder injury: simple extraperitoneal, complex extraperitoneal, or intraperitoneal injury.
3. Whereas simple and small extraperitoneal bladder injuries can be managed with an indwelling Foley catheter, complex extraperitoneal and intraperitoneal injuries usually require exploration and repair.

BLADDER

Introduction

Injury to the bladder can follow blunt, penetrating, or iatrogenic trauma. Most commonly, however, it results as a blowout injury in the context of a pelvic fracture. Gross hematuria in the context of pelvic trauma should warrant an investigation to rule out bladder and urethral injuries, but these injuries can occur without hematuria. Therefore, a high degree of suspicion is necessary. An X-ray cystogram or a computed tomography (CT) cystogram is usually adequate to diagnose bladder injuries.

The distinction between intraperitoneal and extraperitoneal bladder injuries is an important one to make. Extraperitoneal injuries can further be classified as simple or complex. Complex injuries have one or more of the following associated factors: vaginal injury, rectal injury, bony spicule in the bladder lumen, intractable gross hematuria, or the need for exploration for associated visceral or bony injuries.

Simple extraperitoneal bladder injuries can be managed with an indwelling Foley catheter for 10 to 14 days. Complex extraperitoneal bladder injuries are managed like intraperitoneal injuries: exploration with sutured repair and generous bladder drainage remains the mainstay of treatment. Extraperitoneal bladder injuries with associated pelvic fractures requiring hardware fixation are considered complex and therefore require operative repair.

20 URETER AND BLADDER

Anatomy

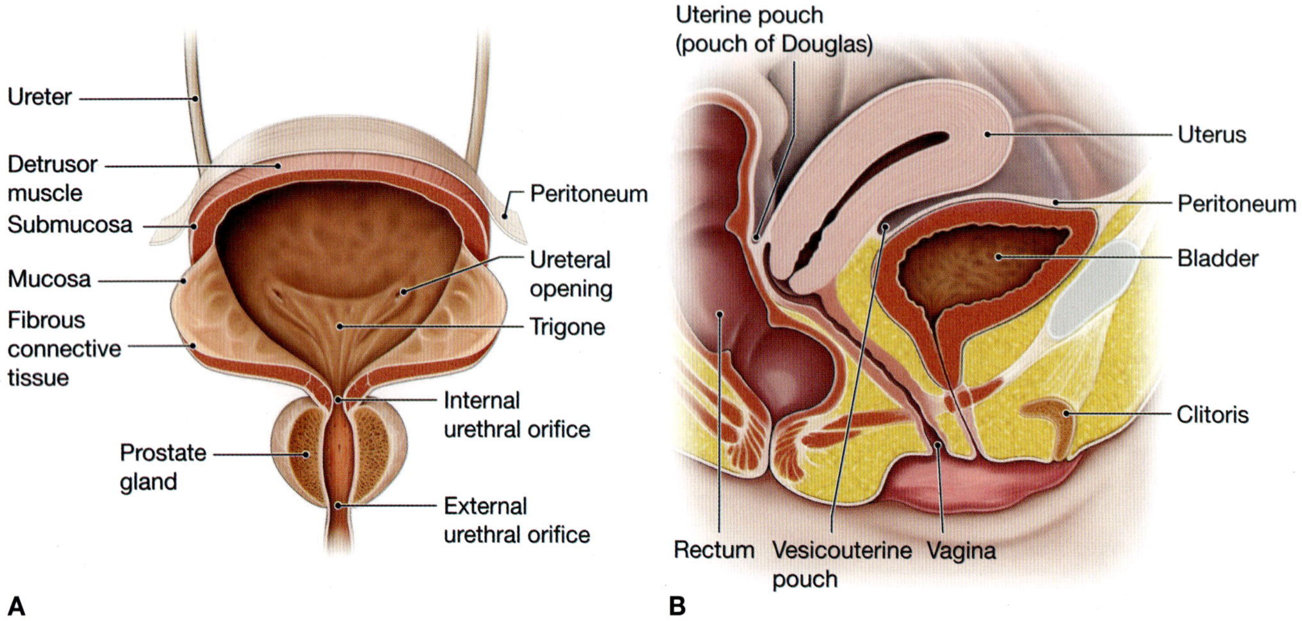

Figure 20-8. A. Anterior view of the bladder. **B.** Lateral view of the bladder.

TABLE 20-2. American Association for the Surgery of Trauma (AAST) Organ Injury Scale: Bladder

Grade*	Injury Type	Description of Injury
I	Hematoma	Contusion, intramural hematoma
	Laceration	Partial thickness
II	Laceration	Extraperitoneal bladder wall laceration <2 cm
III	Laceration	Extraperitoneal (≥2 cm) or intraperitoneal (<2 cm) bladder wall laceration
IV	Laceration	Intraperitoneal bladder wall laceration ≥2 cm
V	Laceration	Intraperitoneal or extraperitoneal bladder wall laceration extending into the bladder neck or ureteral orifice (trigone)

*Advance one grade for multiple lesions up to grade III.

Source: Reproduced with permission from Moore EE, Cogbill TH, Jurkovich GJ, et al. Organ injury scaling. III: Chest wall, abdominal vascular, ureter, bladder, and urethra. *J Trauma.* 1992;33(3):337-339.

Operative Steps

Simple Cystorrhaphy

Intraoperative urology consults are often requested for bladder trauma secondary to iatrogenic injury. It is important to rule out associated urologic injuries to adjacent structures (eg, ureter). Pelvic exposure is usually obtained by extending the midline incision down to the pubic bone, mobilizing the bladder off its ligamentous attachments, and evaluating the injury. The devitalized edges of the bladder injury are debrided, and cystorrhaphy is performed in two layers using running absorbable suture (Figure 20-9). A suprapubic tube can be placed in addition to a urethral Foley in special situations, but its routine use is controversial.

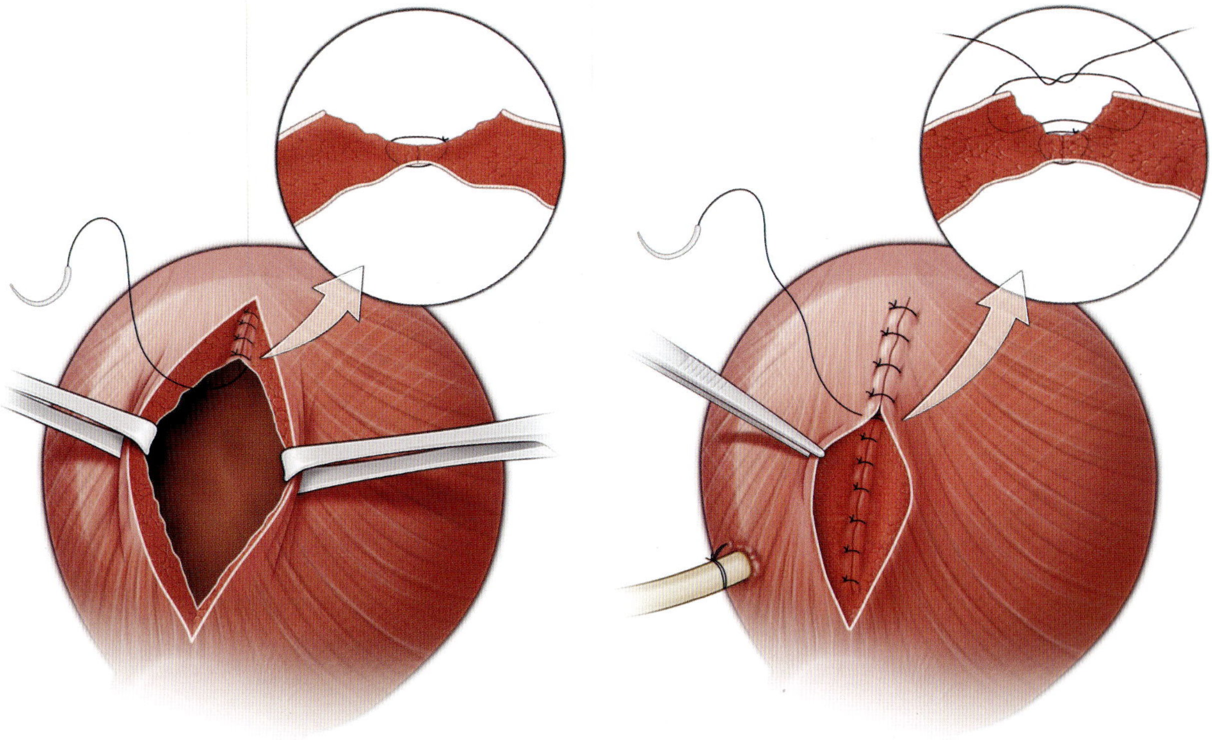

Figure 20-9

Repair of Complicated Extraperitoneal Bladder Injuries

Extraperitoneal bladder injuries can be approached using a lower midline incision. It is important to minimize disturbance to any large pelvic hematomas, and this can be done by avoiding dissection lateral to the bladder. An anterior cystotomy is made, and the injury is identified and repaired in one or two layers. Alternatively, these injuries can be approached through an intraperitoneal approach, followed by an incision at the bladder dome (Figure 20-10). Care should be taken to identify any trigonal injury involving the ureteral orifice or a bladder neck injury.

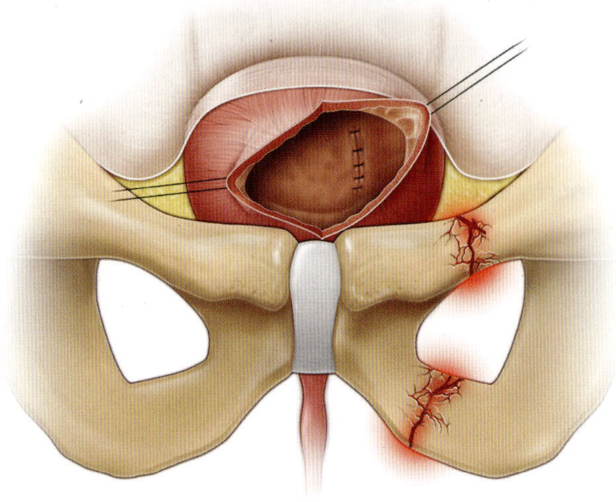

Figure 20-10

Repair of Intraperitoneal Bladder Injuries

Intraperitoneal injuries usually require a longer midline incision. After managing injuries to associated visceral structures, the bladder injury is identified. Allis clamps can be used for traction of the cystotomy edges, and the inside of the bladder is thoroughly evaluated. Sutured repair can be performed in two layers: inner layer of mucosa and muscle followed by an outer layer of muscle, serosa, and overlying peritoneum (Figure 20-11).

An indwelling Foley catheter can be left in place for 10 to 14 days after sutured repair. Routine use of drains or suprapubic tubes is controversial.

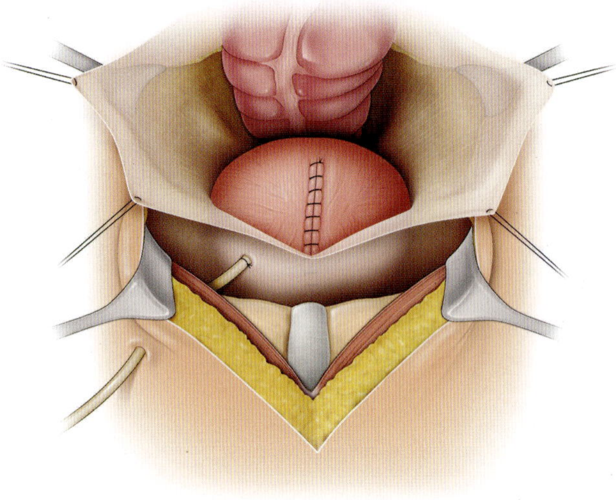

Figure 20-11

Complications

Untreated intraperitoneal or complex extraperitoneal injuries can result in urinary peritonitis and urosepsis. Uncomplicated bladder injuries can be complicated by intractable gross hematuria and clot retention, thereby requiring an operative approach. Complications such as fistula formation or long-term voiding dysfunction are rare.

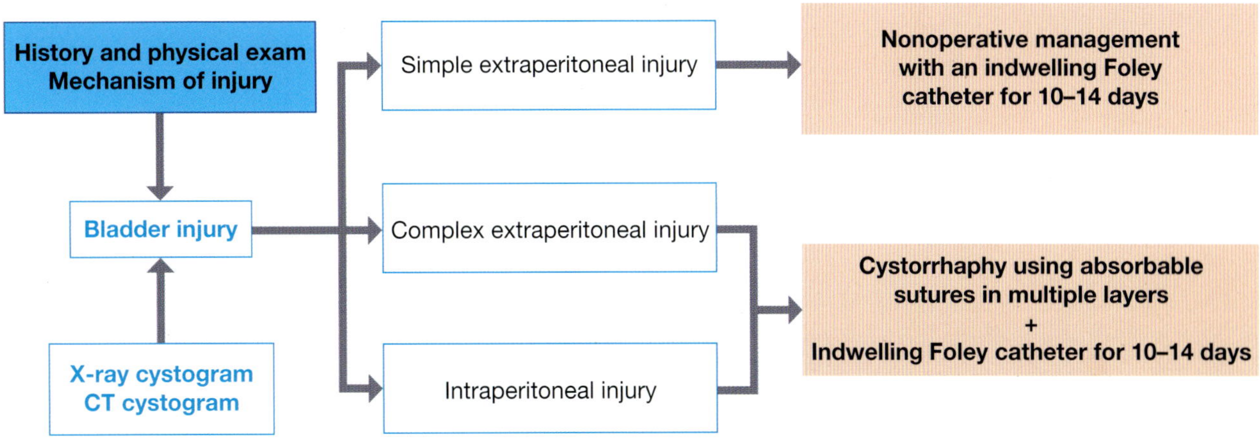

Figure 20-12

21 RETROPERITONEAL AND PELVIC VASCULAR TRAUMA

Todd D. Husty, MD, FACS, CDR, MC, USN
David J. Skarupa, MD, FACS, FCCM, FACHE

TIPS

1. **Remember the basics of dealing with vascular injuries and think about proximal and distal control; direct control with digital pressure can allow for the patient to be stabilized while formulating a plan of approach to the injury.**

2. **In an unstable patient, shunting should be considered.**

3. **Most infrarenal veins, including the inferior vena cava (IVC), can be ligated if necessary in an unstable patient.**

Introduction

Injuries to retroperitoneal vascular structures remain among the most lethal that are encountered by trauma surgeons. These structures include the named vessels in the abdominal cavity: the aorta, IVC, and iliac vessels. The retroperitoneum is divided into three zones: zone 1 (central) extends from the esophageal hiatus to the sacrum and is further subclassified as supramesocolic or inframesocolic; zone 2 (lateral) encompasses the perinephric spaces (bilaterally) from the diaphragm to the iliac crest and contains the renal vessels; zone 3 (pelvic) is defined by the boundaries of the pelvis. Major abdominal vascular trauma may present as free intraperitoneal hemorrhage (rare), large retroperitoneal hematoma, or a combination of both. Management of retroperitoneal vascular injuries depends on the patient's physiology and the zone of injury. Hematomas due to penetrating injuries in any zone found at laparotomy are usually opened and explored. Hematomas found on preoperative CT scan with the trajectory determined could be managed non-operatively. Zone 2 or 3 injuries due to a blunt mechanism are usually left undisturbed unless expanding or pulsatile or if the patient is unstable and there is no other source of hemorrhage. Exceptions to these rules exist, as in cases where the patient's life-threatening physiology may be due to other sources that need to be addressed first (eg, extremity hemorrhage or cardiac tamponade).

Noncompressible torso injury is a leading cause of death in trauma patients. Patients with these injuries can exsanguinate rapidly. The incidence of an injury to the IVC or aorta among patients who have a vascular injury is approximately 3% and 2.5%, respectively, and the injuries are associated with a mortality rate of over 50%. The incidence of iliac vascular injury is relatively rare, being less than 5% of arterial injuries (range, approximately 2%-6.5%), and iliac vascular injury is associated with a mortality rate of over 60%. Familiarity with the anatomy will aid in rapid exposure and control of these injuries, which can be lifesaving.

Anatomy

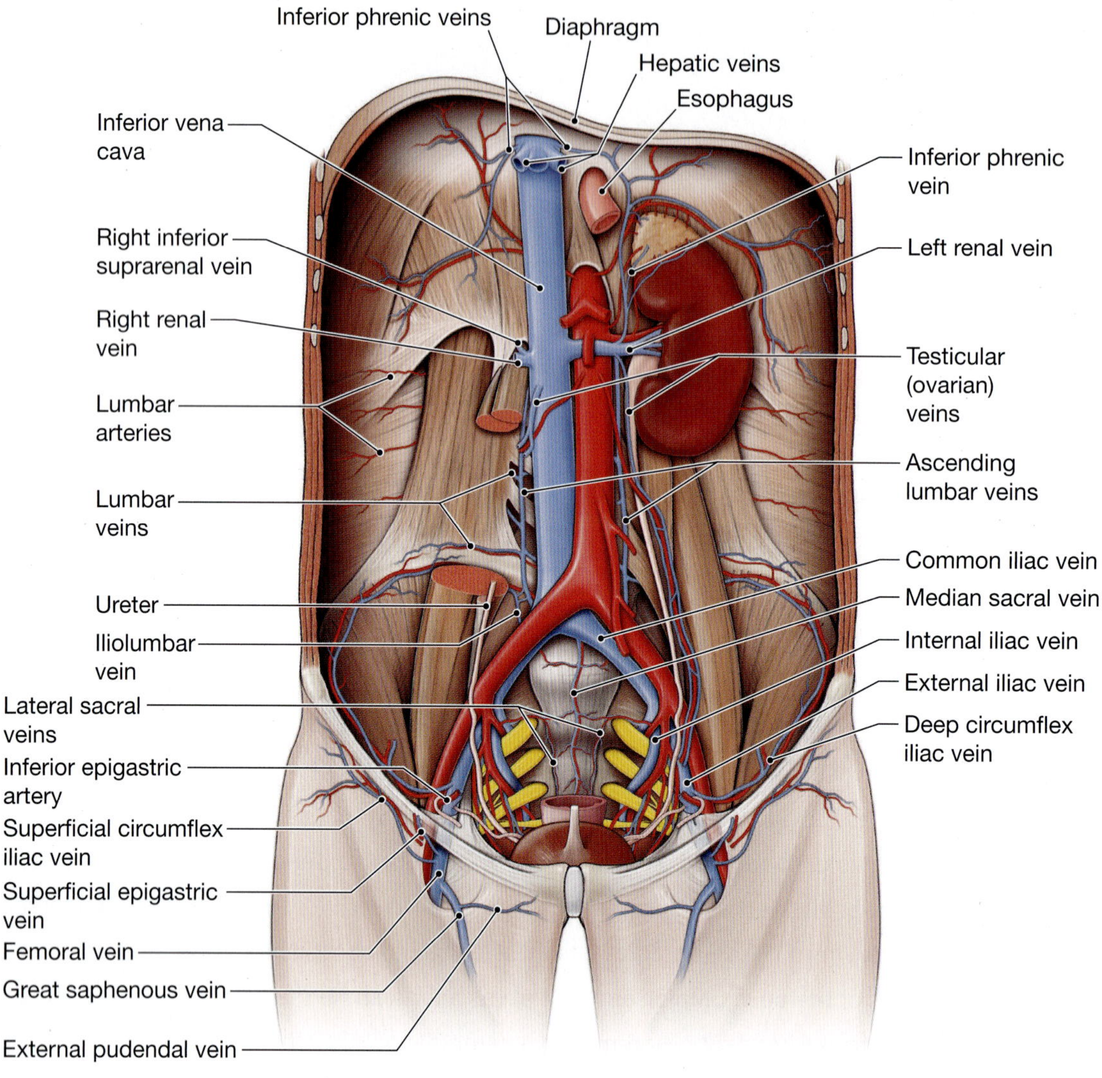

Figure 21-1

Bifurcation of abdominal aorta into left and right common iliac arteries occurs at the level of the fourth lumbar vertebra. The common iliac arteries bifurcate into internal and external iliac arteries at the level of the sacroiliac joints. The ureter crosses over the iliac vessels at this point. The IVC bifurcates at the level of the fifth lumbar vertebra, posterior to the right common iliac artery.

Initial exposure is obtained through a standard midline incision, and all clots and free blood are manually evacuated. An initial inspection is conducted, and the abdomen is packed to control hemorrhage from solid organs. Digital control is more effective than packing or blind clamping for injuries to arterial structures. Following damage control principles, the first priority is

TABLE 21-1. American Association for the Surgery of Trauma (AAST) Injury Table

Abdominal Vascular Injury Scale			
Grade*	**Description of injury**	**ICD-9**	**AIS-90**
I	Nonnamed superior mesenteric artery or superior mesenteric vein branches	902.20/.39	NS
	Nonnamed inferior mesenteric artery or inferior mesenteric vein branches	902.27/.32	NS
	Phrenic artery or vein	902.89	NS
	Lumbar artery or vein	902.89	NS
	Gonadal artery or vein	902.89	NS
	Ovarian artery or vein	902.81/.82	NS
	Other nonnamed small arterial or venous structures requiring ligation	902.90	NS
II	Right, left, or common hepatic artery	902.22	3
	Splenic artery or vein	902.23/.34	3
	Right or left gastric arteries	902.21	3
	Gastroduodenal artery	902.24	3
	Inferior mesenteric artery, or inferior mesenteric vein, trunk	902.27/.32	3
	Primary named branches of mesenteric artery (eg, ileocolic artery) or mesenteric vein	902.26/.31	3
	Other names abdominal vessels requiring ligation or repair	902.89	3
III	Superior mesenteric vein, trunk	902.31	3
	Renal artery or vein	902.41/.42	3
	Iliac artery or vein	902.53/.54	3
	Hypogastric artery or vein	902.51/.52	3
	Vena cava, infrarenal	902.10	3
IV	Superior mesenteric artery, trunk	902.25	3
	Celiac axis proper	902.24	3
	Vena cava, suprarenal and infrahepatic	902.10	3
	Aorta, infrarenal	902.00	4
V	Portal vein Extraparenchymal hepatic vein	902.33 902.11	3 3 (hepatic vein)
			5 (liver + veins)
	Vena cava, retrohepatic or suprahepatic	902.19	5
	Aorta suprarenal, subdiaphragmatic	902.00	4

*This classification system is applicable to extraparenchymal vascular injuries. If the vessel injury is within 2 cm of the organ parenchyma, refer to specific organ injury scale. Increase one grade for multiple grade III or IV injuries involving >50% vessel circumference. Downgrade one grade if <25% vessel circumference laceration for grades IV or V. NS, not scored.

Source: Reproduced with permission from Moore EE, Cogbill TH, Jurkovich GJ, et al. Organ injury scaling. III: Chest wall, abdominal vascular, ureter, bladder, and urethra. *J Trauma.* 1992;33(3):337-339.

hemorrhage control. Basic principles of obtaining proximal and distal control apply. Balloon catheters may be helpful for obtaining temporary vascular control.

Operative Steps for Infrarenal (Inframesocolic) Aortic Injury

Left Medial Visceral Rotation and Anterior Exposures (Modified Approach)

Peritoneal attachments of the left colon are divided. The descending and sigmoid colon are mobilized medially by incising the line of Toldt. Retroperitoneal attachments of the pancreatic tail and spleen are divided to allow for mobilization to the midline staying in a plane anterior to Gerota's fascia. This allows for complete exposure of the aorta from diaphragm aortic hiatus to its bifurcation. Care must be taken to avoid injury to the renal vessels and ureter during this maneuver (Figure 21-2A, B). For anterior infrarenal aorta exposure, an incision is made medial of the duodenojejunal flexure, and the peritoneum is dissected off the aorta. An infrarenal aortic clamp is applied. Slightly higher proximal control can be achieved by ligation of the left renal vein in patients with intact left adrenal and gonadal vessels.

Once the injury is identified, small lacerations are closed with 3-0 or 4-0 polypropylene suture. Larger lacerations may require prosthetic patch or tube graft.

This maneuver gives direct access to the celiac trunk, the superior mesenteric artery, the inferior mesenteric artery, and the left renal pedicle vessels as well as the splenic artery and vein. The dense and fibrous superior mesenteric and celiac nerve plexuses overlie the

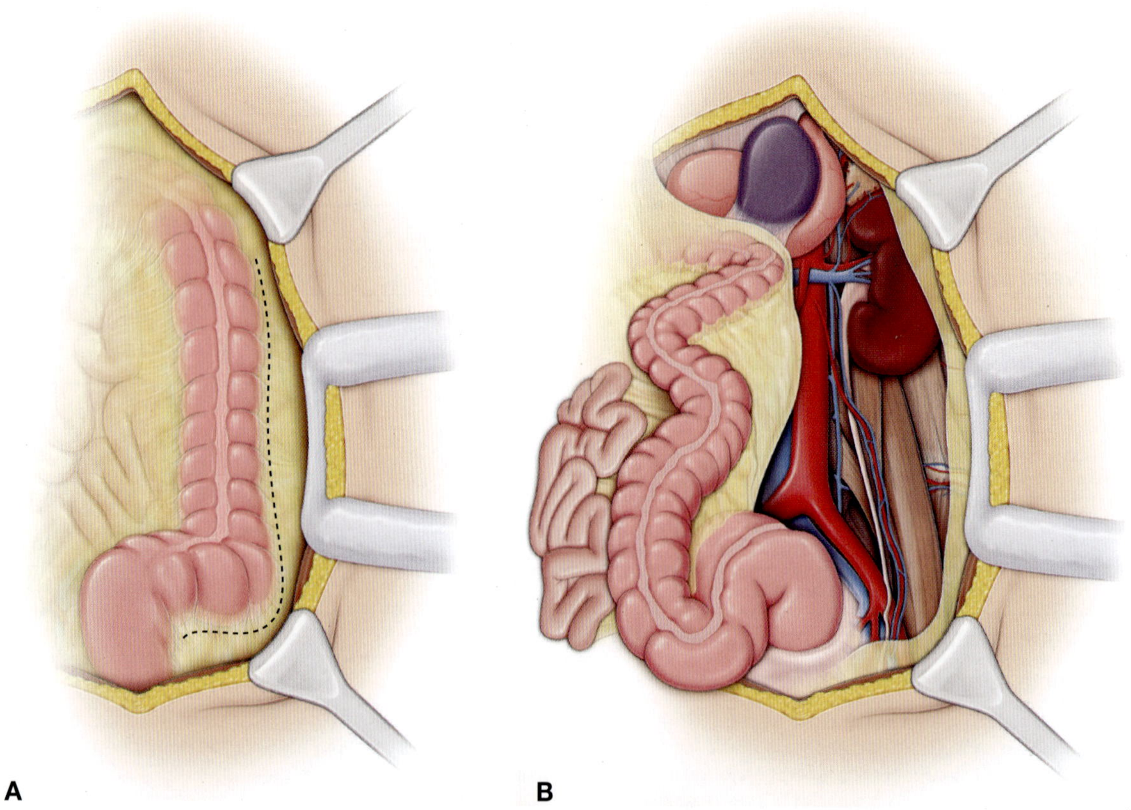

Figure 21-2 A, B

proximal aorta and need to be dissected in order to identify the renal and superior mesenteric arteries.

The classic left medial rotation (Mattox maneuver) involves also mobilizing the kidney out of Gerota's fascia and allows access to the posterior wall of the aorta.

Operative Steps for Suprarenal (Supramesocolic) Aortic Injury

Supraceliac aortic control is used for proximal control. The gastrohepatic ligament is opened, and the stomach is retracted to the left and inferiorly. The left lobe of the liver can be mobilized and retracted superiorly and laterally by incising the left triangular ligaments with electrocautery, although that is not necessary. A window is made in the lesser omentum, and then the peritoneum overlying the crura is divided. The goal is to clamp the descending thoracic aorta to avoid the dense celiac plexus more inferiorly. The fibers of the aortic crura are separated bluntly with a finger or Mayo scissors to expose the anterior surface of the aorta. An atraumatic vascular clamp can then be applied to the aorta at the level of the hiatus for proximal control (Figure 21-3A-D). A vessel loop or umbilical tape can be used through the hole of the clamp to secure the clamp to the drapes superiorly so it does not fall forward into the wound. Temporary compression against the spine using a surgeon's hand or T-bar clamp is an alternative but requires a member of the surgical team to maintain compression for control. The clamp is moved closer to

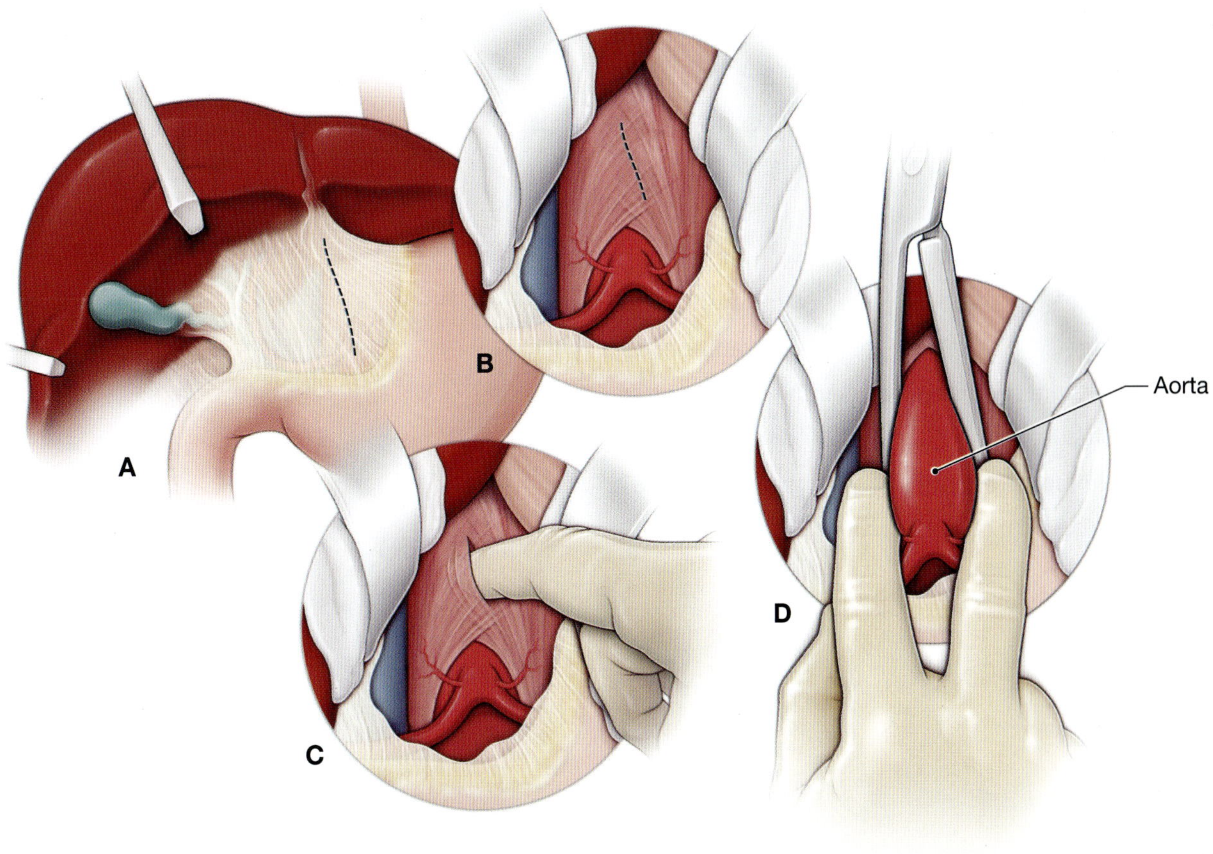

Figure 21-3 A-D

the injury once it is identified in order to limit global visceral ischemic time.

If an injury is identified at this level, more proximal control may be required. The distal thoracic aorta can be clamped via a thoracotomy.

For exposure of the celiac artery, a left medial visceral rotation is used. Alternatively, direct access can be made through the lesser sac (Figure 21-3A-D). All three branches of the celiac trunk can be ligated with impunity. If the common hepatic artery requires ligation, this is done proximal to the origin of the gastroduodenal artery.

Ligation of the left renal vein may aid exposure of the superior mesenteric artery (SMA). The SMA can be exposed immediately under the pancreas from the left by mobilizing the fourth portion duodenum after division of the ligament of Treitz (Figure 21-4). Alternatively, a full right medial visceral rotation (Figure 21-5) to reflect the small bowel cephalad is used to obtain good access to the posterior aspect of the SMA. More distal exposure is obtained at the root of the mesentery (Figure 21-6). The injured SMA is reconstructed using a 6-mm ringed prosthetic graft from the distal aorta or the right common iliac artery. The latter option is advantageous, because it does not require aortic clamping. The suture lines are protected from other surrounding structures that may be injured (eg, injured pancreas, which may jeopardize an arterial reconstruction).

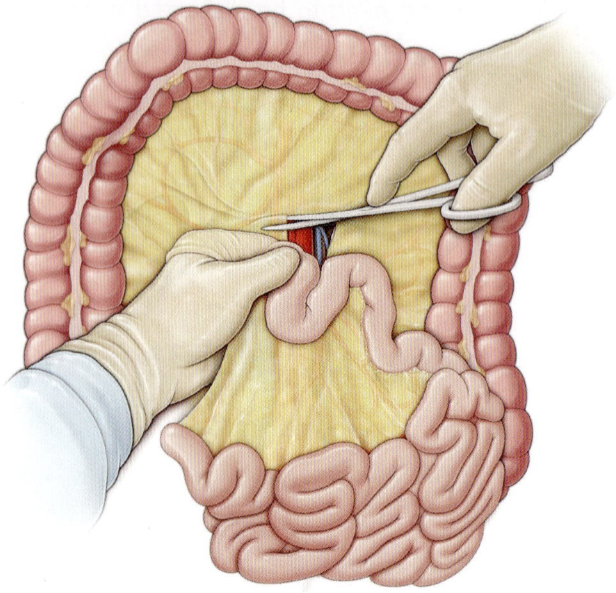

Figure 21-4

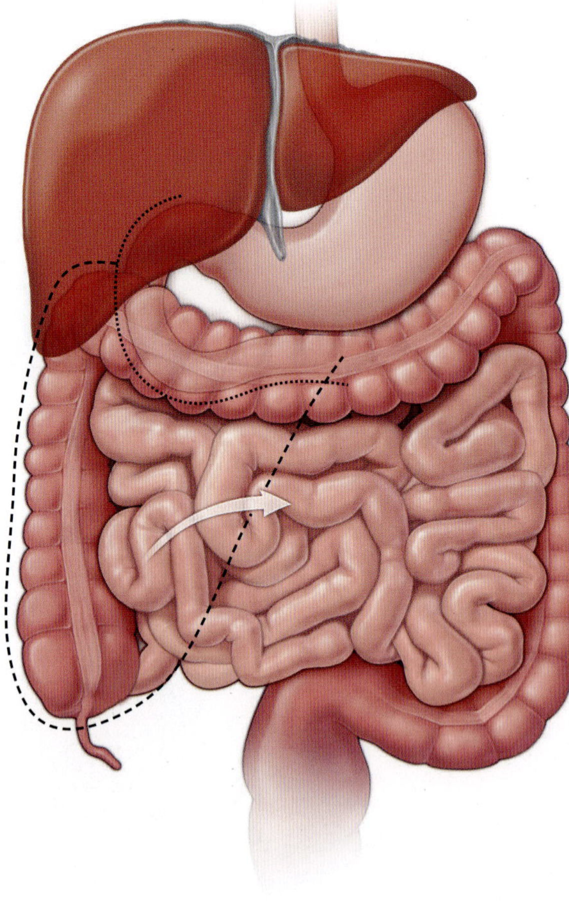

Figure 21-5

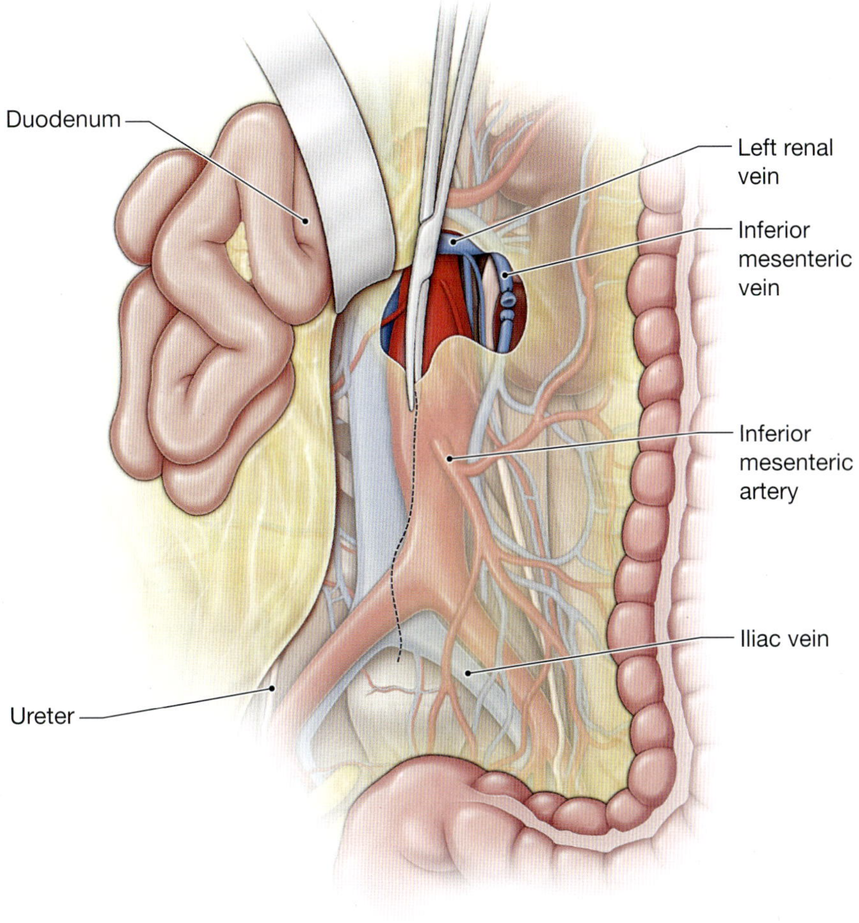
Duodenum
Left renal vein
Inferior mesenteric vein
Inferior mesenteric artery
Iliac vein
Ureter

Figure 21-6

Operative Steps for Infrarenal (Inframesocolic) Vena Cava Exposure

Patients with IVC injuries often have large right retroperitoneal hematomas, which may be contained, may have freely ruptured into the abdominal cavity, or a combination of both. Often, minimal active bleeding is noted as the patient is profoundly hypotensive.

Right Medial Visceral Rotation (Figure 21-7)

The peritoneal reflection lateral to ascending colon is divided. The dissection plane is developed anterior to the right kidney. With medialization of the terminal ileum and right colon, the duodenum is exposed. A Kocher maneuver is performed by dividing the lateral peritoneal attachments and lifting the duodenum and retracting it medially. After the duodenum and pancreatic head are bluntly dissected away from the vena cava and mobilized medially, exposure is gained to the infrahepatic IVC down to the level of the right common iliac vessels (Figure 21-7).

Quick determination of whether the location of the injury is infrarenal or suprarenal is crucial. Once the injury is discovered, rapid proximal and distal control is achieved with sponge sticks or direct digital pressure. Side-biting vascular clamps or Allis clamps placed sequentially on the edges of the injured segment can be used for control (while still allowing venous return) (Figure 21-8). Attempts to circumferentially dissect the IVC to encircle with vessel loops or clamps are avoided, because that can lead to iatrogenic injury to the vena cava itself or lumbar veins, which would

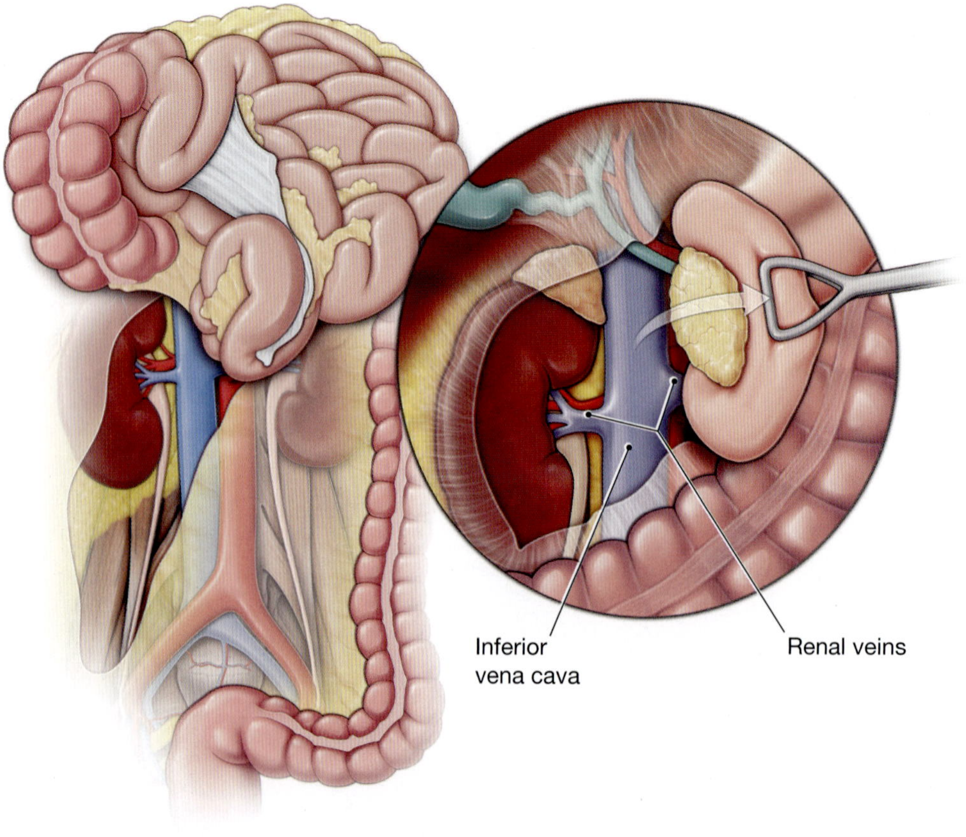

Figure 21-7

lead to troublesome bleeding. If a side-biting clamp is used, a continuous suture is used above the level of the clamp in a back-and-forth fashion along the length of the injury and then brought back in a simple running fashion and tied to itself at the starting point.

The surgeon must be cognizant that complete occlusion of the IVC will sometimes lead to cardiac arrest, particularly in hypotensive patients, because abrupt loss of cardiac filling in a patient in shock will result in cardiovascular collapse. A hemostatic option for temporary control that will preserve some venous return is best.

There often is a second hole just like in bowel injuries. Injuries to the posterior wall of the IVC are closed with a continuous running fashion through the injured anterior wall, which may need to be extended for access. The anterior wall can then be repaired in similar fashion with a 4-0 polypropylene suture. Care is taken to take thin bites to avoid narrowing. Some narrowing is expected. If significant narrowing occurs, patch angioplasty with either autologous vein or synthetic material is performed, although this can be time consuming and more technically challenging.

If the injury is extensive, a quick decision to ligate the infrarenal IVC should be made rather than engage in futile attempts at primary repair. The infrarenal IVC can be ligated without division by encircling the IVC with 0 silk suture. It is preferred to exert some direct pressure to collapse the segment where the ligature is placed to avoid "ballooning" and inadvertent tearing. Some surgeons prefer to place another ligature just inferior to the renal veins to avoid a blind IVC segment that may be a source of a large thrombus burden that could embolize. Collateral venous drainage through the retroperitoneum and the left gonadal vein will provide venous return if the infrarenal IVC is ligated.

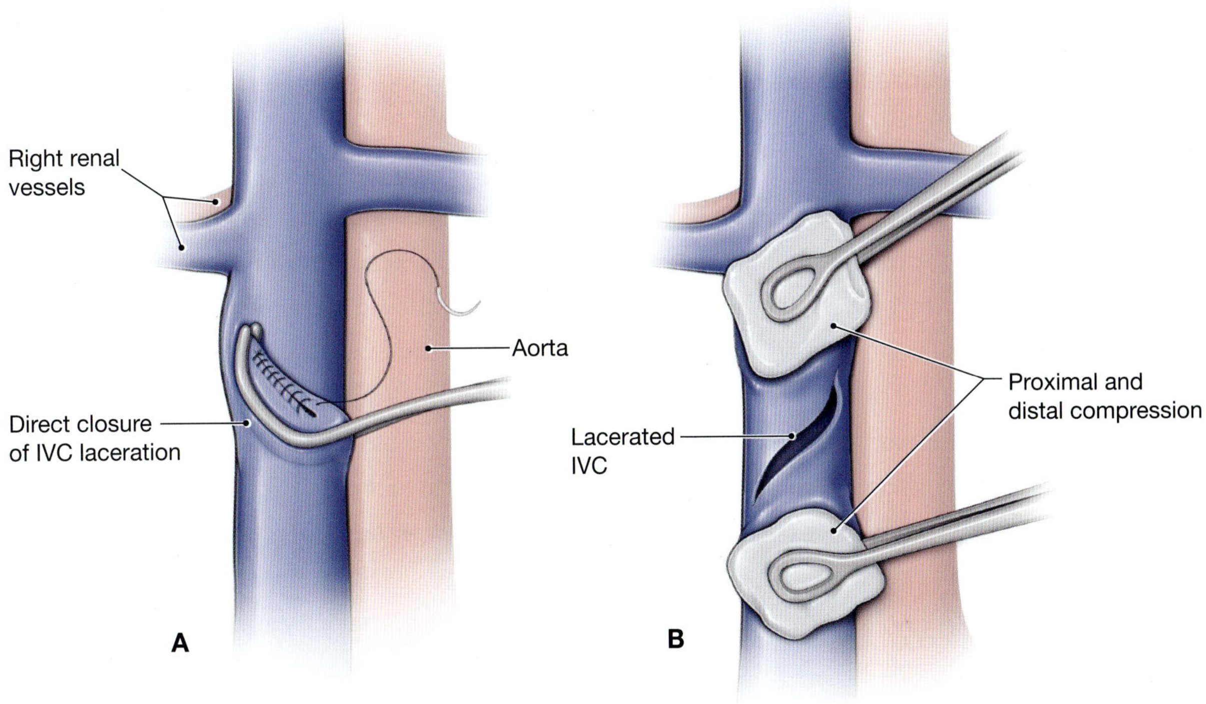

Figure 21-8

Operative Steps for Suprarenal (Supramesocolic) Vena Cava Exposure

A complete Kocher maneuver allows mobilization of the duodenum and the head of the pancreas all the way over across the cava to expose the infrahepatic/suprarenal segment. It is helpful to mobilize the right colon to the proximal transverse colon as described above. Controlling the injury proceeds using one of the techniques described previously.

Primary venorraphy can then proceed. Any small residual bleeding can be repaired with another interrupted suture or generally controlled with a topical hemostatic agent.

Ligation is a viable option in suprarenal IVC injuries if the damage is extensive to preclude primary repair; however, it requires venous reconstruction if possible. Renal function has to be monitored as it may deteriorate.

Retrohepatic IVC Injury

If a retrohepatic IVC injury is suspected, early total vascular isolation with suprahepatic and infrahepatic/suprarenal IVC control is imperative. The infrahepatic IVC is exposed and controlled as described above. Suprahepatic IVC control is more accessible through a median sternotomy and pericardiotomy and by encircling it immediately below the right atrium with a Rummel tourniquet or clamp. Alternatively, the diaphragm can be opened over the suprahepatic IVC and a vascular clamp placed on the suprahepatic IVC from the abdominal approach. Communication with anesthesia colleagues is crucial as preparation with adequate supradiaphragmatic intravenous access is essential (Figure 21-9). Once liver inflow is controlled, the liver is rapidly mobilized by taking down the falciform ligament and the right triangular ligament. Following this, the liver can be reflected medially to expose the retrohepatic cava and hepatic veins for repair.

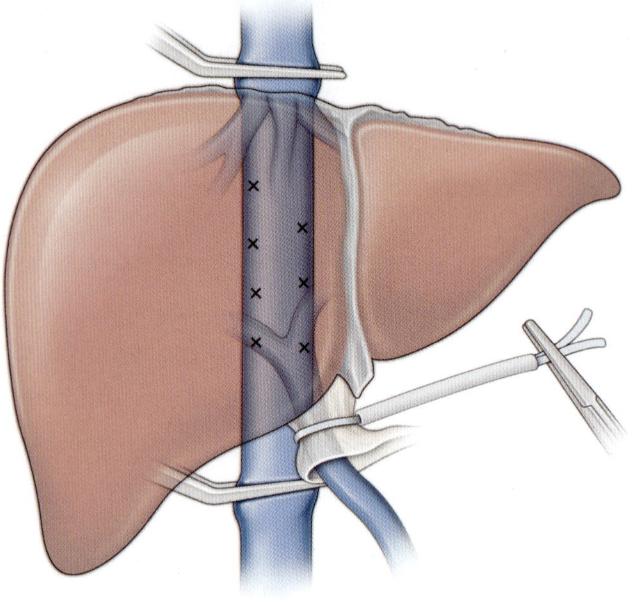

Figure 21-9

Operative Steps for Iliac Exposure

Initial steps of either a left or right medial visceral rotation, depending on the area of concern, are previously described.

Exposure of the right common iliac vein can be challenging because of its location posterior to the common iliac artery.

Formal proximal and distal control can be achieved by opening the retroperitoneum overlying the aortic bifurcation and encircling the common, internal, and external iliac vessels with vascular loops or vascular clamps (Figure 21-10). Ligation of the common iliac and/or external iliac artery is associated with a high rate of limb loss. In patients with multiple injuries or severe shock, a temporary shunt may be placed to allow for damage control. For wounds close to the bifurcation multiple reconstructive options exist. The options include: lateral arteriorraphy, end-to-end anastomosis, interposition with reverse saphenous vein or prosthetic graft (8mm), mobilization and rotation of the internal iliac artery as a replacement

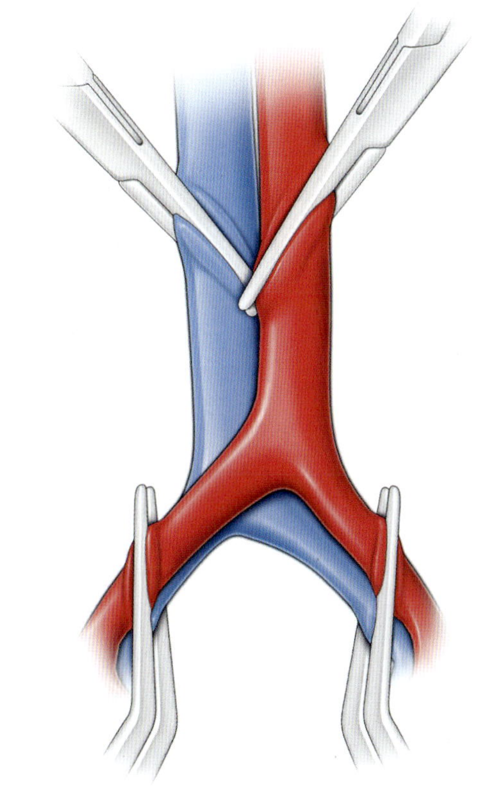

Figure 21-10

(Figure 21-11 C), and transposition of one iliac artery to the side of the contralateral uninjured iliac artery (Figure 21-11 A, B).

If significant fecal or enteric contamination exists, the ends are ligated and an extra-anatomic bypass is performed (femorofemoral crossover graft).

Injuries to the common or external iliac veins can be primarily repaired or ligated. For longitudinal injuries to the vein, using the index finger and the middle finger for venous control and sewing in a running fashion as described above are an efficient method for repair (with 3-0 or 4-0 polypropylene suture). If the iliac veins need to be ligated fasciotomies should be performed. In cases of combined arterial and vein injury, four-compartment fasciotomy of the affected calf should routinely be performed. If narrowed following repair, postoperative anticoagulation should be administered. Four-compartment fasciotomy is strongly considered if the patient is unstable or undergoing ongoing resuscitation or if ischemia time is prolonged.

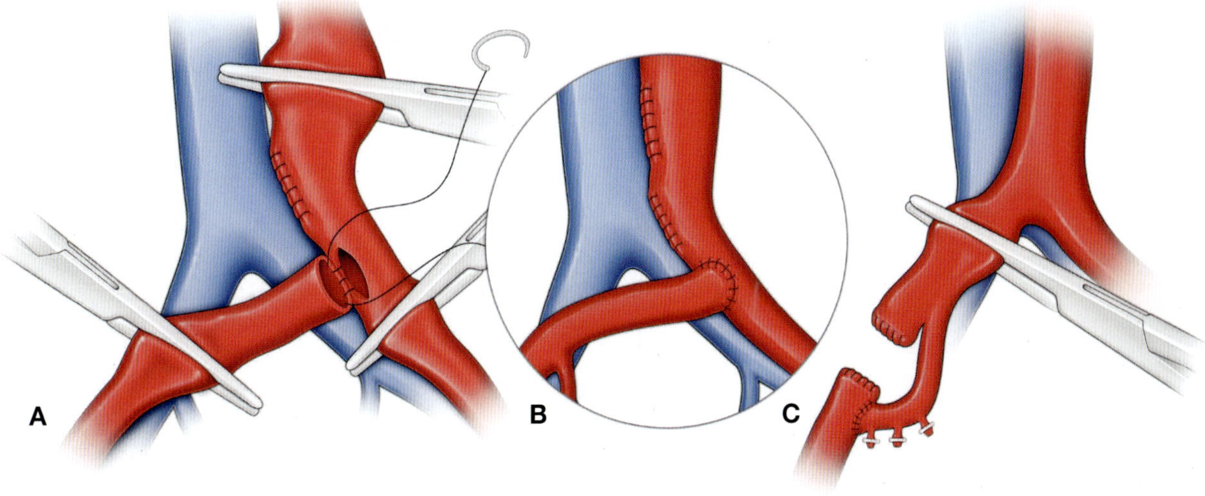

Figure 21-11 A-C

Complications

Morbidities related to patients with injuries to the aorta, IVC, and iliac vessels depend largely on the nature and location of the injury; however, some complications are common to all. The most common early complication following either arterial or venous repair is thrombosis. Postrepair angiography can help to decrease the incidence of thrombosis by potentially identifying any narrowing or dissections.

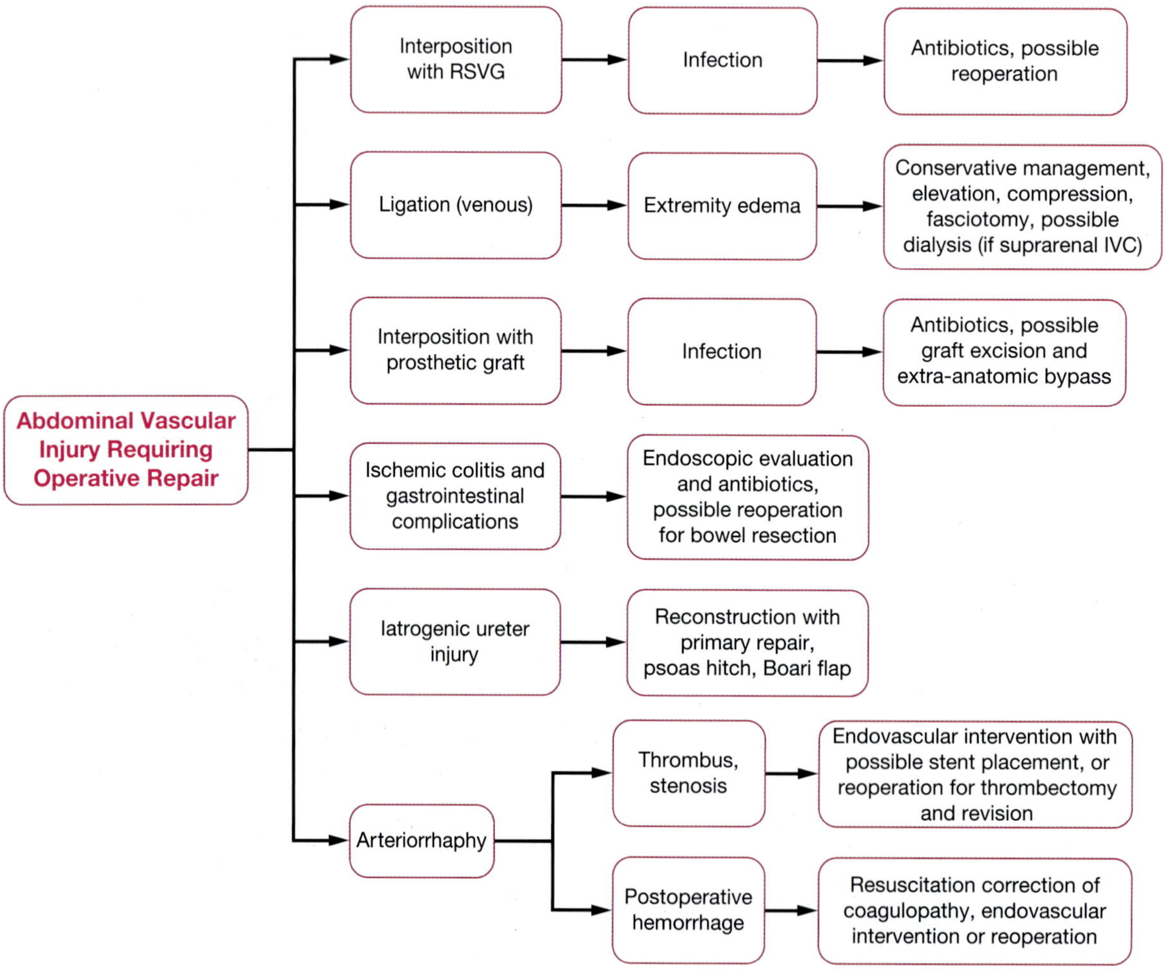

Figure 21-12

DAMAGE CONTROL/OPEN ABDOMEN

22

Laura Velcu, MD
Dale A. Dangleben, MD, FACS

TIPS

1. Damage control resuscitation (DCR = minimizing crystalloids + allowing for permissive hypotension + transfusion in a 1:1:1 ratio of products) significantly decreased the number of open abdomens.
2. Several temporary closures for open abdomen exist; be familiar with what your operating room has, and keep up with newer techniques.
3. Every hour delay in returning to the operating room for initial takeback is associated with a 1.1% reduction in achieving primary fascial closure.

Introduction

As part of damage control laparotomy (DCL) and for the treatment of the abdominal compartment syndrome, the abdomen is frequently left open. DCL allows the surgeon to temporarily halt surgical interventions and focus on the correction of the lethal triad: coagulopathy, hypothermia, and acidosis (Figure 22-1). The indications for DCL are persistent hypotension, acidosis (pH <7.2), hypothermia (temperature <34°F), coagulopathy (blood loss >10 units of packed red blood cells), factors that may lead to abdominal compartment syndrome including injuries requiring packing and planned reoperation, extreme visceral or retroperitoneal swelling, obesity, elevated bladder pressure when abdominal closure is attempted, and aggressive resuscitation.

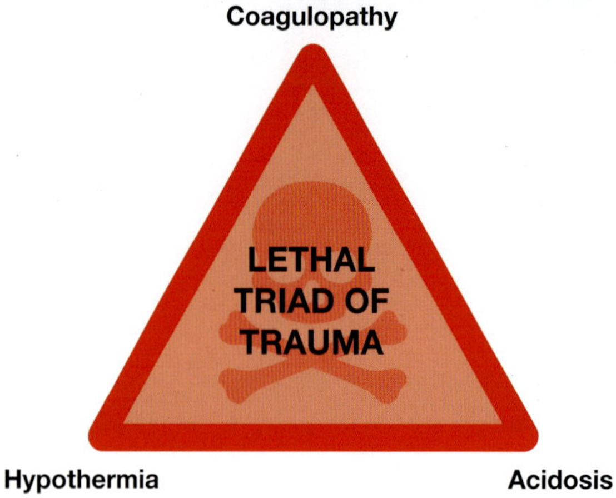

Figure 22-1

DCL has four phases (Table 22-1).

TABLE 22-1. Four Phases of Damage Control Laparotomy

Phase	Description
I	Hemorrhage control and control of gross bowel spillage; vessels are ligated/ repaired/shunted, bowel is resected and left in discontinuity or temporary repaired, solid organs are removed or packed, and a temporary closure device is placed
II	Correction of coagulopathy, rewarming, and reversal of acidosis
III	Unpacking, definitive repairs, reestablishing intestinal continuity and fascial closure
IV	Consists of abdominal wall reconstruction

Source: Data from Godat L, Kobayashi L, Costantini T, Coimbra R. Abdominal damage control surgery and reconstruction: world society of emergency surgery position paper. *World J Emerg Surg.* 2013 Dec 17;8(1):53. doi: 10.1186/1749-7922-8-53. PMID: 24341602; PMCID: PMC3878509.

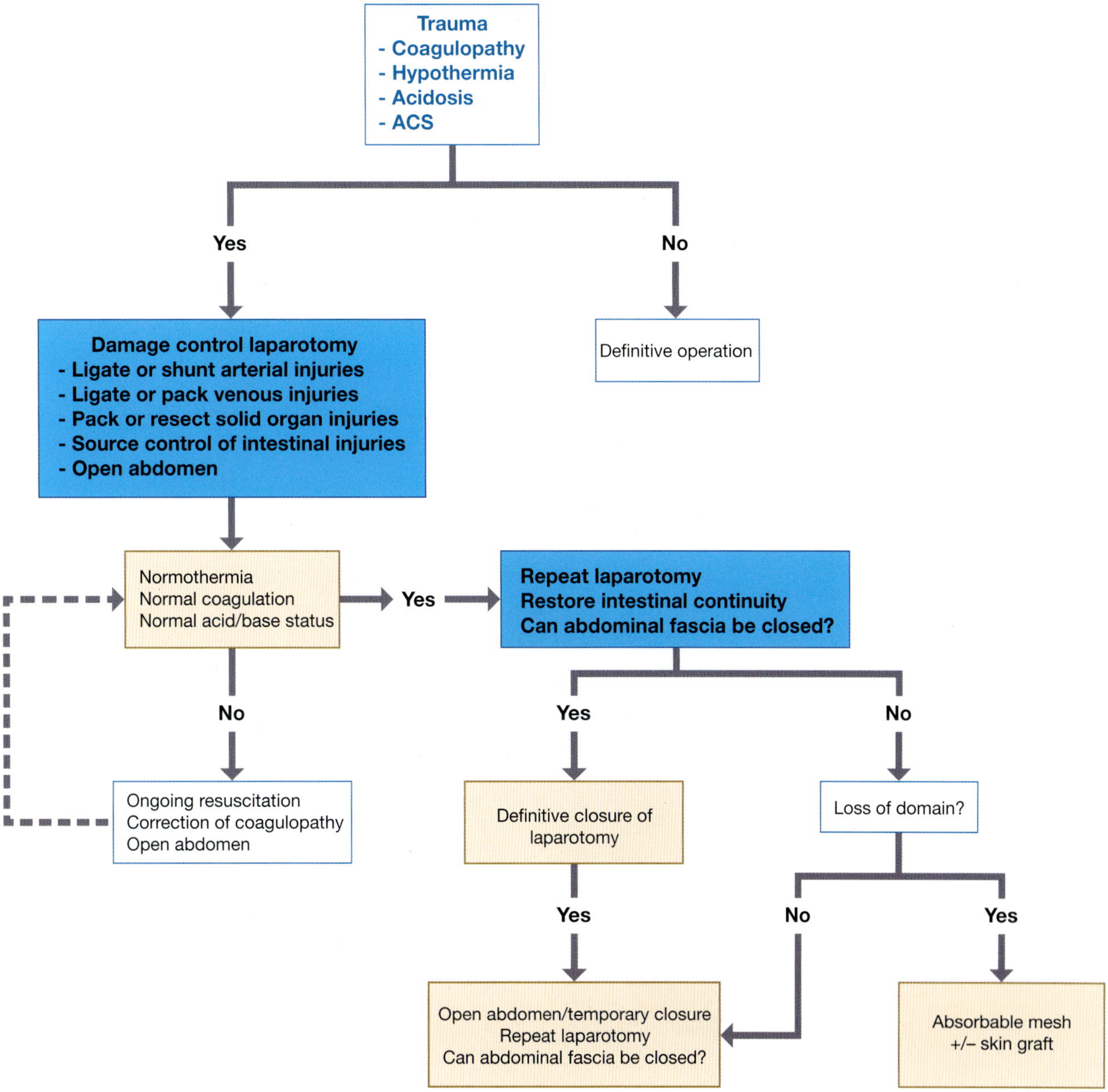
Trauma
- Coagulopathy
- Hypothermia
- Acidosis
- ACS
Yes
No
Damage control laparotomy
- Ligate or shunt arterial injuries
- Ligate or pack venous injuries
- Pack or resect solid organ injuries
- Source control of intestinal injuries
- Open abdomen
Definitive operation
Normothermia
Normal coagulation
Normal acid/base status
Yes
Repeat laparotomy
Restore intestinal continuity
Can abdominal fascia be closed?
No
Yes
No
Ongoing resuscitation
Correction of coagulopathy
Open abdomen
Definitive closure of laparotomy
Loss of domain?
Yes
No
Yes
Open abdomen/temporary closure
Repeat laparotomy
Can abdominal fascia be closed?
Absorbable mesh
+/– skin graft

Figure 22-2

Operative Steps

There are many options in the acute management of the open abdomen. It is advised to use the technique you are comfortable with based on your training. If you have not done one prior, it is recommended that you attend a trauma operative course or ask for assistance. The following are a few examples of methods that exist.

The Vac Pack

A fenestrated 10 × 10 steri-drape is placed over the abdominal contents and guided into the lateral paracolic gutters on either side of the abdomen (Figure 22-3A). A laparotomy sponge is placed over the drape. Two 10-French flat Jackson-Pratt (JP) drains are placed to collect effluent (Figure 22-3B). A sterile towel is shaped to fit over the entire wound. Loban dressing is placed over the entire abdomen. The JP drains are placed to 100-125 mm Hg continuous wall suction (Figure 22-3C).

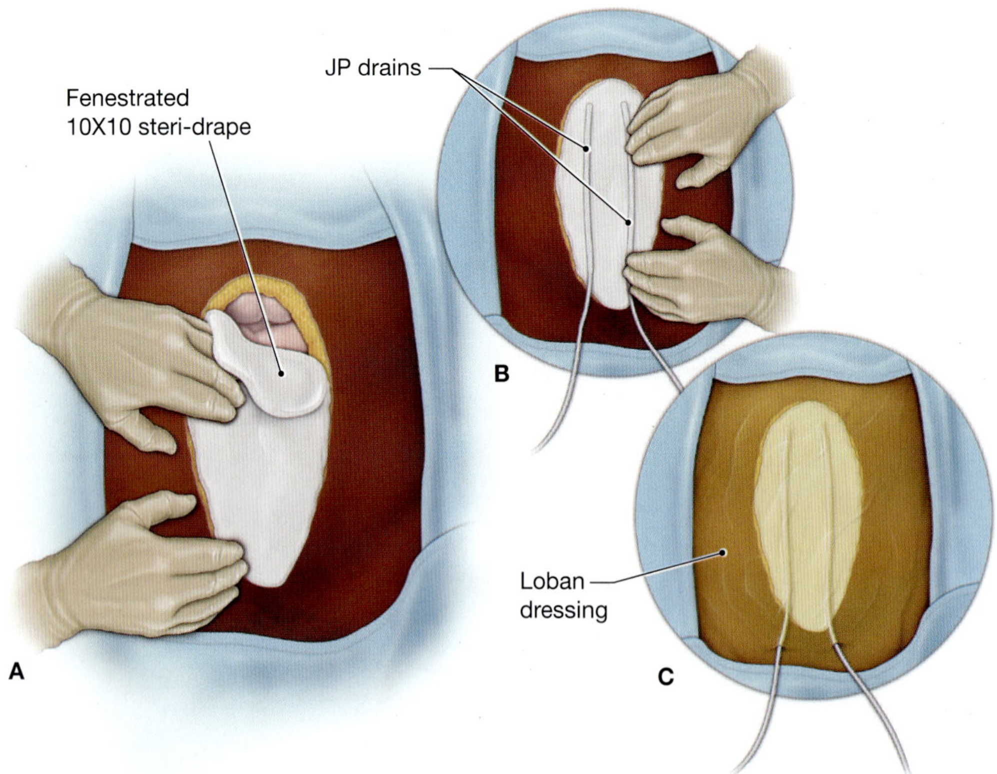

Figure 22-3 A-C

AbThera

This system consists of perforated polyurethane foam encased in a visceral protective layer covered by a drape that is then attached to a negative-pressure therapy unit with a 1-L canister and audible alarms. It actively removes fluid and helps reduce edema, thus providing medial tension, which helps minimize fascial retraction and loss of domain (Figure 22-4A-D).

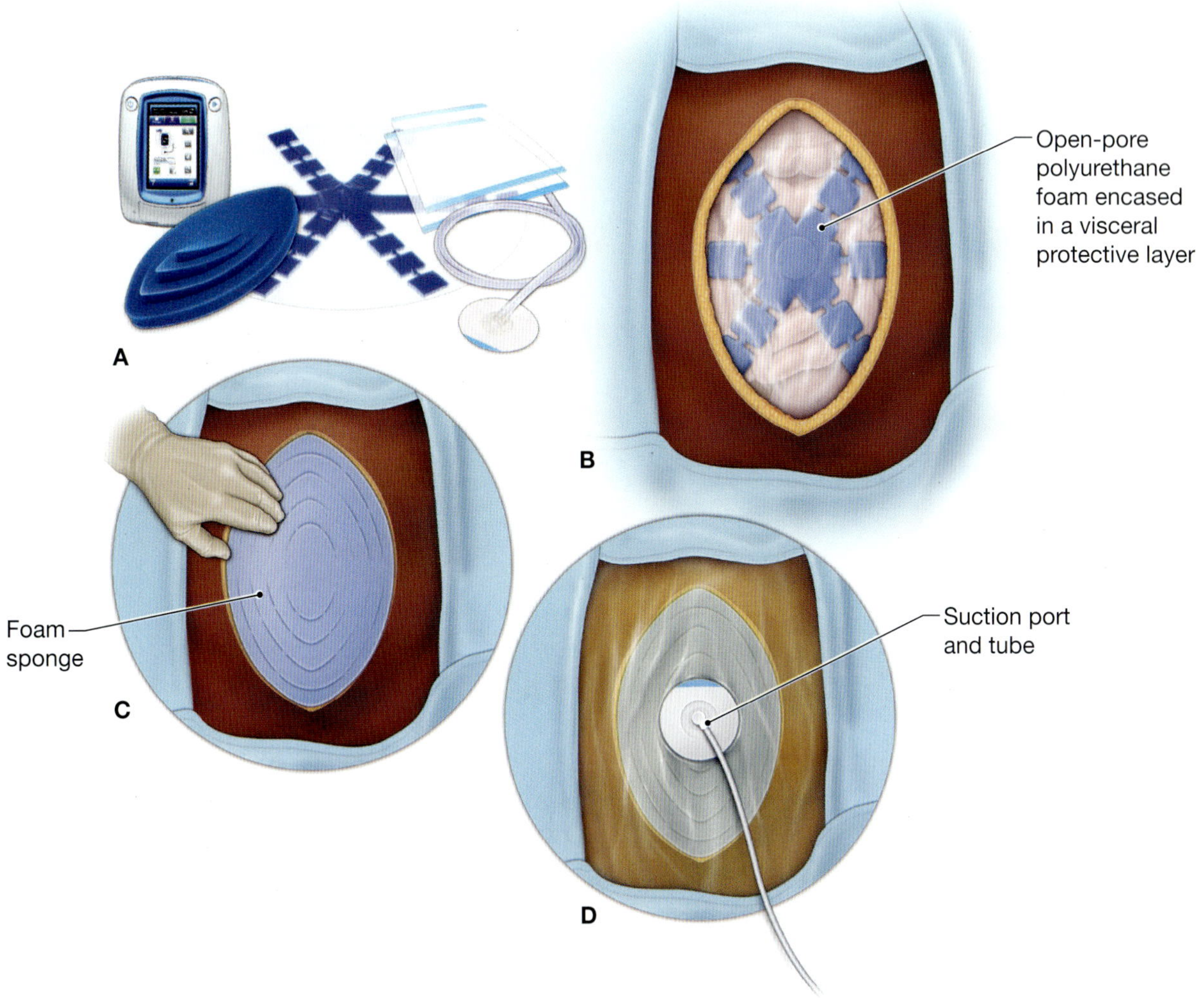

Figure 22-4 A-D

The Wittmann Patch

The technique employs two sheets of Velcro-like prosthetic biocompatible material (propylene) sutured to the fascia and tailored to come together in the midline. The Velcro is then advanced every 4 to 6 hours, bringing the fascia closer together. A major advantage is that the abdomen can be reentered for a definitive procedure by simply unfastening the Velcro at the midline (Figure 22-5A, B).

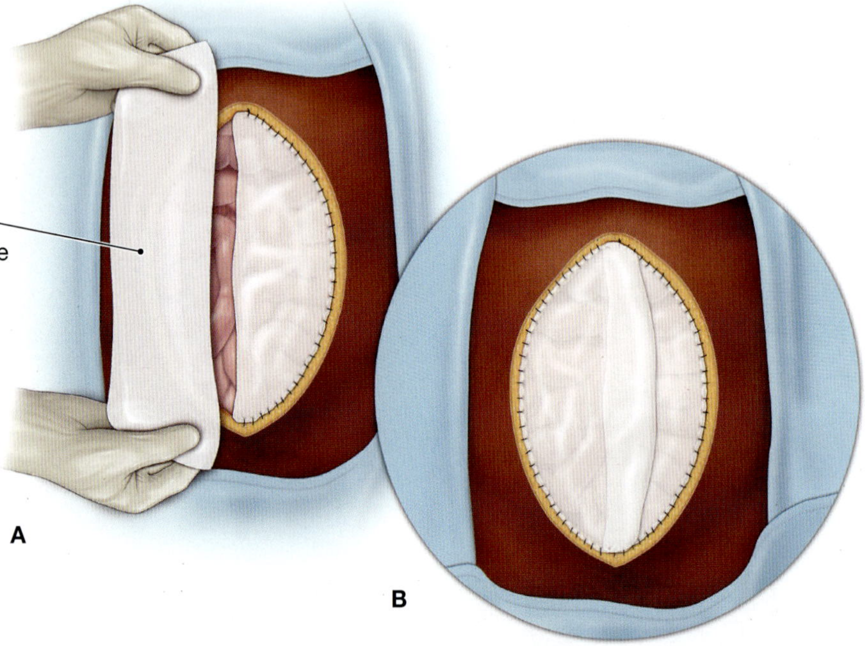

Figure 22-5 A, B

Complications

The complication rate with an open abdomen can be as high as 50% and include wound infections, intra-abdominal abscesses, fistulae (enteroatmospheric, exposed deep fistulae), and ventral hernia.

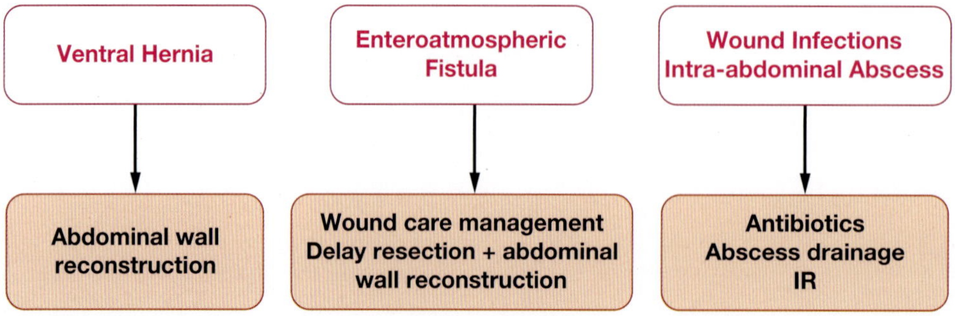

Figure 22-6

INDEX

Page numbers followed by "f" denote figures and "t" denote tables.

INDEX

INDEX